Controlling Cholesterol

FOR

DUMMIES®

2ND EDITION

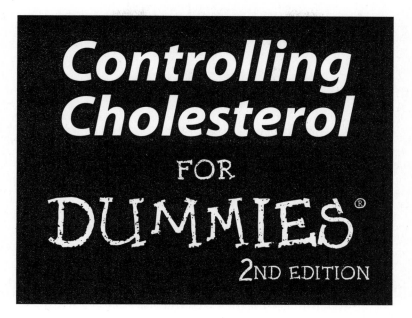

Controlling Cholesterol FOR DUMMIES®

2ND EDITION

by Carol Ann Rinzler

with Martin W. Graf, MD

WILEY

Wiley Publishing, Inc.

Controlling Cholesterol For Dummies®, 2nd Edition

Published by
Wiley Publishing, Inc.
111 River St.
Hoboken, NJ 07030-5774
www.wiley.com

WILEY

About the Author

Carol Ann Rinzler is the author of *Nutrition For Dummies,* now in its 4th edition, as well as *Heartburn and Reflux For Dummies,* and more than 20 other books on food and health. A former nutrition columnist for the *New York Daily News,* Carol lives in New York with her husband Perry Luntz, author of *Whiskey and Spirits For Dummies,* and their amiable cat, Katy.

Dedication

To my husband, Perry Luntz, for all the usual reasons.

Author's Acknowledgments

Every *For Dummies* book is a work of many hands, so I have many people to thank for this one.

First in line, Michael Lewis, my Acquisitions Editor, who moved this new edition of *Controlling Cholesterol For Dummies* from an idea to a reality. Then there's my wonderful project editor, Natalie Harris, whose scientific intelligence and editorial diligence kept things on track. My many thanks to Copy Editor Carrie Burchfield whose keen eye and fine-point blue pen are a writer's delight. And let's not forget Wiley's hardworking proofreaders and page layout technicians.

Like others who write about health and medicine, I am enormously grateful to Martin Graf, MD, and Bonnie Taub-Dix, the experts who've generously taken the time to read the manuscript for accuracy. I also appreciate the assistance of the professionals at the American Heart Association: Aaron Talent, Tagni McRae, and Taylor Morris.

Finally, I would like to put in a word of appreciation for all the anonymous folks at the Food and Drug Administration, the U.S. Departments of Agriculture and Health and Human Services, the Centers for Disease Control and Prevention, and the similar agencies up there in our neighbor to the north, Canada. Without their efforts, you and I would be left without the numbers we need to construct intelligent guidelines for a healthy life. So let's hear it for these guys: Hip! Hip! Hooray!

Publisher's Acknowledgments

We're proud of this book; please send us your comments through our Dummies online registration form located at www.dummies.com/register/.

Some of the people who helped bring this book to market include the following:

Acquisitions, Editorial, and Media Development

Project Editor: Natalie Faye Harris

(Previous Edition: Tonya Maddox Cupp)

Acquisitions Editor: Michael Lewis

(Previous Edition: Natasha Graf)

Copy Editor: Carrie A. Burchfield

(Previous Edition: Mike Baker)

Editorial Program Coordinator: Erin Calligan Mooney

Technical Editors: Martin W. Graf, MD; Bonnie Taub-Dix, MA, RD, CDN, Director of BTD Nutrition Consultants, New York

Editorial Manager: Christine Meloy Beck

Editorial Assistants: Joe Niesen, David Lutton, Leeann Harney

Cover Photos: Daniela Richardson

Cartoons: Rich Tennant (www.the5thwave.com)

Composition Services

Project Coordinator: Erin Smith

Layout and Graphics: Carl Byers, Reuben W. Davis, Alissa D. Ellet, Melissa K. Jester, Christine Williams

Proofreaders: David Faust, Penny Stuart

Indexer: Cheryl Duksta

Special Help
Sarah Faulkner, Alissa Schwipps, Jennifer Tucci

Publishing and Editorial for Consumer Dummies

Diane Graves Steele, Vice President and Publisher, Consumer Dummies

Joyce Pepple, Acquisitions Director, Consumer Dummies

Kristin A. Cocks, Product Development Director, Consumer Dummies

Michael Spring, Vice President and Publisher, Travel

Kelly Regan, Editorial Director, Travel

Publishing for Technology Dummies

Andy Cummings, Vice President and Publisher, Dummies Technology/General User

Composition Services

Gerry Fahey, Vice President of Production Services

Debbie Stailey, Director of Composition Services

Contents at a Glance

Table of Contents

Introduction

*W*hat a difference a day makes. Or, to be more precise, 2,138 days. In the years since the first edition of *Controlling Cholesterol For Dummies* appeared, the medical and nutritional experts have (among other things):

- Changed the numbers that say, "This is a healthy cholesterol level."

- Revised the definition of "bad cholesterol" (low-density lipoproteins, or LDLs) to reflect the discovery that some "bad" cholesterol may actually be just fine.

- Introduced new combo drugs that zap both the cholesterol you get from food *and* the cholesterol your own body makes.

- Re-evaluated the role of hormones in raising or lowering the risk of heart disease.

- Clarified some of the differences between how male and female bodies handle cholesterol.

- Changed the drill on which vitamins, minerals, and other nutrients may (or may not) reduce cholesterol levels.

- Reaffirmed the virtues of the Mediterranean Diet and moderate drinking.

- Added some new items to the list of foods that fight cholesterol.

- Introduced new "functional" foods that fight cholesterol (including a chocolate laced with cholesterol-buster fatty acids).

- Set up some new Web sites to provide cholesterol guidance on everything from defining cholesterol terms (what is a triglyceride, anyway?) to evaluating your own personal risk of a cholesterol-related heart attack.

In other words, the people who rule The World Of Cholesterol Medicine have been very busy little bees. Which is why you are holding this book in your hands. It contains tons of new info to help you control your cholesterol, keep your arteries as clear as a newborn babe's, and thus keep your heart beating merrily along for years to come.

When it comes to solving life's little problems — whether to eat that chocolate cake, whether to dye your hair orange, or whether to lower your cholesterol — I choose to follow the ancient Greek mantra, "Moderation in all things."

In other words, I get to eat the cake about once a week; my hair is gray/

blonde, not orange; and this book is called *Controlling Cholesterol For Dummies* rather than, say, *Knocking Cholesterol Down to Zero For Dummies.*

The simple fact is that no one is perfect, but most people can be much, much better. The same principle holds true for your cholesterol levels. When cholesterol is the topic, lower is almost always better. (I talk about a few exceptions throughout this book.) But if you set a goal you can never reach — dropping 50 points off your cholesterol reading by two weeks from Tuesday — you'll fall off the wagon long before your cholesterol level falls a milligram.

My point? This book is eminently reasonable and moderate; I designed it to help you (working with your doctor, of course) keep your cholesterol within safe boundaries.

About This Book

Controlling Cholesterol For Dummies, 2nd Edition, doesn't ask you to turn yourself into an anti-cholesterol fanatic — the kind of annoying person who sneers at other people's dinner choices while acting superior about his own. (Actually, sneering and acting superior at the same time is a neat trick if you can do it. Just don't try it on your friends at dinner.)

My goal with this book is to lay out the reasons why it makes sense to control your cholesterol and then present reasonable and moderate strategies to help you reach your goal.

Some of the information, like how to translate the cholesterol numbers you get on your annual physical, is simple. Other stuff, such as guidelines you can use to determine whether you're a candidate for a heart attack — or for cholesterol-lowering medication — is more complex.

Throughout this book, the emphasis is on the idea that (here comes another catchy slogan) "Knowledge is power." In this case, it's the power to lower your cholesterol and reduce your risk of heart attack.

Conventions Used in This Book

Don't get me wrong. I write about nutrition, food, and health for a living, but I have to admit that some books and articles about these subjects can be pretty boring. (Unless the author is instructing you how to lose 30 pounds in 30 days or lower your cholesterol by 50 points in 50 minutes. But I deal with non-fiction subjects. Sorry.) I try to remedy this sleepy state of affairs with this book. So, if a few of my jokes don't tickle your funny bone, forgive me. After all, how funny can high cholesterol and plaque-filled arteries be?

To make this book as easy to use as possible, the following conventions are followed throughout:

- ✔ All Web addresses appear in monofont.

  When this book was printed, some Web addresses may have needed to break across two lines of text. If that happened, rest assured that I haven't put in any extra characters (such as hyphens) to indicate the break. So, when using one of these Web addresses, just type exactly what you see in this book, pretending the line break doesn't exist.

- ✔ New terms appear in *italics* and are closely followed by an easy-to-understand definition. I also use italics for emphasis once in a while.

- ✔ **Bold** font highlights keywords in bulleted lists or identifies the action parts of numbered lists.

- ✔ When you find information about the nutrient content of brand-name products in this book, you can assume that what you're reading was right when I wrote it. But here's the catch: Sometimes products change practically overnight. So use the numbers here as a guide, but be sure to check the product label when you shop. As poker players like to say, "Trust your friends — but cut the cards."

What You're Not to Read

Yes, you read that right. You don't have to read everything contained within these snazzy black and yellow covers. Any text in a gray box is a sidebar. Sidebars contain "nice to know" (and may I add, pretty interesting) material, but skipping them won't take away from your understanding of the subject at hand.

Additionally, anything marked with a Technical Stuff icon deals with nuts-and-bolts medical info that simply provides background information and in-depth scientific explanations about various subjects. You may skip these bits of text as well (although they provide some great info, if I do say so myself).

Foolish Assumptions

A writer has to make a few assumptions about her audience, and I've made a few assumptions about you. If you've picked up this book, I'm guessing that you fall into one or more of these categories:

- You've been told by your doctor that your cholesterol levels aren't up to par, and you have to do something about it.

- You've heard all the talk about high cholesterol in recent years, and you want to find out what all the fuss is about.

- You routinely buy every *For Dummies* book that hits the shelf, and this one is next on your list.

- You're a health-conscious individual.

- You're concerned about heart disease, and controlling the ol' cholesterol levels has become very important to you.

I've also assumed that you don't have a level of health-related knowledge to rival the U.S. Surgeon General's. If this assumption is correct, you've come to the right place. Easy-to-follow explanations are a hallmark of this book.

But if you approach the subject of controlling cholesterol with some information already tucked away in that brain of yours, don't worry — I've included plenty of info in this book for you as well.

How This Book Is Organized

This summary aims to whet your appetite for cholesterol control by giving you a glimpse of what's ahead in the 14 regular chapters, four — count 'em, four — Part of Tens chapters, and one bang-up, nutrition-chart appendix. Use this section as a thumbnail guide to what you want to read first.

Part 1: Getting Up Close and Personal with Cholesterol

Chapter 1 is, well, the first chapter. It explains why you should read this book — to reduce your risk of heart attack. Chapter 2 explains the good side of cholesterol (yes, cholesterol has a good side), as well as the problems it can cause. Chapter 3 says, "Okay, now figure out your own personal risk of cholesterol-related heart disease."

Don't skip Chapter 3: The news may be better than you think. And hey, if it isn't, the rest of the book tells you how to reverse the picture and improve your odds for a long, healthy life.

Part II: Eating Your Way to Lower Cholesterol

Yes, your diet pulls some weight when it comes to your cholesterol numbers. Actually, your diet matters big time. Chapter 4 lays out principles for a cholesterol-lowering diet proposed by all the usual suspects, oops, I mean experts. Chapter 5 tells you how to assemble a cholesterol-lowering diet. Chapter 6 tells how to apply the information in chapters 4 and 5 to real life.

Part III: Leading a Cholesterol-Lowering Lifestyle

Diet matters, but so does your lifestyle. Chapter 7 is a *very* important explanation of the relationship between your weight and your cholesterol levels. Chapter 8 describes how movin' your bod can help push down your cholesterol.

Chapter 9 is *not,* repeat *not,* a both-sides-of-the-issue type of chapter. Smoking does many bad things, including lifting your cholesterol levels, so this chapter pulls no punches.

In Chapter 10, I head back into moderate territory — moderate drinking that is. In study after study, sober researchers have found that moderate drinking — one drink a day for a woman, two drinks a day for a man — appears to increase your "good" cholesterol and lower your risk of heart attack. Check it out.

Part IV: Cutting Cholesterol with Nutrients and Medicine

Chapter 11 is all about nutritional supplements, including vitamins and how they affect your cholesterol, sometimes in surprising ways. Chapter 12 is a primer on cholesterol-lowering prescription drug products — the good, the bad, and (sorry about this) the truly ugly. Chapter 13 is a guide to medicines that may adversely affect your cholesterol (and your heart). Chapter 14 is filled with recipes for fun, heart-healthy party foods so that you can continue to control your cholesterol while celebrating special occasions.

Part V: The Part of Tens

I just love this part of the book because it lets me draw up lists of odd and unusual factoids that I may not otherwise be able to include.

Chapter 15 lists ten good Web sites for heart and cholesterol info. Chapter 16 has ten nifty nutrition Web sites. Chapter 17 is one of my favorites — ten cholesterol myths. Chapter 18 tickles my historical fancy with ten really important moments in cholesterol history.

This part also includes an appendix, which contains a chart of more than 500 foods and the cholesterol, fat, and fiber content for common servings. The material, from my old friend, the U.S. Department of Agriculture (USDA), is invaluable when you're putting together heart-friendly meals. So use it.

For even more info on even more foods, check out the USDA Nutrient Database (which I discuss in Chapter 16) on the Web at www.nal.usda. gov/fnic/cgi-bin/nut_search.pl.

Icons Used in This Book

Throughout this book you find a collection of handy icons in the margins. These icons highlight particularly useful information and can help you get the most out of your copy of *Controlling Cholesterol For Dummies,* 2nd Edition.

This icon makes your life easier. It signals an activity that saves you time or a bit of knowledge that I've gained from experience.

Think danger! This icon warns you to tread carefully. Pay close attention: Your health could turn out worse for the wear if you don't follow this advice.

I use this important icon to call out basic rules and information that you can file away for future reference whenever you encounter related situations.

You can skip this stuff if you want, but if you want to get really down and dirty with cholesterol details, dive in.

Where to Go from Here

No, you don't have to start at Chapter 1 and read straight through this book. As with all *For Dummies* books, this one is set up so you can read any chapter, in any order, and still come out ahead.

Sound good? Then keep on reading (starting wherever you want, of course).

Part I

Getting Up Close and Personal with Cholesterol

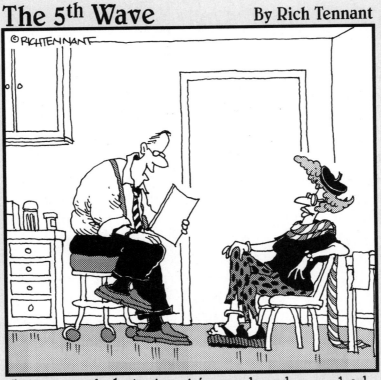

The 5th Wave — By Rich Tennant

©RICHTENNANT

"Your good cholesterol is good, and your bad cholesterol isn't so much bad as it is charmingly irreverent."

In this part . . .

To do the best job of controlling your cholesterol, you need to have a handle on the basics — info such as what cholesterol is, where it comes from, what it does, and why some varieties are more threatening than others. And being a Serious Seeker of Knowledge, you probably want to be able to perform a realistic evaluation of your own risk of developing cholesterol-related problems. The info you need is right here in this part. Go for it.

Chapter 1

Mapping the Heart Land

Heart disease is America's number one health killer; it's ahead of every type of cancer combined and every infectious and degenerative disease. Heart attack is the most common form of heart disease, and one significant risk factor for heart attack is high cholesterol or, more specifically, a high level of certain kinds of *low-density lipoproteins* (LDLs) — the "bad" fat and protein particles that ferry cholesterol into your arteries.

If you already know all this introductory stuff, feel free to skip Chapter 1 and head right into Chapter 2 where I describe cholesterol's dual nature (yes, cholesterol has two sides).

But, then again, this chapter does lay out a statistical picture of heart disease and heart attack and explain the role cholesterol plays in placing you at risk. In fact, come to think of it, this chapter is a darn good intro to *Controlling Cholesterol For Dummies,* 2nd Edition.

No surprise there!

Ladies and Gentlemen, Meet Your Heart

Your heart is a pretty spectacular organ — a four-chambered, hollow muscle right smack in the middle of your chest. The heart's job is to pump the blood that carries life-giving oxygen and other nutrients to every body tissue. To show how this works, the clever *For Dummies* artists have drawn a cross section of your heart in Figure 1-1 tracing the path of blood flowing in and out and in and out and in . . . you get the idea.

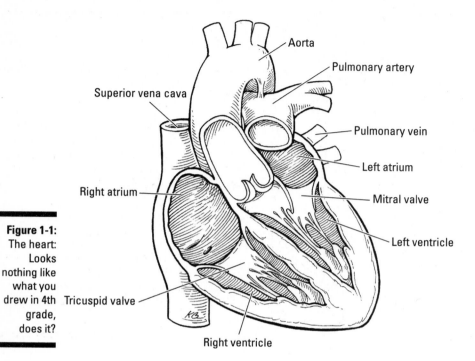

Figure 1-1:
The heart:
Looks
nothing like
what you
drew in 4th
grade,
does it?

Every second of every minute of every hour of every day, blood flows out from your heart to carry oxygen and other nutrients to every tissue and organ in your body, and then comes back to your heart to pick up more oxygen and nutrients. In other words, blood *circulates,* which is why your heart and the vessels through which blood travels are called the *circulatory system.*

The best way to explain this process is to begin at the beginning, the point at which blood flows back from your body, into your heart:

1. **The blood enters your heart from the superior *vena cava,* a large vein that opens into the *right atrium,* the first chamber of your heart.**

Yes, the *vena cava* and the right atrium are on the left side of the picture above. In this picture, you're looking at the front of the heart as it sits in the chest of the person to whom it belongs. If he were to turn around so that you were looking at him from the back, the vena cava and the right atrium would be in the correct position, on the right side of his body. Got it? Good. Onward.

Naming the blood vessels

Blood vessels are grouped according to the job they perform in your body, which means they're grouped in terms of whether they carry blood *to* your heart or *away* from your heart. This list explains how the groupings work:

- ✔ **Veins:** Blood vessels that carry blood toward your heart. The word *vein* comes from *vena,* the Latin word for hollow.

- ✔ **Venules:** Small veins.

- ✔ **Capillaries:** Teensy, little veins that connect arteries to veins right under the skin. When blood flows into your capillaries, the red liquid under the skin gives you a rosy glow — a blush.

- ✔ **Arteries:** Blood vessels that carry blood away from your heart. The word *artery* comes from *arteria,* the Latin word for windpipe.

- ✔ **Arterioles:** Very small arteries.

I have no idea why the person who named the blood vessels picked a word that means hollow for veins and a word that means windpipe for arteries. If it were up to me, I would've used a word that means "bring to" for veins, and a word that means "go away from" for arteries.

In fact, the words *afferent* (from the Latin *ad* = toward and *ferro* = carry) and *efferent* (*ferro* plus the Latin *ex* = away*)* are used to describe, respectively, nerves that carry impulses to or away from the central nervous system. Maybe whoever named the blood vessels picked *veins* and *arteries* because *afferent* and *efferent* were already taken. Works for me.

2. From the right atrium, blood spills down through a one-way "trapdoor" called the *tricuspid valve* and into the *right ventricle.*

3. When the right ventricle contracts (squeezes together), the blood is sent out of your heart through the *pulmonary artery* and into your lungs where it picks up a plentiful supply of oxygen.

4. The newly oxygenated blood flows back into your heart through the *pulmonary vein* into the *left atrium.*

5. Then the blood spills down through a second one-way trapdoor called the *mitral valve* and into the *left ventricle.*

6. When the left ventricle contracts, blood is pushed up through the large artery called the *aorta* and out into your body.

In real life, as opposed to a drawing, the right atrium and the left atrium receive blood simultaneously from the vena cava and the pulmonary vein respectively. The right and the left atria (plural for atrium) contract simultaneously to send blood down through the tricuspid valve and the mitral valve respectively. And the right and left ventricles contract simultaneously to push blood up into the pulmonary artery and the aorta respectively. All this without missing a beat. Hey, I told you this was a spectacular organ!

Talking heart disease

The phrase *cardiovascular disease* (CVD) means "all medical conditions affecting the heart and blood vessels." CVD includes heart attack, high blood pressure, stroke, rheumatic heart disease, congenital defects, and congestive heart failure.

Coronary artery disease (CAD) or *coronary heart disease* (CHD) means "conditions affecting the heart and its major blood vessels" — heart attack and *angina pectoris* (chest pain due to narrowed blood vessels).

Myocardial infarction (*myo* = muscle, *cardio* = heart, *infarction* = blockage) is the formal name for a heart attack. The name pretty much describes what happens, but you can read all the truly excruciating details in Chapter 2.

Attack of the Killer Heart Disease

Heart disease is the leading killer of Americans, and heart attacks are the most common form of heart disease. But you don't have to take my word for it. Many U.S. government agencies, including the Centers for Disease Control and Prevention and the National Center for Health Statistics, have piled up a ton of stats and translated all the numbers into dozens of charts to show exactly how lethal heart disease can be.

Heart disease versus everything else

First things first. Table 1-1 lists the ten leading causes of death in the United States for 2004. See what's in first place? Check it out. *Note:* Stroke, a form of cardiovascular disease known medically as *cerebrovascular disease,* is counted as a separate category.

Table 1-1	Ten Leading Causes of Death in the U.S. in 2004
Condition	*Number of Deaths*
Heart disease	654,092
Cancer (all kinds)	550,270
Stroke	150,147

Condition	Number of Deaths
Chronic respiratory disease	123,884
Accidents (unintentional injuries)	108,694
Diabetes	72,815
Alzheimer's disease	65,829
Influenza/pneumonia	61,472
Kidney disease	42,762
Blood poisoning	33,464

Source: Arialdi M. Minino, Melonie P. Heron, Betty L. Smith, Deaths: Preliminary Data for 2004, National Vital Statistics Reports, 54, 19, June 28, 2006.

Heart disease versus heart attack

The United States isn't alone in its battle with cardiovascular disease (CVD) and coronary heart disease (CHD) — heart attack. According to the World Health Organization (WHO), CVD and CHD are the Numero Uno nasties around the globe. Grouping the rich countries, poor countries, and countries in-between, WHO statisticians discovered one common thread: Heart disease kills more people every year than any other illness or medical condition.

Table 1-2 lays out the WHO statistics for causes of death in 2002 and the predicted figures for 2005. Some points of interest in these figures are as follows:

- ✔ Yes, as you read this, 2005 is already several years in the past, and 2002 is practically ancient history. But as every math major knows, in the statistics game, several years must pass before you can gather all the numbers you need to draw a firm conclusion. Hence the lag time.

- ✔ Yes, the percentage of the world's population that succumbs to the various forms of cancer is lower than the percentage in the United States. Why? Because in many poor countries, so many infants die at birth or expire young of preventable illnesses that there are fewer people who grow old enough to develop and eventually die of illnesses of older age, such as cancer or Alzheimer's disease.

Table 1-2	The Ten Leading Causes of Death Worldwide	
	2002	*2005 (projected)*
Cardiovascular disease/ Coronary heart disease	7,210,000	7,570,000
Respiratory infections	3,890,000	3,680,000
Stroke	3,807,000	5,740,000
HIV/AIDS	2,760,000	8,550,000
Chronic obstructive pulmonary disease (COPD)	2,750,000	3,010,000
Causes linked to birth	2,430,000	1,780,000
Cancer (breast, colorectal, lung & throat, stomach)	2,160,000	4,050,000
Diarrheal diseases	1,540,000	1,480,000
Malaria	1,240,000	870,000
Diabetes mellitus	220,000	240,000

Source: *World Health Organization, Fact Sheet #310, March 2007.*

Getting to the Point of This Book

Congratulations! By plunking down some of your hard-earned cash for a copy of *Controlling Cholesterol For Dummies,* 2nd Edition, (or borrowing it from a smart friend), you've made a commitment to, well, try to control your cholesterol before it controls you.

And, by slogging your way through a discussion of how your heart works and a slew of charts with figures proving what I bet you already knew — heart disease and heart attack send a great many folks to their ultimate reward — you've shown just how serious you are about getting a handle on those nasty cholesterol numbers. As a reward, now, by gosh, you've reached the heart of the matter: cholesterol.

Why counting cholesterol numbers counts

In the past half century, literally hundreds of well-run scientific studies, run by thousands of different researchers in dozens of different countries, have shown beyond a shadow of a doubt that having high cholesterol — specifically, high levels of LDLs, particularly the smaller ones described in Chapter 2 — is a strong warning that Mr. Heart Disease and Ms. Heart Attack are lying in wait somewhere in the future. Luckily, a similar long list of studies shows that what you eat and how you live your life to stay fit and relatively trim can help reduce your risk

How to control your cholesterol risks

What you eat and drink plays an important role in controlling your cholesterol, as I explain in Part II of this book. So does maintaining a healthful weight, engaging in a realistic exercise program, and avoiding tobacco (in all its ugly forms) — three subjects covered in Part III. And if these basic first steps don't do the job, cholesterol-lowering medications, discussed in Part IV, offer yet another option.

Each of these methods for lowering your cholesterol — diet, weight control, exercise, and medicines — has its own chapter (or two or three) in this book. As a health-conscious consumer, you get to pick and choose among them — like a gourmet at a gorgeous buffet table. A low-fat, low-cholesterol buffet table, of course. After which you can relax with the grab bag of factoids and funny stuff in Part V — the well-known *For Dummies* Part of Tens.

Go for it. Your heart will thank you.

Chapter 2

Comparing Cholesterol's Risks and Benefits

In This Chapter

▶ Locating the cholesterol in the human body

▶ Proving that cholesterol has a good side

▶ Confirming cholesterol's risks

▶ Identifying other harmful compounds in your blood

▶ Mastering CPR

_T_his chapter starts off by covering the ways in which your body uses cholesterol for everything from powering your brain to building your sex hormones. Then — fair is fair — you can find out why something so good can also be hazardous to your heart health.

Finally, because cholesterol isn't the only bad guy to be found in your blood, I provide you with a short description of some of the other unhealthy criminals floating through your bloodstream.

After you've made your way through the heavy stuff, reward yourself with a bit of fun by taking the heart art quiz at the end of this chapter. The quiz asks you to match literary, musical, and other heart-related titles with their authors.

Shaking Hands with Cholesterol

Cholesterol is the Dr. Jekyll and Mr. Hyde of the nutrition world. This fat-like substance is both essential for your healthy body and potentially hazardous to your heart.

Double trouble

The split-personality title character in Robert Louis Stevenson's novel, *The Strange Case of Dr. Jekyll and Mr. Hyde* (1886), embodies both good and evil — the two sides of human nature. (Pop quiz: Which personality is the good guy? Which one isn't? See the end of this sidebar for the answers.)

This sort of duality isn't uncommon in religion, philosophy, and literature. For example, the Aztec god Quetzalcoatl was both male and female. And Janus, the Roman god of doors, had two faces, one in the front of his head and one in back, because every door faces two ways — in and out. By the way, Janus is the namesake of January, the door to the New Year.

The Chinese symbol of two-sidedness is the yin and the yang. The yin symbolizes the female, and the yang stands for the male. The yin and yang also symbolize the coexistence of other opposing concepts, such as life and death, good and evil, black and white, and love and hate. What makes this even more interesting is the fact that the word *yin,* which sounds totally non-Western, is a variant on the Scottish word for *one.*

So, you can see that cholesterol has some company when it comes to having two sides to a story. And Jekyll is the good guy; Hyde isn't.

Making the most of cholesterol's Jekyll-like good characteristics while counteracting its Hyde-like bad impulses can be a delicate but not impossible balancing act. The task begins with understanding how and where cholesterol does its good work and how and where it can cause problems. Begin your mission, in the true scientific spirit, at the beginning.

Where cholesterol comes from

Yes, you get some cholesterol from food, but the curious fact is that most of the cholesterol in your blood and body tissues is produced right in your very own liver. Your liver uses the proteins, fats, and carbohydrates in food to manufacture and churn out about 1 gram (1,000 milligrams) of cholesterol a day.

How cholesterol travels around your body

Whether your cholesterol comes from food or your liver, it travels through your bloodstream in particles called *lipoproteins,* a name derived from *lipos* (the Greek word for "fat") and *protos* (Greek for "first" or "most important").

The fatty substances in lipoproteins include cholesterol and *triglycerides,* the most common fatty substance in the human body (more about triglycerides in the section "Focusing on Other Blood Baddies"). The proteins that combine with fats to produce lipoproteins are called *apolipoproteins,* often abbreviated as *apo.*

Lipoproteins develop through five distinct phases as they mature into the particles that carry cholesterol around your body:

- **Phase 1:** Chylomicrons
- **Phase 2:** Very low-density lipoproteins (VLDLs)
- **Phase 3:** Intermediate-density lipoproteins (IDLs)
- **Phase 4:** Low-density lipoproteins (LDLs)
- **Phase 5:** High-density lipoproteins (HDLs)

How does a chylomicron become a VLDL, then an IDL, then an LDL, and finally, maybe, an HDL? The following roadmap marks the route.

Bringing up baby lipoproteins

A lipoprotein is born as a *chylomicron,* a particle that your intestinal cells assemble from the proteins and fats you eat. Chylomicrons are very, very low-density particles.

Why are some lipoproteins called *low-density* and others *high-density?*

- The term *density* refers to a lipoprotein's weight.
- Protein weighs more than fat.
- Lipoproteins containing proportionately less protein than fat are low-density lipoproteins, also known as LDLs. LDLs are the "bad" particles that carry cholesterol into your arteries.
- Lipoproteins containing proportionately more protein than fat are high-density lipoproteins, also known as HDLs. HDLs are the "good" particles that ferry cholesterol out of your body.

Now, back to chylomicrons. These lipoproteins start out with very little protein and a lot of light and fluffy fat and cholesterol. But as they flow through your bloodstream from your intestines on their way to your liver (your body's lipoprotein factory), the chylomicrons release their fats, known as *triglycerides,* into your blood.

The stripped-down chylomicron, also known as a *chylomicron remnant,* still has its cholesterol and protein. Now, the remnant slides into your liver, and fat comes back into the picture.

Moving through the fat factory

As anyone who has ever read a nutrient chart knows, liver (as a food) is very high in fat and cholesterol. In fact, *your* liver is a veritable fat and cholesterol factory that collects fat fragments from your blood and uses them to make cholesterol and new fats that your body can use to build tissue and perform other physiological functions.

The next few sections explain exactly how lipoproteins are made.

Putting the fats in lipoproteins (and taking them out again)

When the chylomicron hits the liver, it picks up fat particles and mutates into the largest kind of lipoprotein, a fluffy particle called a *very low-density lipoprotein* (VLDL).

Then your liver sends the VLDL out into the wide world — your body. As the VLDL travels far and wide, it drops globs of fat, picks up globs of cholesterol, and changes into a slightly smaller, heavier particle called an *intermediate low-density lipoprotein* (IDL), and then a slightly smaller, heavier *low-density lipoprotein* (LDL).

The last step in the transformation of the baby lipoprotein (the chylomicron) occurs when an LDL has dropped so much fat and cholesterol into body tissue that it's mostly protein. Now, you're looking at a *high-density lipoprotein* (HDL).

Naming the proteins in lipoproteins

The primary proteins in VLDLs, IDLs, and LDLs belong to a class of apolipoproteins called *apoB.* The primary proteins in HDLs belong to a class of apolipoproteins called *apoA.* Other less prominent apolipoproteins found in lipoproteins are *apoC* and *apoE.*

You may have heard about a blood test for apoA; this test is interesting because a high level of apoA indicates a high level of protective HDLs (the "good" particles that haul cholesterol out of your body).

Pinning a blue ribbon on good lipoproteins

HDLs truly deserve the name "good cholesterol." These particles don't carry cholesterol into your arteries for the simple reason that they're so compact and dense that they can't squeeze through the spaces in the walls of your arteries. As a result, HDLs — and their cholesterol — travel away from your arteries and out of your body with the rest of your, um, solid waste.

What a neat set of facts to park in the back of your brain for the next time you're at a party and someone asks you to explain the differences between VLDLs, IDLs, LDLs, and HDLs. "Well," you can say, "it's all a question of density, which, as you know, means. . . ." Don't you just love being the smartest kid in class?

The good news about HDLs

You can think of HDLs as scavenger molecules that remove cholesterol from the arteries. Having a lot of HDLs reduces your risk of heart attack regardless of your total cholesterol levels.

In fact, X-ray studies have shown that people who raise their HDLs by exercising, stopping smoking, or taking medication not only reduce the cholesterol in the arteries but also remove the plaque — thus opening the arteries.

Having read that paragraph carefully, you may assume that all LDLs are bad guys, right? Wrong.

With LDLs, size may make all the difference

For years, everyone — that is, all the experts evaluating your cholesterol — conversely believed that a person with a lot of light and mushy LDLs (which *can* squeeze through your artery walls) inevitably had a higher risk of heart attack. The fact that some people with high levels of LDLs sailed happily into old age without experiencing heart problems was dismissed as plain good luck.

Maybe not, says a group of researchers at Albert Einstein College of Medicine in New York City. In 2003, looking for clues to longevity, the team, which included members from the University of Maryland School of Medicine, Tufts University, Boston University School of Medicine, and Roche Molecular Systems, ran various tests, including cholesterol tests, on 213 senior citizens, plus 216 of their children and grandchildren. For comparison, they ran the same tests on a control group of non-blood relatives, such as the children's husbands and wives.

The tests showed something really surprising: The long-lived oldsters were three times more likely than other people to have a mutation in a gene that regulates *cholesteryl ester transfer protein* (CETP), an enzyme that affects the size of lipoproteins. As a result, compared with other people, including those non-related husbands and wives, even the oldsters who had high levels of LDLs had relatively larger low-density lipoproteins. (Their HDLs were also relatively bigger.)

According to the Einstein team, led by Dr. Nir Barzilai, the level of LDLs doesn't predict heart disease; it's the size of the LDLs in the mix. In other words, having many small LDLs may raise the risk of heart attack even if your overall cholesterol level is low. Definitely more to come on this one.

Believe It or Not, You Need Cholesterol

Your healthy body needs cholesterol, but I haven't told you the reasons why. Let me list them now:

- ✔ Cholesterol directs the development of some cells in the growing fetus.
- ✔ Cholesterol is part of the membrane that surrounds and protects each cell in your body.
- ✔ Cholesterol comprises a major portion of your brain, which is composed of mostly fatty tissue.
- ✔ Cholesterol contributes to the construction of *synapses,* structures through which nerve cells transmit messages.
- ✔ Cholesterol is a building block for hormones, including the male sex hormone testosterone and the vital adrenal hormone cortisone.
- ✔ Cholesterol is an ingredient in digestive juices, such as bile.
- ✔ Cholesterol is used as a building block for vitamin D, which is made when sunlight hits the fatty tissue just under your skin.
- ✔ And, oh yes, cholesterol is part of body fat.

Is that an impressive list or what? I think it's impressive as all get out, so I'm going to take some time to explain exactly how cholesterol performs each of these incredibly important jobs.

Cholesterol helps your body develop

Cholesterol begins to influence your body even before you're born. According to a 1996 report in the journal *Science,* cholesterol enhances an embryo's healthy development by triggering the activity of the specific genes that instruct embryonic cells to become specialized body structures — arms, legs, spine, and so on. Sadly, as *Science* reported, approximately one in every 9,000 babies is born with a birth defect linked to the fetus's failure to make the cholesterol it needs.

In 2003, researchers at the U.S. National Human Genome Research Institute linked a pregnant woman's cholesterol deficiency to a defect in the fetal brain called HPE (the failure of the brain to divide normally into two halves). Ninety-nine percent of embryos with HPE are spontaneously aborted; those born live experience severe mental retardation, are unable to walk or talk, and usually die within the first year of life.

To prevent these problems, pregnant women are often advised not to take cholesterol-lowering drugs.

Cholesterol holds your cells together

Think back to your first chemistry or physics class. Never took chemistry or physics? Well, then imagine being in class where one of the first things your teacher wants you to know is that there's no such thing as a solid substance.

Things that look solid — this book, that lamp, you, and me — are actually gazillions of individual atoms, molecules, and cells whirling around in space, held together only by an exchange of electrical charges. If you can't remember much chemistry or physics, check out the "Recognizing the difference between an atom, a molecule, and a body cell" sidebar in this chapter. Mark your place, read the sidebar, and then come right back.

Okay, as I was saying, some things that look solid aren't solid. They're simply groups of cells held together by electrical charges that keep the cells in place so that a piece of this page or a piece of your finger doesn't go spinning off into space. Individual cells stay intact because they have a *cell membrane,* an outer skin that serves as neat and tidy packaging for the cell.

One requirement for healthy cell membranes is — drumroll please — cholesterol. A whopping 90 percent of all the cholesterol in your body is in your cell membranes. The cholesterol protects the integrity of the cell membrane, helping to keep it flexible and strong.

If you were to diet so stringently or use so many cholesterol-lowering drugs that your cholesterol level fell to zero (an impossibility by the way), your cell membranes would be very dry and easily torn. The stuff inside the cells would leak out, and cells would die all over the place. That would sort of put an end to the whole darn shootin' match. Every healthy body cell needs some cholesterol, and so does every healthy brain.

Recognizing the difference between an atom, a molecule, and a body cell

Atoms are the basic building blocks of elements — hydrogen, oxygen, carbon, and all their chemical cousins.

Each atom carries the name of the element it represents (such as *hydrogen*). In addition, each atom has a shorthand symbol — call it a nickname — such as *H* for hydrogen. Sometimes, an atom's shorthand name seems totally divorced from its full name. For example, lead atoms are called, well, lead atoms, but the symbol for a lead atom is *Pb*, from *plumbum*, the Latin word for lead. There are also elements and atoms named for human beings. For example, seaborgium is named for Nobel Laureate Glenn T. Seaborg; its shorthand symbol is *Sg*.

Individual atoms form bonds with other atoms to create clusters of atoms called *molecules*. To write the name of a molecule — its formula — you write the symbols of the different atoms that the molecule contains and the number of each type of atom right after the symbol. For example, if I write H_2O, the formula for the water molecule, you know immediately that a water molecule has two hydrogen atoms and one oxygen atom.

A *body cell,* the smallest independent unit of a living creature, is a collection of molecules. And you, wonderful reader, are a collection of cells.

Cholesterol builds your gray matter

As French philosopher René Descartes so eloquently wrote in 1637, "I think, therefore I am." The organ that enables you to think — and therefore, to be — is your brain, a marvelous structure composed primarily of water and fat.

The average human brain weighs about 3 pounds. Up to 78 percent of that weight is water. Some of the weight is protein (8 percent), some is carbohydrates (1 percent), and some is a grab bag of organic and inorganic compounds (3 percent). The rest (up to 12 percent) is fat, including — surprise, surprise — cholesterol.

Cholesterol on the brain? You bet. As I explain in the next section, without cholesterol, your brain cells can't send the messages that power every other organ in your body and, most importantly, make it possible for you to think. To paraphrase Descartes, "Wow!"

Cholesterol revs up your nerve cells

The fact that you have cholesterol in your brain tissue isn't a new discovery, but the knowledge of what the cholesterol actually does up there is new. In November 2001, a group of French and German researchers at the Max-Delbruck Center for Molecular Medicine in Berlin reported something extraordinary, so extraordinary that the lead researcher told fellow scientists at a meeting of the Society for Neuroscience, "We were definitely shocked."

Before getting to the shocking part, take a timeout for a short but important lesson in neurology. About 90 percent of the cells in your brain are non-nerve cells called *glial cells.* Glial cells aren't the cells through which brain cells communicate, so they have always seemed sort of blah.

Now comes the shocking part. The guys at Max-Delbruck discovered that glial cells contain cholesterol, which enables them to secrete a molecule that encourages the formation of *synapses,* teensy junctions in the brain where messages are exchanged among nerve cells. The molecule secreted by the glial cell is called *apolipoprotein E* (apoE). When the Berlin researchers added plain cholesterol to nerve cells in a laboratory dish, the nerve cells began to form synapses like crazy.

So should you start stuffing yourself with cholesterol-rich foods to jump-start your brain? In a word, no. Your glial cells make all the cholesterol your brain requires. The point of this section is just to let you know what cholesterol is doing up there in your head.

Cholesterol is part of your hormones

What else can one wonder fat do? "What else?" you ask? How about, it helps make you sexy?

Chemically speaking, cholesterol is a *sterol,* a compound made of hydrogen and oxygen atoms arranged in a series of ring-like structures with chain-like attachments of atoms hanging off the sides. Your body uses cholesterol to synthesize other sterol compounds, such as the adrenal hormone *cortisol,* the fat-soluble nutrient vitamin D, and — yes, indeed — the male sex hormone, testosterone.

Figure 2-1 shows the structure of the cholesterol molecule, and Figure 2-2 shows the structure of the molecule for testosterone. See how similar they are? Didn't expect that, did you?

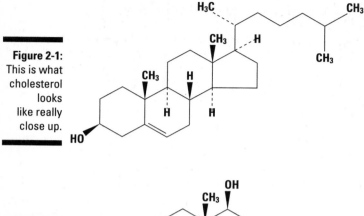

Figure 2-1: This is what cholesterol looks like really close up.

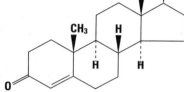

Figure 2-2: And here's a close-up of testosterone.

Cholesterol powers up your digestive system

The gallbladder is a small organ that sits atop your small intestine. In pictures of the digestive system, the gallbladder is often colored green because it secretes a greenish liquid called *bile* or *bile acids,* digestive compounds based on — you got it — cholesterol.

On their own, fats — including the fats in food — don't mix with water. Fat molecules and water molecules lack the chemical hooks-and-eyes (the proper electrical charges) needed to form bonds between their molecules. As a result, when you swallow fat-rich foods, the fat floats on top of the watery food and liquid mixture in your stomach, which means that fat-busting digestive enzymes in the mix below can't reach it. But as fatty food moves through your digestive tract into your small intestine, an intestinal hormone called *cholestokinin* beeps your gallbladder, signaling it to release bile.

Bile is an *emulsifier,* a substance that makes it possible for fat to mix with water so you can digest and absorb dietary fats and fat-soluble nutrients such as vitamins A, D, E, and K.

Without cholesterol, you wouldn't be able to make bile or bile acids. Without bile and bile acids, you wouldn't be able to absorb fats. Without fats, you wouldn't be able to manufacture fatty tissue, which cushions your organs, keeps your body warm, and serves as a base for various body chemicals. And that state of affairs isn't compatible with a healthy, comfortable life. So thank your lucky stars that you have the cholesterol you need to make the bile and bile acids that process fat.

Breaking the Bad News

By now, you may be convinced that everything you've ever read about cholesterol is wrong, wrong, wrong. In fact, you may be muttering to yourself, "Hey, where can I get some more of this great stuff?" Well, hold your horses, cowboy. I hate to be the one to break this to you, but cholesterol can be a villain as well as a hero.

Yes, cholesterol protects your cells, maintains your brainpower, helps make hormones and vitamins, and on, and on, and on. But under certain circumstances, it can block your arteries and trigger — Oh no! — a heart attack. It's all in the lipoproteins. This section focuses on cholesterol's not-so-good effects on your body.

Cholesterol may endanger your heart

LDLs are the most common fat-and-protein particles in your body. Like their parents, the VLDLs and their cousins the IDLs, LDLs are soft enough to squeeze between the cells of your blood vessel walls, dragging cholesterol into your coronary arteries (the blood vessels leading away from your heart).

Once inside an artery, cholesterol particles may get caught on the infinite number of chinks in the artery wall. Stuck in place, the cholesterol now snags other particles floating by, eventually creating deposits called plaque. In time, the plaque on the artery wall may grow thick enough to block the flow of blood through the blood vessel, or a piece of plaque may break off, triggering the formation of a blood clot that can also block the artery. Either way, the sequence is called a heart attack.

As a general rule, heart docs assume that the more cholesterol you have floating through your bloodstream — especially the "bad" LDL cholesterol — the higher your risk for plaque build-up in your arteries and the higher your risk of a heart attack. In other words, to lower your risk of heart attack, you must lower your cholesterol, particularly those "bad" LDLs.

But this simple equation may not be the solution for *every* human body. In December 2007, the results from a clinical trial of the new drug ezetimibe (Zetia) showed that taking the medicine, either alone or in combination with the statin drug simvastatin (Zocor), definitely lowered "bad" cholesterol, but also hastened the buildup of arterial plaque for some of the people in the trial.

In other words, simply lowering their LDLs did not protect these people from a heart attack. Something else, such as an individual tendency to pile up arterial plaque, also seemed to be at work. (Conversely, people with high cholesterol but clear arteries may have the opposite attribute — an inherent ability to resist plaque — that explains the puzzle of why some people with high cholesterol do not have heart attacks.)

You can read more about the ezetimibe trial in Chapter 12, which lays out the facts on various cholesterol-buster meds. Right here, the take-away point is that when you're talking medicine, never assume that one size — or one theory — fits all.

Cholesterol can clog your brain

This is a very short section because everything you need to know about how cholesterol may be hazardous to your brain can be summed up in one word — *ditto*.

That's *ditto* to what you've just read about cholesterol and your coronary arteries. Having high levels of cholesterol may also increase the risk of plaque in a cranial artery. Plaque can block the flow of blood traveling through a cranial artery to your brain, triggering a stroke.

Prevention is another ditto. The preventative steps that you can take in relation to your coronary arteries and your heart can also benefit your cranial arteries and your brain.

Cholesterol can build boulders in your gallbladder

Cholesterol is a building block for the bile you need to digest fats. This side of cholesterol behaves like the good Dr. Jekyll. But every yin has its yang, and the bad Mr. Hyde is gallstones.

A gallstone is a rock-like lump that forms when the normal percentages of fat in bile change so that the fat (in this case cholesterol) clumps in a lump in your gallbladder or in the duct leading from the gallbladder to your intestines. Approximately 80 to 95 percent of all gallstones are made primarily of cholesterol. (The rest are made primarily of calcium.)

According to the National Institute of Diabetes and Digestive and Kidney Disease (NIDDK), as many as 42 million Americans have gallstones. Many of the risk factors for cholesterol gallstones are the same as those for heart disease, such as the following:

- ✔ Diabetes
- ✔ High-cholesterol diet
- ✔ Obesity
- ✔ Smoking

But here's an odd fact: Yes, being overweight raises your risk of gallstones, but so does going on a diet and losing weight very rapidly.

When your body is deprived of its normal quota of calories and fat, your liver is likely to increase its natural production of cholesterol (see the "Where cholesterol comes from" section back toward the beginning of this chapter). Sometimes you can't win for losing, which includes the symptoms, signs, and consequences of gallstones: pain, nausea, belching, vomiting, fever, chills, and, maybe, surgery to remove your gallbladder.

If your doctor recommends yanking out the offending organ, not to worry. Or at least not too much. True, all surgery has potential risks, but modern gallbladder surgery is performed laparoscopically (translation: through very small incisions that heal quickly).

Once the gallbladder is out, you probably won't notice much change in your ability to eat what you want. Your gallbladder is just a storage bin where bile produced by the liver is parked until your body yells, "Yo! Send down some bile." After surgery, your liver still produces bile, which still makes its way into the intestine to help you digest fats.

While some people do develop gastric rumbles, okay, diarrhea, after eating a large, very fatty meal, most patients do just fine so long as they stick with food/meals containing moderate amounts of fat. What's moderate varies from person to person. If you exceed your own personal limit, trust me, you will know.

Tick. Tock.

According to Yasuko Rikihisa, professor of veterinary biosciences at Ohio State University, people with high cholesterol may be more susceptible to human granulocytotropic anaplasmosis (HGA), a disease transmitted by *Ixodes scapularis* (deer tick), the little buggers that spread Lyme disease.

HGA attacks granulocytes, cells the immune system uses to knock out infectious agents such as bacteria. In Rikihisa's lab, mice with high cholesterol were less able than mice with normal cholesterol levels to fight off HGA.

Should you worry about those mice? Maybe. The United States experiences up to 1,000 cases of HGA a year, but the symptoms of HGA are so similar to those caused by flu that many cases may go undetected. Once diagnosed, HGA can be treated with antibiotics; left untreated, HGA, like flu, may be fatal for those who are very young, very old, or have a weakened immune system. In other words, watch your cholesterol and never ignore a tick bite. But you knew that already, right?

Focusing on Other Blood Baddies

Although cholesterol gets most of the buzz, it isn't the only substance in your blood that increases your risk of heart disease. Two other problematic compounds discussed in this section are homocysteine and triglycerides. The first is an amino acid; the second is a thoroughly useful fat.

Hunting homocysteine

Amino acids are the building blocks of protein. Most amino acids are friendly to your body, but homocysteine is a potentially hostile amino acid released when you digest protein foods. Researchers have conducted about a dozen important homocysteine studies in recent years, and most of the studies have demonstrated a clear link between high homocysteine levels (called *hyperhomocysteinemia*) and an increased risk of heart attack. The reasons for this connection are still a mystery. The current theory is that homocysteine may chew up cells in the lining of your blood vessels, trigger blood clots, or produce debris that blocks the arteries.

The American Heart Association (AHA) hasn't yet labeled hyperhomocysteinemia a major risk factor for cardiovascular disease. But the AHA does recommend that people who have at least one other known risk factor for heart disease, such as high blood pressure, high cholesterol, smoking, obesity, or a family history of heart disease, attempt to lower their homocysteine level.

How do you lower homocysteine? No problem. The good news is that consuming adequate amounts of the B vitamins — folic acid (also known as folacin or folates), vitamin B6 (also known as pyridoxal, pyridoxine, and pyridoxamine), and vitamin B12 — efficiently lowers the amount of homocysteine in your blood.

If you're at high risk, check with your doctor to see how you can include foods high in B vitamins in your diet. Table 2-1 lists the homocysteine fighters and some of the foods you can find them in. It hasn't been shown, however, that lowering homocysteine levels in the blood reduces the incidence of heart disease.

Table 2-1	Homocysteine Fighters
Vitamin	_Contained in_
Folic acid	Beans, citrus fruits, fortified wheat flour, grains, tomatoes, green leafy vegetables
Vitamin B6	Asparagus, bananas, beans, bok choy, cauliflower, grains, tuna, turkey, mustard/turnip greens
Vitamin B12	Fish, milk, poultry, red meat

Source: U.S. Department of Agriculture.

Tracking triglycerides

Ninety-five percent of the fats in foods are _triglycerides_, compounds that contain one molecule of glycerin and three (tri) molecules of fatty acids. Triglycerides are also the most common fats in your body. You use them to

- Build _adipose_ (fatty tissue)
- Build cholesterol
- Fuel your energy

Chapter 5 has a complete definition of the different kinds of fats and fatty acids in your food. For the moment, just take my word for the fact that triglycerides are made of one unit of glycerol and three fatty acids.

Glycerol is a small, water-soluble carbohydrate that carries fats through blood; fatty acids are chains of carbon atoms with hydrogen atoms attached.

You get some triglycerides from food. You also manufacture them in your liver using carbohydrates, alcohol, and some of the cholesterol in food. Either way, high levels of triglycerides are a risk factor for heart disease because, like cholesterol, triglycerides — which travel in lipoproteins — can rough up the lining of your arteries, which enables floating particles to get stuck and begin to build plaque that can clog the artery, leading to a heart attack.

How high is high? Check out Chapter 3 where you can also find a whole bunch of tests designed to rate your risk of heart disease.

Clearly, you want to keep your triglycerides in the normal range, which means watching what you eat. But here's an interesting fact: A diet that's very low in fat and very high in carbohydrate foods, such as veggies, fruits, and grains — the quintessential "good heart" diet — may actually raise your triglycerides rather than lower them.

To lower your triglycerides, the AHA recommends eating a reasonable amount of polyunsaturated fats. No kidding. Read all about fats in Chapter 5. So much reading, so little time.

Warning! Heart Attack in Progress!

You say, "Heart attack." Your doctor says, "Myocardial infarction." Either way, heart attacks occur when the blood supply to your heart muscle is suddenly reduced or completely shut off. This reduction in blood supply is most commonly caused by a piece of plaque that breaks off from an artery wall, triggering the formation of a blood clot. That is why a coronary artery filled with a lesser amount of soft plaque (which can break off easily) is more dangerous than an artery filled with hard plaque.

The damage caused by a heart attack is due directly to how long the artery is blocked and how long your heart muscle and your brain don't get the oxygen they need. Clearly, the faster a heart attack victim gets medical attention, the better his or her chances of surviving with minimal damage.

Knowing the symptoms

To get help, you need to recognize the classic symptoms of a heart attack:

✔ Pressure or pain in the center of your chest that lasts longer than a few minutes. Some people describe the pain as feeling like an elephant is sitting on their chests.

✔ Pain that starts in your chest and spreads out to your shoulders, up your neck, to your jaw, or down your arms.

✔ Pain in your chest plus

- Feelings of lightheadedness

- Nausea or heavy sweating

- Shortness of breath

- All of these symptoms, all at once

This list sounds definitive, but it isn't. Diagnosing a heart attack is tricky business because any one of the symptoms listed above — on its own, without any pain — may also be a heart attack alert.

Sometimes, simple lightheadedness (what an awkward word) or nausea is the body's way of saying, "Listen up! We're in trouble here!" This is especially true for women who, as a group, are likely to experience much less severe heart attack symptoms than men do. The lesson? Better safe than sorry.

Chest pain or a feeling of "tightness" (sometimes described as a rubber band tightening around your chest) or pressure (sometimes described as "an elephant sitting on your chest") that comes on with exertion such as walking up a slight hill, especially in cold weather, or climbing an ordinary flight of stairs that hadn't caused problems in the past is a suspicious symptom. You should see your doctor or go to the emergency room immediately lest your symptoms signal an imminent heart attack.

As soon as you suspect that someone is having a heart attack, the American Heart Association recommends taking (or giving) one 325-milligram aspirin. The aspirin is a blood thinner. According to the AHA, taking the aspirin at the onset of symptoms lowers the risk of dying by 23 percent. Would you believe that only 20 to 40 percent of all heart attack victims follow this simple recommendation that the AHA insists could save 10,000 lives a year?

Never, ever ignore signs of a problem. Don't panic, but do move quickly. Dial 911 or your local emergency medical service (EMS) to summon an ambulance staffed by EMS technicians who are trained to treat heart attack victims. The ambulance is likely to get to you faster than you can get to the hospital, especially if you're the one having the heart attack and would have to drive yourself.

Yes, yes, yes. If the hospital is right across the street, you should just go. But will you go? Will your friend? Maybe not. According to the AHA, denial is common. Many heart attack victims refuse to believe that they're having a heart attack. That attitude can be a killer, robbing you (or your friend) of precious time.

Never ignore signs of a heart attack. If you're with someone who's having symptoms, don't take *no* for an answer. Your friend may protest now, but she'll thank you later when she's still alive.

Becoming a coronary lifeguard

One type of heart attack is due to a cholesterol-related blockage of an artery. A second type of heart attack is *cardiac arrest,* a sudden interruption in the heartbeat that effectively stops the circulation of blood and oxygen throughout the body, leading fairly quickly to the phenomenon called *sudden death.*

The American Heart Association estimates that more than half the people who experience cardiac arrest outside a hospital setting can be saved if someone in the immediate vicinity knows how to perform cardiopulmonary resuscitation, commonly called CPR.

CPR uses physical compression of the patient's chest along with breathing into his mouth to restart the heart while providing desperately needed oxygen. If you don't already know CPR, get familiar with it. The life you save won't be your own — even if you're so flexible that you can wrap your legs behind your ears, you can't do CPR on yourself — but your skill may someday save someone near and dear to you.

The following sections cover three ways to discover how to perform CPR.

Join a CPR class

The absolutely best way to master CPR is to take classes from a live instructor in a room with live people. You practice on an inflatable dummy and not the person standing next to you, but being in class gives you the opportunity to ask questions that can help perfect your technique.

To find classes in your area, do an Internet search for the American Heart Association. After you reach the home page, slide your mouse down the left side of the page and click "Local info." Then click the name of your state to get the phone number for your local AHA chapter.

You may also find CPR classes at your local YMCA/YWCA, a police precinct, or a firehouse. In addition, many businesses now conduct classes on site for their employees. If yours doesn't, maybe this is one suggestion to drop in the work comment box.

Heart art

Once upon a time, poets, authors, playwrights, and just about everyone else thought of the heart as the seat of some of our warmest emotions, not as an organ in distress. Some of this sentiment is still around — consider the late 20th-century illustration, "I ♥ you." So, as promised in the intro, I end this chapter on a warm and fuzzy note.

Heart art is an opportunity to revisit this simpler point of view. Match the heart-related story, play, song, and film titles with their authors. While scoring high isn't necessarily the point, getting seven or more answers correct qualifies you as a heart specialist. If you fall on the younger side of this book's audience, check it out with Mom and Dad. Grandparents are good sources, too.

Film, Song, Story, or Play	Responsible Individual(s)
1. "Heart and Soul" (song)	a. Carson McCullers
2. *Heartburn* (film)	b. Edgar Allen Poe
3. "Don't Go Breaking My Heart" (song)	c. Elaine May
4. "The Telltale Heart" (short story)	d. Frank Loesser (lyrics) Hoagy Carmichael (music)
5. "Piece of My Heart" (song)	e. Ned Washington (lyrics) Victor Young (music)
6. *The Heartbreak Kid* (film)	f. Robert Hunter (lyrics) Jerry Garcia (music)
7. "Foolish Heart" (song)	g. Elton John
8. *Heart of Darkness* (long short story)	h. Joseph Conrad
9. "My Heart Belongs to Daddy" (song)	i. Janis Joplin
10. *The Heart Is a Lonely Hunter* (play)	j. Cole Porter
11. "My Foolish Heart" (song)	k. Robert Dunn, Paul Guay, Stephen Mazur
12. *Heartbreakers* (film/2001)	l. William Goldman/Stephen King
13. *Hearts in Atlantis* (film)	m. Nora Ephron

Answers: 1. d, 2. m, 3. g, 4. b, 5. i, 6. c, 7. f, 8. h, 9. j, 10. a, 11. e, 12. k, 13. l

Study CPR at home

You can study CPR with the American Heart Association's CPR Anytime kit. Check out www.cpranytime.org online and order CPR Anytime Today! You can choose between adult and child models, and the $29.95 kit includes a CPR Anytime Skills Practice DVD, a CPR for **Family and Friends** resource booklet, and — among other things — your very own personal inflatable manikin (medical dummy).

Read about CPR

In a pinch, until you can get to a class or order a DVD, one excellent online site for CPR techniques is *Learn CPR*. The URL address is www.depts. Washington.edu/learncpr. This site, supported by the University of Washington School of Medicine, is a real treasure with pictures and diagrams and FAQs and facts and links and quizzes and CPR history.

The site is a great place to start, but eventually you need to polish your technique with a live instructor.

Chapter 3

Rating Your Cholesterol-Related Risk

- -

In This Chapter

▶ Running through the tests to count your cholesterol and check your arteries

▶ Explaining why your cholesterol level is where it is

▶ Adapting adult cholesterol goals for kids

▶ Explaining how cholesterol's effects change with age

▶ Figuring your own personal chance for heart attack

- -

*T*his chapter is totally straightforward. The information here has just one purpose: to provide answers to three basic questions and make it possible for you to evaluate your own cholesterol-related risk of heart disease (the whole range of heart problems) and heart attack (the 800-pound gorilla). As for those three basic questions, here they are:

✔ **Question #1:** What's the real definition of high cholesterol?

✔ **Question #2:** Who's likely to have high cholesterol?

✔ **Question #3:** Are you at risk for high cholesterol?

My editors remind me that I should tell you to grab a pencil before you start reading this chapter because I include several tests for you to fill out at the end. Meanwhile, *avanti*! (That's Italian for, "Let's get to it!")

Categorizing Cholesterol as a Risk Factor

Generally, medical risk factors fit into one of three basic categories:

- Risk factors you can't control
- Risk factors you can control
- Risk factors whose effects you can lessen but not entirely eliminate

High cholesterol is an interesting risk factor because it fits into all three of these categories. Take a look at the evidence:

- Your genes determine how much cholesterol your body produces naturally, so high cholesterol may be a risk factor you can't control.
- You can take one of several different cholesterol-lowering drugs designed to pull your cholesterol down to safe levels, so high cholesterol may be a risk factor you can control. (For more about cholesterol-lowering drugs, check out Chapter 12.)
- You can change your diet, lose weight, and exercise to increase your "good" cholesterol, *high-density lipoproteins* (HDLs), while lowering your "bad" cholesterol, *low-density lipoproteins* (LDLs), so high cholesterol (or at least high "bad" cholesterol) may be a risk factor whose effects you can soften.

My point? Although high cholesterol is an important risk factor for heart disease — and decreasing your longevity — you have a leading role to play in controlling the risk. What you eat, how you spend your leisure time, and how you work with your doctor have much to do with determining where your rank is on the cholesterol scale. Interesting proposition, eh?

Adding Up Your Basic Cholesterol Numbers

Before you decide what to do about your cholesterol, you need to know how much cholesterol you actually have. So get up, march over to your doctor's office, and hold out your arm so your doctor can stick a hollow needle into the vein in the crook of your elbow and draw about 20 milliliters (ml) of bright, red blood. Then when you go home, the little glass tube holding your blood goes off to a medical laboratory where a technician counts the cholesterol particles. The results you get back look like this: 225 mg/dL. Translation: You have 225 milligrams of total cholesterol in every deciliter (⅒ liter) of blood.

But these numbers don't paint the whole picture. The figures for your low-density lipoproteins (VLDLs, IDLs, LDLs) and high-density lipoproteins (HDLs) are still missing. Shaky on the details? You can read all about these little fellas in Chapter 2, which explains that lipoproteins are fat-and-protein particles that carry cholesterol into your arteries (LDLs) or out of your body (HDLs), which is why HDLs are "good" and *some* of the LDLs are "bad."

The problem with simple *finger-stick tests* such as those found in cholesterol home-testing kits is that they only measure *total* cholesterol levels — no HDLs and no LDLs. An incomplete result (total cholesterol alone) can scare you to death if it shows you have high total cholesterol without letting you know that you — lucky girl! lucky boy! — also have high HDLs. The finger-stick test can also provide false reassurance if it shows a low total cholesterol level without letting you know that your LDLs are also very low.

Now that you know all this and have an accurate, complete doctor's report in hand, what do the results say about you? How can you tell if the numbers are high, low, or in-between?

Defining Higher, Lower, Medium — and Just Right

The information you need to grade your cholesterol levels comes from the usual suspects — I mean the usual experts: the National Cholesterol Education Program (NCEP) at the National Heart, Lung, and Blood Institute (NHLBI), an arm of the National Institutes of Health (NIH).

In 2001, the NCEP issued a report called *ATP III*, short for *The Third Report of the Expert Panel on the Detection, Evaluation, and Treatment of High Blood Cholesterol in Adults.* In this report, the NCEP said:

✔ A total cholesterol level higher than 240 mg/dL translates into a "high risk" for heart disease.

✔ A total cholesterol level between 200 and 239 mg/dL means there's a "moderate risk" for heart disease.

✔ A total cholesterol level below 200 mg/dL is "desirable."

Regardless of total cholesterol levels, the risk of heart attack is highest among men whose HDLs are lower than 37 mg/dL and women whose HDLs are lower than 47 mg/dL. Conversely, the risk of heart attack is lowest among men whose HDLs are higher than 53 mg/dL and women whose HDLs are higher than 60 mg/dL.

Table 3-1 shows the current descriptions of various levels of total cholesterol, LDL cholesterol, and HDL cholesterol.

Table 3-1	Characterizing Cholesterol Levels
Total Cholesterol	
<200 mg/dL	Desirable
200–239 mg/dL	Borderline high
>240 mg/dL	High
LDL Cholesterol	
<100 mg/dL	Optimal
100–129 mg/dL	Near optimal/Above optimal
130–159 mg/dL	Borderline high
160–190 mg/dL	High
>190 mg/dL	Very high
HDL Cholesterol	
<40 mg/dL	Low
>60 mg/dL	High

Source: National Cholesterol Education Program, www.nhlibi.nih.gov/huide lines/cholesterol/atglance.htm.

But in July 2004, just when everyone thought they had the numbers down pat, the experts at the NCEP added a footnote: People at high risk should push their LDLs down below 100 mg/dL, a task that requires taking one or more of the cholesterol-busting drugs described in Chapter 12.

Are these recommendations final? Probably not. Experience shows that precise numbers for healthful cholesterol levels can change at any moment. What doesn't change are the basics: Higher HDLs are good. Lower LDLs are good. Sooner or later, like Goldilocks and the Three Bears, someone will figure out exactly how low and how high is *just right.*

Blood simple

Blood circulates through a system of vessels called arteries and veins. *Arteries* carry blood away from the heart; *veins* carry blood back to the heart. The average human body has about 5 quarts of blood. Large people may have slightly more; small people may have slightly less. Every 60 seconds, about ⅕ quart of blood flows out of your heart through your coronary arteries. Sixty seconds after that, the blood zips through your entire circulatory system and heads back to your heart.

The life span of one red blood cell is about 120 days for a man and about 14 days less for a woman. Men have more red blood cells — about 4.5 to 6.2 million per cubic microliter of blood compared to 4 to 5.5 million for women. Because males have more red blood cells, they also have higher values of *hemoglobin,* the pigment in red blood cells that carries oxygen throughout the body. They also have higher levels of iron, an important element in hemoglobin.

White blood cells play a primary role in your immune system as avengers that zero in on invaders, such as bacteria, to chew them up and spit them out. The normal number of white blood cells is exactly the same for men and women — 4,100 to 10,900 per microliter of blood.

Blood is a vehicle for nutrients, medications, and other circulating particles such as — what a surprise — the lipoproteins that carry cholesterol. By the way, the blood for a cholesterol test always comes from a vein, not an artery. Blood from a vein is easier and safer to obtain, and it's a representative sample of what's in your body. And yes, clenching your fist does make your vein pop up so it's easier to puncture.

Listing Other Risk Factors

According to the American Heart Association, as you read this chapter an estimated 105,200,000 Americans have total cholesterol levels higher than 200 mg/dL, putting them all into the *borderline high* category; 36.6 million of those have *high* total cholesterol levels above 240 mg/dL. Who are all these people? What puts them into these special high-risk categories?

Age and gender

Among people younger than 50, men are more likely to have high cholesterol. After age 50, women edge into the lead. Either way, a woman's blood vessels are more elastic than a man's blood vessels. As a result, women have a little more protection than men throughout their lives against a blood clot that may block their blood vessels and trigger a heart attack.

Pregnancy — strictly a female activity — lowers a woman's levels of good HDLs, but a study of 1,051 women conducted by researchers at Kaiser Permanente in Oakland, California, showed that nursing the newborn for longer than three months is protective and reduces the decline of HDLs.

Counting kids' cholesterol

The cholesterol levels shown in Table 3-1 earlier in this chapter are for grown-ups. (Translation: *Adults* are people between the ages of 20 and 74.) The recommendations for children are a different story. A child's total cholesterol level rises slowly from age 2 to age 10 and then begins to rise and fall in a gender-related pattern. According to University of Texas (Houston) researcher Darwin R. Labarthe, a girl's cholesterol level is likely to peak around age 9, a boy's around age 16. Conversely, a girl's cholesterol level goes down for a while around age 16; a boy's cholesterol goes down for a while around age 17.

All adults should be tested at least once to establish a baseline cholesterol reading; if the level is higher than it should be, more frequent testing may be required. But as of this writing, the American Academy of Pediatrics (AAP) only recommends cholesterol testing for a relatively small number of children:

- Kids with a parent or grandparent who had a heart attack, suffered a stroke, or received a diagnosis of coronary artery disease before age 55

- Children whose parents have high cholesterol (above 240 mg/dL)

The recommendations of the American Heart Association (AHA) are similar to those of the AAP. The AHA suggests only testing children older than the age of 2 who have a family history of coronary artery disease — a parent or a grandparent with high cholesterol or a history of heart disease.

Table 3-2 shows the AHA-recommended cholesterol levels for children and adolescents between the ages of 2 and 19.

Table 3-2	Kids' Cholesterol Levels	
	Total Cholesterol	*LDL*
Acceptable	<170 mg/dL	<110 mg/dL
Borderline	170–199 mg/dL	110–129 mg/dL
High	>200 mg/dL	>130 mg/dL

Source: *American Heart Association,* www.americanheart.org/presenter.jhtml?identifier=4499.

Lower isn't always safer

You get your blood test back from your doctor and — wonder of wonders — your cholesterol has dropped! Time to celebrate? Not necessarily.

A steady, gradual decrease in cholesterol due to a cholesterol-control diet (see Chapter 4) or one of the new cholesterol-lowering medications (see Chapter 12) is great. But a sudden, unexplained decline in total cholesterol — *hypocholesterolemia* in doctor-speak — may be a pre-clinical sign (something that shows up before disease is evident) of malnutrition, an overactive thyroid, cirrhosis of the liver, certain forms of cancer, or genetic mutations. All of these factors can drop total cholesterol levels to the basement (<100 mg/dL).

And get this: According to a 2007 report on a 2,000-person study at the Aging Research Center at the Karolinska Institute in Stockholm, Sweden, a sudden unexplained drop in cholesterol levels at mid-life, around age 50, may be a risk factor for cognitive problems (translation: dementia) later on. Sometimes it seems you can't win for losing!

Gilding the golden years

Pssst! Come over here. I have a secret to share with you. As people turn 70 and sail into their eighth decade, their cholesterol level becomes a less important predictor of death by heart disease.

What should you make of this?

- ✔ Perhaps people who die of cholesterol-induced coronary artery disease simply check out earlier in life. After all, cholesterol is often described as a risk factor for an early heart attack.
- ✔ Perhaps, as you age, your cholesterol level becomes less important than your overall health.
- ✔ Perhaps total cholesterol levels aren't as important as LDL and HDL levels, which aren't reflected in studies that show the decreasing importance of cholesterol levels as a predictor of death by heart disease as people age.

Should you rush out to tell grandma and grandpa to toss out that salad and start gorging on high-fat, high-cholesterol foods? Not yet. But you can send them a postcard with this comment from the American Heart Association: "The issue of cholesterol levels in the elderly is still unclear."

Ethnicity

The cholesterol stats on ethnic groups in the United States are, to put it mildly, incomplete. Many stats exist for non-Hispanic Blacks, non-Hispanic Whites, and Mexican Americans. Scattered statistics exist for Native Americans, but there are no numbers for other ethnic groupings. As a result, given the variety of human beings in the U.S., it's hard to figure out exactly which ethnic groups are most at risk of high cholesterol.

Nonetheless, Table 3-3, Table 3-4, and Table 3-5 provide useful — though, *repeat,* incomplete — guides. The tables show the percentage of 99,900,000 Americans (48,400,000 men and 51,500,000 women) age 20 and older whose cholesterol, LDL, or HDL levels put them at increased risk of heart disease in 2003.

Yes, this study predates the American Heart Association estimate of 105,200,000 adults with cholesterol levels above 200 mg/dL cited above (see "Listing Other Risk Factors" earlier in this chapter). That's life in statistics-land.

Table 3-3	Percentages of U.S. Males with Specific Cholesterol Levels, 2003			
Population	*Total Cholesterol >200 mg/dL*	*Total Cholesterol >240 mg/dL*	*LDL Cholesterol >130 mg/dL*	*HDL Cholesterol <40 mg/dL*
All men	50.1%	17.0%	40.8%	31.7%
Non-Hispanic Whites	47.9%	16.1%	31.7%	26.2%
Non-Hispanic Blacks	44.8%	14.1%	32.4%	15.5%
Mexican Americans	49.9%	16.0%	39.0%	27.7%

Source: American Heart Association, American Stroke Association, Heart Disease and Stroke Statistics – 2007 Update At-a-Glance.

Table 3-4	Percentages of U.S. Females with Specific Cholesterol Levels, 2003			
Population	*Total Cholesterol >200 mg/dL*	*Total Cholesterol >240 mg/dL*	*LDL Cholesterol >130 mg/dL*	*HDL Cholesterol <40 mg/dL*
All women	55.2%	19.7%	38.6%	12.3%
Non-Hispanic Whites	49.7%	18.2%	33.8%	12.3%
Non-Hispanic Blacks	42.1%	12.5%	33.8%	6.9%
Mexican Americans	50.0%	14.2%	30.7%	13.0%

Source: American Heart Association, American Stroke Association, Heart Disease and Stroke Statistics – 2007 Update At-a-Glance.

Table 3-5	Percentages of Asian/Pacific Islanders and Native American Men and Women, Cholesterol Levels Higher than 240 mg/dL, 2003
Group	*Total Cholesterol >240 mg/dL*
Asian/Pacific Islanders	27.3%
Native Alaskans	26.0%
Native Americans	28.6%

Source: Heart Disease and Stroke Statistics – 2000 Update, Circulation, January 11, 2006, 113: e85-e151, `http://circ.ahajournals.org/cgi/content/full/113/6/e85/TBL13.`

Evaluating Your Own Risk Factors File

Now that you know what's high and what's low in the wide world of cholesterol and who's likely to have high cholesterol and who isn't, you can turn your attention to the specifics for one person: you. This section helps you figure out your very own personal risk of having high cholesterol. Begin at the beginning: your family.

When the "A" list rates a "B"

According to Ronald M. Krauss of the University of California (Berkeley), not everyone is created equal when it comes to LDL (the "bad" cholesterol) production. First in 2001 and then in follow-up studies in 2004 and 2005, Krauss proposed that genes tend to divide people into two groups of LDL-makers.

Some people — the A list — make big, bouncy LDLs. Others — the B list — make smaller, denser LDLs. (Need to know more about density — as in low-density lipoproteins? See Chapter 2.)

The B people tend to get better results when they go on low-fat, carb-based diets to reduce overall cholesterol levels, dropping levels of both the big LDLs and the little LDLs, which results in an overall reduction in LDL cholesterol. The A people lose a lot of big, non-threatening LDLs, but their overall level of small, dense LDLs (the bad guys) rises. The catch is that nobody has yet identified the gene that determines whether you are an A or a B. Stay tuned.

The family

Your family history says a lot about your future. Your genes are a family trait, so if your first-degree relatives — father, mother, brothers, and sisters — have high cholesterol, you may too. If your father or brother had a heart attack when he was younger than 55 or your mother or sister had a heart attack before she turned 65, you need to watch your other risk factors.

But, all things being relative, your relatives' cholesterol levels may not mirror yours. In my family, my mother has high cholesterol, and so do I. My father had low cholesterol, and so does my sister who, I might point out, also got the good nails and curly hair. Life can be sooooooo unfair!

You, yourself, and you

Some medical conditions either affect your risk of having high cholesterol or intensify cholesterol's bad effects. If you have one of these conditions, you probably already know about the risks. But it never hurts to be sure, so here's the scoop.

High blood pressure (hypertension)

Blood pressure is the force exerted by your heart when it pushes blood out into your arteries. When your arteries are clear and clean, your heart has an easy job: The blood flows easily into the arteries, and your blood pressure is normal.

But if your arteries have been narrowed — perhaps by cholesterol plaque buildup on the inside walls — your heart must contract more strongly and push harder to get the blood out into the vessel. As a result, blood is pushed out of the heart at higher-than-normal pressure. The high-pressure stream of blood bouncing against arterial walls can worsen the damage caused by cholesterol and plaque. (The damage is called *arteriosclerosis* or "hardening of the arteries.")

How can you tell if you have high blood pressure? Look at your blood pressure reading. You'll see two numbers written like this: 130/90 or 130/90 mm/Hg. The first number, the *systolic* reading, is the pressure exerted by your heart when it contracts (beats) to pump out blood. The second number, the *diastolic* reading, is the force exerted by your heart between beats.

The letters *mm/Hg* stand for millimeters/mercury. (Hg is the chemical symbol for mercury.) These terms are part of the reading because your doctor measures blood pressure by how high (in millimeters) mercury rises on the little gauge attached to the blood pressure cuff wrapped around your arm. Reading the gauge is similar to reading the temperature on a thermometer as the mercury inside the thermometer's glass tube rises or falls when warmed or cooled.

For years and years, doctors considered an adult's blood pressure normal when the systolic reading was lower than 130 mm/Hg and the diastolic reading was lower than 90 mm/Hg (130/90), but the newest numbers from the experts at the National Institutes of Health now put normal at 120/80. And as with cholesterol, there are varying degrees of normal when it comes to describing blood pressure.

Table 3-6 shows the most recent categorization of blood-pressure levels from the National Institutes of Health, starting with *optimal* (translation: the best possible result), and running up (or down) through *normal* and *high normal* to the various stages of *hypertension* (higher than high, and potentially hazardous to your health).

Table 3-6	Pressure Points	
Category	*Systolic Pressure*	*Diastolic Pressure*
Optimal	<120 mm/Hg	<80 mm/Hg
Normal	<130 mm/Hg	<85 mm/Hg
High normal	130–139 mm/Hg	85–89 mm/Hg
Mild hypertension	140–159 mm/Hg	90–99 mm/Hg
Moderate hypertension	160–179 mm/Hg	100–109 mm/Hg
Severe hypertension	>180 mm/Hg	>110 mm/Hg

If you already have high blood pressure, your doctor has no doubt told you about the basic strategies you can use to control it:

- ✔ Lose weight.
- ✔ Change your diet.
- ✔ Exercise.
- ✔ Take a pill.

Strangely enough, these steps sound just like the ways to control cholesterol. Think of them as a medical two-for-one coupon!

Diabetes

People with diabetes often have frighteningly high cholesterol levels. I'm not talking your piddling 240 mg/dL reading here. No, what I mean is a cholesterol level hovering around — hold your hat — 500 mg/dL.

People with diabetes also have high blood-levels of insulin, the hormone produced by the pancreas and used to digest food. Yes, I know, you may have thought that people with diabetes have low levels of insulin. Actually, people with diabetes do produce less insulin than healthy people do, but they also have a problem using insulin to digest food, so the unused insulin continues to circulate in their blood until it is excreted from the body.

Type 2 diabetics are usually overweight adults. Being overweight leads to insulin resistance. Insulin resistance means that the cells in the body require a greater amount of insulin to push the glucose (sugar) into the cells so it can be used for energy. This is why they have higher levels of circulating insulin.

The best way to control diabetes? Lose weight, change your diet, exercise, and take your medicine. Good ways to control cholesterol? Lose weight (Chapter 7), change your diet (Chapter 4), and — sometimes — take your medicine (Chapter 12). Are you beginning to see a pattern here?

Previous heart attack

If you've already had a heart attack, you know your cholesterol numbers, and your doctor has probably already prescribed one of the cholesterol-lowering medications I talk about in Chapter 12. No need to dwell on this one.

Obesity

No, you don't have to be rail thin. No, you don't have to spend your life on a diet. Your body was created to be at a good weight for your size and shape. This weight may not be the same for you as for your best friend or that model over there in the who-is-she-kidding slinky dress or the painted-on swim trunks. Just turn to Chapter 7, which explains exactly how excess pounds raise your cholesterol level and how staying in reasonable shape or losing as few as 3 to 5 pounds can lower your cholesterol.

Lifestyle

Are you a couch potato? Do you smoke? Shame on you! Don't wait another minute — turn to Chapters 8 and 9. Read about the hazards of inactivity and smoking. You can decide to change these risk factors by the time you finish reading this sentence. So do it.

Heart Attack Risk Factors at a Glance

High LDLs and low HDLs are only two of the heart attack risk factors on the list compiled by the National Cholesterol Education Project, a group with more statistical information than you can shake a stick at. (I have no idea why anyone would want to shake a stick at these stats — or even what the saying means. Inquiring minds want to know!) Table 3-7 gives you a quick rundown on a whole bunch of risk factors. What a handy guide!

Table 3-7	Risk Factors for a Heart Attack
Risks You Can't Control	
Being a man	
Being older than 45 (for men) or 55 (for women)	
Family history of heart attacks	
Risks You Can Control	
Being overweight or obese	
Inactivity	
Smoking	
Risks You Can Reduce	
High blood pressure	
Diabetes	
High levels of low-density lipoproteins	
Low levels of high-density lipoproteins	
High levels of triglycerides	
High levels of homocysteine	

Source: *National Cholesterol Education Project.*

Cultural math: When 13 = 4

Westerners often turn shivery when they see the number 13. The number that spooks some Asians is 4. In Mandarin, Cantonese, and Japanese, the word for the number *four* sounds exactly like the word for *death,* a linguistic oddity that may have serious implications for some Asian-American heart attack victims.

A recent report in the *British Medical Journal* compared death statistics from 1973 to 1998 for more than 200,000 Asian Americans and 47 million White Americans living in the United States. The data shows that Chinese-American and Japanese-American heart attack victims who die of their heart disease are most likely to die on the fourth day of the month.

The highest number of fourth-day deaths occurred among hospitalized heart attack victims (versus people who had a heart attack at home or somewhere else). One possible conclusion is that the power of suggestion may play an important role in deciding whether a person survives a heart attack. Another possible conclusion is that being able to leave the hospital quickly after a heart attack increases the chances of survival.

By the way, there was no similar link between the 13th day of the month and the incidence of death among non-Asian heart attack patients, perhaps because the word *thirteen* doesn't sound like *death.*

Checking for Plaque Buildup

A cholesterol blood test is definitely valuable because it tells you exactly where you stand, cholesterol-wise. But the test doesn't tell you whether you already have plaque — the technical term for cholesterol deposits — in your arteries or whether the plaque deposits are serious enough to set a heart attack in motion. That's a job for other tests specifically designed to determine the condition of your arteries. You can group these tests into two handy categories: blood tests and physical tests.

Blood tests

Blood tests are simple to do. Just stick out your arm and . . . well, if you've had your cholesterol tested, you know the drill.

Catching C-reactive proteins

C-reactive proteins (CRP) are substances released into your bloodstream when tissues, including the blood vessels leading to your heart, are damaged and inflamed. As a result, measuring levels of cardiac CRP in your blood can serve as a guide to the condition of your arteries and predict your risk of heart attack or stroke.

In 1998, a team of researchers from Brigham and Women's Hospital and Harvard Medical School rated the risks linked to CRP levels in blood samples from nearly 40,000 healthy, post-menopausal female nurses participating in the legendary *Nurses' Health Study.* The result? Women with the highest levels of CRP were five times more likely than women with very low levels to develop cardiovascular disease and seven times more likely to have a heart attack or stroke.

One year earlier, the Boston team noted similar results in an ongoing study of 22,000 healthy male doctors. These results led them to conclude that using "high-sensitivity" or "ultrasensitive" tests to measure cardiac CRP is a good way to "predict the risk of future heart attack and stroke events." (Check out Chapter 8 for info on the connection between exercise and reducing CRP levels.)

Measuring MPO

White blood cells are the body's natural defense against inflammation and infection. When the white blood cells sense trouble, they release *myeloperoxi-dase* (MPO), a protein that can knock the heck out of the bugs causing the inflammation and infection.

But MPO may also irritate arteries and short-circuit natural body chemicals that keep "bad" cholesterol particles from glomming on to artery walls, thus contributing to the buildup of plaque inside your blood vessels. In July 2007, the *Journal of the American College of Cardiology* published data from a study of more than 1,000 healthy Brits showing that, over the years, those with the highest blood levels of MPO had the highest risk of coronary artery disease (CAD).

In other words, high blood levels of MPO may signal artery trouble ahead, even when other indicators, such as LDL levels, are fine. Naturally, the researchers want to see more studies before they stick an MPO test onto your yearly lab tests, but, as one of the researchers said, "MPO looks like a 'keeper' that will one day become part of clinical care."

Many insurance companies, including Medicare, may not pay for CRP or MPO blood tests because they argue that if you have elevated levels, you need to make all the necessary lifestyle changes (lose weight, treat high blood pressure, stop smoking, eat a healthy diet, and so on). You should be doing this anyway! However, sometimes demonstrating to people that their risk of a heart attack in the next five years is great can stimulate them to become more serious about making lifestyle changes.

Physical tests

You don't stick out your arm for these tests; you warm up the muscles on treadmills and other such devices.

Stress tests

For a *simple stress test,* your doctor sticks electrodes on various parts of your anatomy, mainly your upper torso, and reads the results as you march on a treadmill or push the pedals on a stationary bike . . . No, no, no — come back. Electrodes aren't needles. They're round, flat gizmos that are "pasted" on to you with sticky fluid. The electrodes transmit electrical impulses to a machine. The machine then translates the impulses into numerical measurements of the flow of blood through your cardiovascular system as you do the treadmill or bicycle thing.

Sometimes a simple stress test delivers *false positives* (suggesting you have heart disease when you don't) or *false negatives* (suggesting you're risk-free when you're not). For more accurate results, your doctor relies on a *thallium stress test* or *sestamibi stress test.*

The thallium or sestamibi stress test begins with an injection containing radioactive thallium or sestamibi. After the shot, your doctor asks you to wait for about three hours while the radioactive substance circulates through your blood vessels. Then you get fitted with electrodes, climb on the treadmill or bike, and your doctor monitors your blood flow via those electrodes. Next you lie on a table while a special low-dose X-ray machine tracks the radioactive substance as it flows through your heart and blood vessels. As you can imagine, trouble spots — a narrowing here and buildup there — are clearly visible.

By the way, if you have a medical condition, such as arthritis, that makes it difficult for you to walk on the treadmill or ride the bike, your doctor can use a special medication called *persantium,* rather than exercise, to speed up your heartbeat and blood flow.

ECBT

No, *electron-beam-computed tomography* (ECBT), sometimes called *ultrafast CT,* isn't the machine that beams Captain Kirk up to the Enterprise. It's an injection-free CAT scan that provides snapshots of your heart, lungs, and coronary arteries to uncover the presence of calcium deposits, a warning sign of plaque buildup in your arteries.

The ECBT is about seven times faster than a conventional CAT scan. The test, which takes about five minutes to run, is a super way to catch plaque problems very early or (think positively) to show that you're plaque-free. Unfortunately, the test costs $300 to $500, and although doctors consider it basic medicine, some insurance plans haven't yet adopted this view. Bummer.

Angiogram

Having an *angiogram* isn't an everyday walk in the medical park. This procedure is reserved for people with chest pain or other signs of an imminent heart attack.

To perform the test, your cardiologist or radiologist (by this time, you're way past the primary-care-physician stage) inserts a very small tube called a *catheter* into an artery, sends dye through the tube into your bloodstream, and watches an X-ray monitor to see how freely the dye flows. If the dye suddenly slows or stops, blocked by a clot or narrowed area, your doctor may perform immediate *angioplasty,* the surgical procedure that removes the blockage and clears the blood vessel. In most cases, after clearing the vessel, the surgeon inserts a *stent* — a tiny spring — into the artery to hold it open, hopefully forever. The stent is designed to prevent *restenosis,* the technical term for blocking an artery after it has been cleared out. If the artery is blocked again, the treatment is a new angioplasty and a new stent.

In order to be able to do an angioplasty, the blockage must not be too far down the coronary artery or else the balloon won't be able to fit in there. If you have multiple blocked arteries or an angioplasty can't be performed, a cardiac surgeon can perform coronary bypass surgery whereby he takes arteries from one place in your body, such as the internal mammary arteries, and attaches them to your coronary circulation.

I certainly hope you never need an angiogram. But, if you do, the good news is that it can save your life and keep you alive for years and years to come, which gives you plenty of time to work on controlling your cholesterol.

Calculating Your Heart Attack Risk

Now you know all there is to know about the risk factors associated with high cholesterol and your risk of having high cholesterol. In this section, you can use all the info you've picked up to calculate your personal risk of having a heart attack in the next ten years.

The NCEP calculator

Luckily, you don't have to be a calculus whiz to do the math. The National Cholesterol Education Project has created an interactive "Risk Assessment Tool for Estimating Your Ten-Year Risk of Having A Heart Attack." You can find this tool at the following Web site: `http://hp2010.nhlbihin.net/atpiii/calculator.asp?usertype=pub`.

On the online form, type in the appropriate numbers, click the proper boxes, and hit the appropriate button (the one labeled "Calculate Your Ten-Year Risk"). What you get back may surprise you. For example, my total cholesterol is high, but my HDLs are also high. My blood pressure is normal, and I haven't smoked in years, so the calculator puts my ten-year risk of heart attack at 5 percent (meaning 5 of every 100 persons with my particular numbers will experience a heart attack in the next ten years).

Try it. You, too, may be pleasantly surprised at the answer. On the other hand, if your number is higher than you want, move on to the next section, a calculator with a point system.

A second numbers game

The multi-part Risk Predictor Score Sheet created by the National Heart, Lung, and Blood Institute, a division of the National Institutes of Health (NHLBI/NIH, for short), calculates the ten-year risk of heart attack by assigning specific points for the following six specific risk factors:

- Age
- Total cholesterol
- HDL cholesterol
- Blood pressure
- Diabetes
- Smoking

Because men and women have different bodies and, thus, different levels of risk, there are two score sheets based on gender:

- **Women:** `www.nhlbi.nih.gov/about/framingham/risktwom.pdf`
- **Men:** `www.aafp.org/fpm/20040100/coronarydiseaserisk_men.pdf`

You can simply grab a pencil and walk through the following steps, which are as simple as one, two, three, four . . . or, more accurately, Table 3-8 all the way up through Table 3-12.

Follow these steps:

1. **Score yourself from the following five tables.** Yup. This is where the pencil pushing starts.

Table 3-8	Risk Points for Age (Men/Women)		
Age	*Points (Men/Women)*	*Age*	*Points (Men/Women)*
30–34	–1/–9	55–59	4/7
35–39	0/–4	60–64	5/6
40–44	1/0	65–69	6/8
45–49	2/3	70–74	7/8
50–54	3/6		
Your score:_____			

Source: NHLBI/NIH.

Table 3-9	Risk Points for Total Cholesterol (Men/Women)	
Total Cholesterol	*Points for Men*	*Points for Women*
<160 mg/dL	–3	–2
160–199 mg/dL	0	0
200–239 mg/dL	1	1
240–279 mg/dL	2	1
>280 mg/dL	3	3
Your score:_____		

Source: NHLBI/NIH.

Table 3-10	Risk Points for HDL Levels (Men/Women)	
HDLs	**Points for Men**	**Points for Women**
<35 mg/dL	2	5
35–44 mg/dL	1	2
45–49 mg/dL	0	1
50–59 mg/dL	0	0
>60 mg/dL	−2	−3
Your score:_____		

Source: NHLBI/NIH.

Table 3-11	Risk Points for Blood Pressure (Men & Women)				
Systolic Pressure	**Diastolic Pressure**				
	<80 mm/Hg	**80–84 mm/Hg**	**85–59 mm/Hg**	**90–99 mm/Hg**	**>100 mm/Hg**
<120 mm/Hg	0	–	–	–	–
120–129 mm/Hg	–	0	–	–	–
130–139 mm/Hg	–	–	1	–	–
140–149 mm/Hg	–	–	–	2	–
>160 mm/Hg	–	–	–	–	3
Your score:_____					

Source: NHLBI/NIH.

Table 3-12	Risk Points for Diabetes & Smoking (Men/Women)	
Diabetes/Smoking Status	**Points for Men**	**Points for Women**
I have diabetes	2	4
I don't have diabetes	0	0
I smoke	2	2
I don't smoke	0	0
Your score:_____		

Source: NHLBI/NIH.

2. **Add up your scores from Table 3-7, Table 3-8, Table 3-9, Table 3-10, Table 3-11, and Table 3-12 to get your total score.**

   Your total score: _____

3. **Check your total against Table 3-13, which estimates your risk for heart disease in the next ten years due to blocked arteries.**

   For example, a man with a total point score of 9 has a 20 percent risk of heart attack in the next ten years. With a point score of 14 — where the count for men stops — the odds of his having a heart attack in the next ten years zoom all the way up to 53 percent. For a woman, the equivalent risks are 8 percent and 19 percent.

Table 3-13		Estimated 10-Year Risk for Heart Attack			
Total Score	**Male Risk**	**Female Risk**	**Total Score**	**Male Risk**	**Female Risk**
>−2	—	1%	8	16%	7%
>−1	2%	2%	9	20%	8%
0	3%	2%	10	25%	10%
1	3%	3%	11	31%	11%
2	4%	3%	12	37%	13%
3	5%	3%	13	45%	16%
4	7%	4%	14+	>53%	19%
5	8%	4%	15	—	20%
6	10%	5%	16	—	24%
7	13%	7%	17	—	>27%

Source: NHLBI/NIH.

Part II

Eating Your Way to Lower Cholesterol

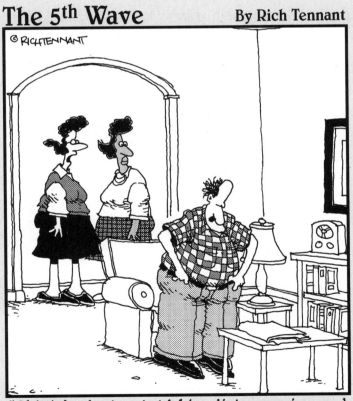

The 5th Wave — By Rich Tennant

"Phillip's doctor told him diet, exercise, and genes can effect your cholesterol levels, so he cut out fatty foods, walks everyday, and switched to chinos."

In this part . . .

Remember the old maxim, "A few seconds on your lips, a lifetime on your hips?" Well, here's a new one: "A few seconds on your plate, a lifetime in your blood." The simple fact is that all plans to rejigger your cholesterol levels start with reforming your diet. Okay, it may sound boring, and it may lack a certain zip. But trust me — tweaking what you eat with an eye toward improving your cholesterol profile is worth the effort. You can get started by taking a look at that page right over there to your right.

Chapter 4

Writing Rules for a Cholesterol-Lowering Diet

*O*kay. You've been to the doctor. She ran a blood test for cholesterol (check out Chapter 3), and your numbers are high. Her first recommendation is likely to be a cholesterol-lowering diet. What's that? The answer is in this very short chapter; so short, in fact, that you may be tempted to skip past it and go right on to Chapter 5, which explains how to put the strategies listed here into action to create a meal plan of your own.

But in the words of the golden-hearted lady of the evening played by Shirley McLaine in *Sweet Charity:* "Hey, Big Spender, spend a little time with me." It won't take long. I won't waste words. As a result, you can head into Chapter 5 armed with a better understanding of why your doctor is pushing a low-fat, high-fiber diet to control your cholesterol. What's to lose?

Being Prudent

The first people to say, "Hey, we can prevent heart attacks by changing what people eat," were almost certainly the guys at the New York City Department of Health who created the Diet and Coronary Heart Disease Study Project of the Bureau of Nutrition, commonly known as the Anti-Coronary Club, on February 19, 1957. Their goal was to track a group of overweight, middle-age men who'd either had a heart attack or looked like they were about to experience one.

By the way, you may notice that I said *men*. No women were in the club because before the days of women's lib, nobody considered women to be at risk for a heart attack. Gee.

Anyway, the nutrition docs enlisted the Anti-Coronary Club members as volunteers in a trial of a new controlled-fat, low-cholesterol diet. Half of the participants got the experimental diet, and half were allowed to eat whatever their little, bursting hearts desired.

Within four years, it was clear that the incidence of heart attack among the men on the controlled-fat, low-cholesterol diet was much lower than incidence among men in the other group. By cutting back on fats, cholesterol, and calories, the project turned modern heart-disease prevention in a new direction. Thus the Prudent Diet — the very first cholesterol-lowering regimen — was born.

By the way, not only was the first cholesterol-lowering diet created right here in my hometown, The Big Apple, the cardiologist-in-charge was my uncle, Seymour H. Rinzler, MD, one really good reason for my continuing interest in this subject. And make a note: Although being in The Big Apple raises some people's blood pressure, apples, the food, are great little cholesterol busters. Check it out in Chapter 5.

Doing the Diet Two-Step

By the 1980s, Americans had pretty much accepted the idea of a link between high cholesterol and an increased risk of heart disease. In addition, they were now living long enough so that medical problems of older age — think heart attack — were becoming more common, and therefore more worrisome.

To confront the heart issue, sorry, *head* on, in 1984, the National Heart, Lung, and Blood Institute (NHLBI), a division of the National Institutes of Health (NIH), convened a Consensus Development Conference to deal with *hypercholesterolemia* (high cholesterol to you and me).

Fourteen experts, meeting for two days, issued two important edicts (as in "do this or you'll be really sorry"):

✔ **Edict Number One:** Henceforth, Americans will be divided into three risk groups for heart attack based on their total cholesterol levels:

• The lowest quarter of cholesterol levels (below 200 mg/dL) is "low." People occupying the low quarter are at low risk of heart attack.

- The two middle quarters (200–239 mg/dL) are "normal." Those folks in the middle quarters are at moderate risk for heart attack.

- The top quarter (240 mg/dL and above) is "high." Folks sitting in the high quarter are at high risk for heart attack.

Mg stands for *milligrams,* and *dL* is the abbreviation for *deciliter* (1/10 of a liter).

✔ **Edict Number Two:** Sticking to a low-fat, controlled-cholesterol diet is a person's best bet for reducing the risk of heart attack, so cut your total fat intake and cut back on animal foods (the source of dietary cholesterol). Or else.

The authoritative food plan was — surprise! — the Prudent Diet, which NHLBI's brand-spanking-new National Cholesterol Education Project (NCEP) had magically transformed into something called The Step I and Step II diets.

Step I (notice the Roman numerals which somehow make this title look very important) was meant for healthy people with cholesterol readings in the 200–239 mg/dL range. Step II was for people who'd already had a heart attack or had a cholesterol reading above 240 mg/dL. Here's what each diet mandated:

Step 1

✔ No more than 30 percent of your total daily calories from fat.

✔ No more than 10 percent of your total daily calories from saturated fat. Chapter 5 explains saturated fats (versus unsaturated, polyunsaturated, and monounsaturated fats) in detail.

✔ No more than 300 milligrams of cholesterol per day, regardless of how many calories you consume.

Step 11

✔ No more than 30 percent of your total daily calories from fat.

✔ No more than 7 percent of your total daily calories from saturated fat.

✔ No more than 200 milligrams of cholesterol per day, regardless of how many calories you consume.

No, you're not entitled to 30 percent of your calories from fat *plus* 10 percent or 7 percent of your calories from saturated fat. The percent allowed for saturated fat is part of the 30 percent allowed for total fat.

Table 4-1 does the math to show how the Step I/Step II formulas apply to 1,600-calorie, 2,000-calorie, and 3,000-calorie daily diets.

Table 4-1	The Step I & Step II Diets in Action		
Calories per Day	*Calories from Fat (Step I/Step II)*	*Calories from Saturated Fat (Step I/Step II)*	*Cholesterol per Day (Step I/Step II)*
3,000	900/900	300/210	300 mg/200 mg
2,000	600/600	200/140	300 mg/200 mg
1,600	480/480	160/112	300 mg/200 mg

Adding TLC

No, TLC doesn't stand for Tender Loving Care. The letters are the abbreviation for Therapeutic Lifestyle Changes (TLC) diet, the food facts recommended in May 2001 when NCEP released a whole new set of guidelines for managing cholesterol. Which, come to think of it, may actually be Tender Loving Care for your heart.

The document in question is the *Third Report of the Expert Panel on Detection, Evaluation, and Treatment of High Blood Cholesterol in Adults,* commonly known as *ATP III.* (For more about *ATP III* and its recommendations on cholesterol-lowering meds, check out Chapter 12.)

Step I (see the preceding section) was still okey-dokey, but TLC replaced Step II as the must-use diet for people with specific medical conditions and risk factors such as

✔ High level of LDLs

✔ A previous heart attack or cardiovascular disease, such as blocked arteries

✔ Type 1 diabetes (insulin-dependent diabetes, diabetes mellitus) or *metabolic syndrome,* also known as insulin resistance syndrome, a cluster of risk factors that includes Type 2 diabetes (non-insulin dependent diabetes), high blood pressure, excess weight, elevated LDLs ("bad" cholesterol), and low HDLs ("good" cholesterol)

Table 4-2 shows the daily rules for the TLC diet. As you read them, notice that this diet allows slightly more total fat than you got with the Step II diet. Why? To give people with diabetes the option to replace some calories from carbs with calories from fat. Are these guys considerate, or what?

Table 4-2	The TLC Diet Rules
Nutrient	**Recommended Intake**
Calories	Balanced with physical activity to prevent weight gain
Total fat	25%–35% of total calories
Saturated fat	Less than 7% of total calories
Polyunsaturated fat	Up to 10% of total calories
Monounsaturated fat	Up to 20% of total calories
Carbohydrates	50%–60% of total calories
Protein	About 15% of total calories

Source: National Cholesterol Education Project, ATP III.

Finding Diet Aids

Some people have no trouble adapting to a cholesterol-lowering diet. Others find it pure torture. The following resources may relieve some of the pain:

✔ **Healthcare professionals and groups:** These fine folks can show you how to adapt your menus to your diet or send you to other fine folks who can get the job done:

- **GPs:** Your general practitioner (your family doctor) is your first stop on the way to lower cholesterol. She can give you menu plans and tips to ease your way into low-cholesterol eating.

- **HMOs and PPOs:** Yes, mangled care, I mean managed care, can be annoying, frustrating, and — let's not mince words — downright loathsome. But once in a while the system works. Many managed-care plans now include some options for alternative medicine, such as nutrition therapy and consultations with registered dietitians. If your plan is among the innovators, that's good news for your pocketbook — and your cholesterol.

✔ **The local YMCA or YWCA:** Ask about diet classes. There's bound to be a heart-healthy one on the list. Just be sure that anyone who hands out personal advice for your very own body has the proper credentials, like the letters *RD* (for registered dietitian) after his or her name.

✔ **The Internet:** They don't call it the Information Age for nothin'. Try these Web sites:

- **www.eatright.org:** The American Dietetic Association. Follow the prompts to the feature that enables you to find a registered dietitian/personal nutritionist right in your neighborhood (or at least close to home).

- **www.americanheart.org:** The American Heart Association.

- **www.nhlbi.nih.gov:** The National Cholesterol Education Project. Reach it through the National Heart, Lung, and Blood Institute site.

When in doubt, just search www.google.com, type **cholesterol diet**, and surf. What? You're reading this book on a boat drifting up the Amazon? In a balloon-tire, all-terrain vehicle on your way to the Alaska pipeline? No nutritionist in sight? No excuses, please. If The Person In Charge of Everything didn't want you to check out your diet wherever you are, would she have

---

The low-fat surprise

Just when you think you've heard it all, somebody springs a surprise. This time I'm the surprise springer, and this is my surprise: Not everyone benefits from a low-fat diet. Who are the exceptions?

✔ **Newborns and infants:** In the early 1980s, just as cholesterol-mania was hitting its first peak, some conscientious parents decided to cut back on fat and cholesterol right from the beginning in order to give their baby a head start in preventing a heart attack later in life. It sounds reasonable — a low-cholesterol diet in infancy equals high heart protection later on — but in this case, one and one don't add up to two.

Unlike an adult whose body is completely developed, an infant is still making new tissue and new connections in the wiring of his brain — an organ packed with cholesterol. As a result, newborns and infants require whole-fat foods.

As the low-fat infant diet spread, hospitals began to see otherwise healthy infants who didn't thrive — a medical way of saying that

they didn't develop properly. When doctors identified the cause of the problem — these low-fat baby diets — and parents added fats back into their baby's diet, some damage was reversed.

Today, the American College of Pediatrics recommends that a full 50 percent of an infant's calories should come from fat. The organization also says that children absolutely shouldn't be on a low-fat diet until they are at least past their second birthday and then only on the advice of a physician. Babies are not little adults; they're complicated organisms complete with (invisible) handle-with-care tags!

✔ **People with diabetes:** Some experts have suggested that a diet high in carbohydrates and low in fat is less beneficial for people with diabetes than a diet high in fat and relatively low in carbohydrates. This claim hasn't been nailed down yet to anyone's complete satisfaction. If you have diabetes, you know better than to change your diet without talking to your doctor first.

Rating your risk

One way to estimate your risk of heart attack is to calculate the ratio of your total cholesterol to your HDLs. To do this, you divide the number for your total cholesterol by the number for your HDLs. For example, if your total cholesterol is 240 mg/dL and your HDLs are 59 mg/dL, divide 240 by 59 to get a ratio of 4.06. Oh, call it 4.1

$$240 \div 59 = 4.06 = 4.1$$

This ratio is used because standard lab tests only measure your total cholesterol and your HDL levels. LDL and VLDL levels are estimated. Triglycerides are used to estimate the VLDL, and LDL levels are discerned by subtracting the HDL readings and VLDL estimates from your total cholesterol numbers. But what does this tell you about your risk?

The following table lists the risk associated with specific total-cholesterol-to-HDL ratios. I found these descriptions on a laboratory report for one of my own annual checkups. Consider these numbers to be guesstimates for your risk of heart attack. Only use them as a rough guide until you and your doctor draw some blood and crunch some numbers. Health risk assessments are always a work in progress, so the numbers on your annual report may be different.

Cholesterol-to-HDL Ratios

Heart Attack Risk Level	Women	Men
Lowest	3.8 and below	2.9 and below
Low	3.9–4.7	3.0–3.6
Moderate	4.9–5.9	3.7–4.6
High	6.0–6.9	4.7–5.6
Highest	7.0 and above	5.7 and above

invented GPS (global-positioning satellite) cell phones, or wireless laptops? Give me a break! Better still, give yourself a break, and check out the Real Rules for yourself.

You can also buy a really reliable cookbook, such as

- ✔ *The American Heart Association Cookbook*
- ✔ *Low-Cholesterol Cookbook For Dummies* by Molly Siple (Wiley)
- ✔ *Lowfat Cooking For Dummies* by Lynn Fischer and W. Virgil Brown (Wiley)

Each recipe comes with a nutrient analysis listing the amount of the following nutrients in a single serving:

- ✔ Calories
- ✔ Protein
- ✔ Carbohydrates
- ✔ Cholesterol
- ✔ Sodium
- ✔ Total fat
- ✔ Saturated fat
- ✔ Polyunsaturated fat
- ✔ Monounsaturated fat

Armed with these nutrition numbers, you can put together menus that fit the requirements of a cholesterol-lowering diet. Can't wait for another trip to the bookstore? Check out the hearty-healthy recipes in Chapter 14.

Chapter 5

Building a Cholesterol-Lowering Diet

*P*op quiz: Who said, "A journey of a thousand miles must begin with a single step"? No, it wasn't John F. Kennedy, although he used it in a speech. No, it wasn't Condoleeza Rice. No, no, no, it wasn't Jon Stewart. The actual author of the quote was the ancient Chinese philosopher Laotzu.

Clearly, ol' Laotzu, who lived 26 centuries before cholesterol was identified, wasn't an expert on dietary fats and fiber, but he sure had a handle on human nature. And his admonition to just get going — take that first step — is great advice for anyone who wants to lower his or her cholesterol.

As you read this chapter, remember that the very first step in this particular journey is to set a diet strategy. Cut back on fats. Increase your consumption of foods high in dietary fiber. And put this all together so you can look forward to smiling as your doctor says, "Wow! Your cholesterol is down." Frankly, I think Laotzu would approve. Don't you?

Making Your Game Plan

I say, "Diet." You think, "Calories." No surprise there — for most people, *diet* is synonymous with *weight-loss plan*. But if I add *cholesterol control* to *diet,* the picture changes.

In Chapter 4, I discuss all the people who helped create the authoritative cholesterol-control diet, a regimen that delivers one simple message: Eat less fat and more dietary fiber. Not that calories don't count: As you can see in Chapter 7, losing weight is an excellent way to improve your cholesterol numbers. But the pleasant surprise is that if you manage your fat and fiber, the calories take care of themselves, and your diet takes care of your cholesterol. What a great deal.

Choosing the Fat That Fits

All fats, including the fat on your bod and (more to the point) the fats in your food, are composed of *fatty acids* — long chain-like molecules of carbon and hydrogen atoms plus an oxygen atom or two. Folks in the know about fats put fatty acids into one of three categories:

- ✔ Saturated
- ✔ Monounsaturated
- ✔ Polyunsaturated

The chemical differences between these fats are described in the "Demystifying saturation" sidebar later in this chapter. For the moment, the important thing to keep in mind is that a diet high in saturated fats raises cholesterol levels, and a diet high in unsaturated fats lowers them.

Dealing up close and personal with cholesterol

Eating a lot of foods high in dietary cholesterol increases the amount of cholesterol in your blood and raises your risk of heart attack. So, controlling the cholesterol in your diet reduces the risk of two potential problems in your arteries.

Cholesterol is a saturated fat found only in foods from animals: meat, dairy products, and eggs.

- ✔ **Dietary-cholesterol problem #1:** As I explain in Chapter 2, cholesterol and perhaps *homocysteine* (an amino acid produced when you digest food — the jury is still out on this amino acid) can rough up the linings of your arteries, creating teensy little crags that snag cholesterol particles as they float by. The trapped cholesterol particles snag other debris floating through your blood, producing small piles of gunk (technical term: *plaque*) that narrow and may eventually block the artery, leading to the unpleasant event called a heart attack.

Fat entries in the name game

The chemical family name for fats and related compounds, such as cholesterol, is *lipids,* which comes from *lipos,* the Greek word for fat. Now that you know that little factoid, you're likely to see the *lipo-* (or *lipe-*) prefix popping up everywhere you look.

For example, the correct scientific term for your cholesterol numbers is *lipid profile.* And your lipid profile includes *lipoproteins,* the fat-and-protein particles that carry cholesterol around and sometimes out of your body. Here are a few more lipo-licious words:

✔ **Lipases:** Enzymes that enable you to digest fats

✔ **Lipemia:** Excess amounts of fat in your blood

✔ **Lipoblasts:** Embryonic fat cells

✔ **Lipomas:** Fatty tumors

✔ **Liposuction:** Surgical removal of body fat

Just about the only "lip" that doesn't come from *lipos* is your lip, the one that covers your teeth. That lip is descended from *labium,* the Latin word for, you guessed it, lip. As Sigmund Freud, he of the mysterious unconscious, once said, "Sometimes a good cigar is just a smoke."

✔ **Dietary-cholesterol problem #2:** Extra cholesterol in your diet may also increase the amount of *low-density lipoproteins* (LDLs) in your blood. LDLs, also known as "bad" cholesterol, are the fat and protein particles that ferry cholesterol into your arteries, leading to problem #1.

Conclusion? Adding foods high in cholesterol can mess up any diet, which certainly explains why every description of a cholesterol-lowering diet calls the diet *low cholesterol* and *controlled fat.* You keep the cholesterol low and you control the kinds of fat by following the 30-10-300 formula described in Chapter 4:

✔ Less than 30 percent of your total calories each day from fat — predominantly unsaturated fats

✔ Less than 10 percent of your total calories each day from saturated fat

✔ Less than 300 milligrams of cholesterol per day, regardless of your calorie count

Showing fat who's boss

After you decide to control your cholesterol by controlling the amount of fat in your diet, the question is, which foods work best and which foods aren't that hot?

Unconfusing a confusing cholesterol calculation

In 2000, nutrition scientists at the U.S. Department of Agriculture Human Nutrition Research Center on Aging at Tufts University (Boston) fed volunteers one of two diets. Both diets derived 30 percent of their total calories from fat, but one diet used polyunsaturated fat from corn oil, and the other got its saturated fat from beef. And don't let me forget to mention that both diets included extra cholesterol.

Ordinarily, a diet high in unsaturated fats reduces the amount of cholesterol circulating in your blood, and a diet high in saturated fat does the opposite, increasing the amount of cholesterol circulating in your blood. In addition, a diet high in unsaturated fatty acids is generally assumed to inhibit a chemical reaction called *oxidation* that makes LDLs more likely to slip into your arteries and start the downhill slide toward a heart attack. But guess what?

✔ Adding cholesterol to the diets high in polyunsaturated fatty acids (corn oil) *increased* LDL oxidation by 28 percent.

✔ Adding cholesterol to the high-saturated beef-fat diet *increased* oxidation of LDLs by 15 percent.

✔ Both diets *increased* the volunteers' cholesterol levels.

Time out! How come the people on the polyunsaturated fat had a greater increase in LDL oxidation than the people on the saturated beef-fat diet? Because — any math majors in the room? — the amount of oxidation associated with the unsaturated fat diet is *much* lower to begin with, and any actual increase in oxidation creates a larger percentage increase relative to diets high in saturated fats.

Oh, what an easy one to answer! (Either skip ahead to the section titled "Building a nutritional pyramid" or take a slightly longer way through the following text.)

✔ **Grains:** Grains have very small amounts of fat — just about 3 percent of their total weight — and most of the fats in grains are unsaturated. In addition, grains are filling, and they have dietary fiber, which I talk about a bit later in this chapter. The *Dietary Guidelines for Americans* from the U.S. Department of Agriculture and the U.S. Department of Health and Human Services (USDA/HHS) says that a healthy diet is based on grain foods. Who am I to argue?

✔ **Fruits and veggies:** Fruits and vegetables have only traces of fat, and most of it is unsaturated. Your diet should have a lot of fruits and veggies. But you knew that, right?

✔ **Dairy products:** Dairy products are a varied lot. For example, sweet cream is a high-fat food. Whole milks and whole-milk cheeses are moderately high in fat. Skim milk and skim-milk products are low-fat foods. And for the record, most of the fats in any dairy product are saturated, but milk products are your best source of calcium, so balance the fats and get your calcium by sticking to low- or no-fat dairy products — and don't forget the yummy low- or no-fat frozen desserts.

✔ **Meat and poultry:** Meat is moderately high in fat, and most of its fats are saturated. Some poultry — chicken and turkey — are relatively low in fat. Other poultry — duck and goose — have higher fat contents. You can lower the fat content of any poultry serving by removing the skin. I know; I know. That's the good part! But your cholesterol levels will thank you.

✔ **Fish and shellfish:** Fish and shellfish are special cases. Some fish, such as salmon and herring, are high in fat, but guess what? Those are the best fish from a cholesterol standpoint because their fats are rich in omega-3 fatty acids (more about them in the sidebar titled, "Omega-3 me"), polyunsaturated fatty acids credited with lowering your risk of heart disease.

Your body converts *alpha-linolenic acid,* the most important omega-3, to hormone-like substances called *eicosapentaenoic acid* (EPA) and *docosa-hexaenoic acid* (DHA). EPA and DHA appear to protect your heart by reducing inflammation, preventing blood clots, and — get this! — preventing other fats like cholesterol from injuring artery walls.

Omega-6 polyunsaturated fatty acids, found in beef, pork, and several veggie oils (corn, cottonseed, safflower, and sunflower), are chemical cousins of omega-3s, but they don't protect your heart.

✔ **Fats and oils:** Vegetable oils, butter, and lard are high-fat foods, but their actual fat content varies from heart healthy to are-you-kidding-me! This info is the subject of the "Linking fatty acids and dietary fat" section later in this chapter.

✔ **Proteins:** Protein is an essential nutrient — so important that its name comes from the Greek word *proteios,* which means "holding first place." A protein molecule is a chain of other molecules called amino acids, the building blocks of protein. *Amino acids* are molecules made of carbon, hydrogen, and oxygen atoms, plus a nitrogen unit called an *amino group.*

The amino group is essential for *synthesizing* (creating) specialized proteins, including the enzymes and hormones that make it possible for you to perform such basic functions as working your muscles and digesting food. So, when people talk about how much protein they need, what they really mean is how much nitrogen they need to synthesize specialized proteins.

Your body also uses proteins to build new cells and maintain tissues. Considering all that, you may be puzzled as to why it has taken me so long to get around to talking about protein. The reason is simple. Some protein foods are positively loaded with cholesterol and saturated fatty acids:

- **Animal protein:** The only foods that add cholesterol to your diet are foods from animals — meat, poultry, fish, milk products, and eggs. Most of these foods are also high in saturated fatty acids. True, some animal foods have less cholesterol than others. True, some animal foods are lower in saturated fats. True, you can cut

Omega-3 me

It's clear that laboratory pigs and monkeys have cleaner arteries when their feed includes omega-3 fatty acids, and studies suggest human beings may also benefit. In the Diet and Reinfarction Trial (DART), a 2,033-man study run by the Medical Research Council Epidemiological Unit in Cardiff, Wales, in the late 1980s, men who ate two servings of fatty fish a week had a lower rate of heart attack than men who either cut their fat to no more than 30 percent of their total calories or increased their dietary fiber (from grains) to 16 grams a day. Yo, bring on the salmon!

But don't forget the chocolate or at least the very special new chocolate form Canada. In the summer of 2007, Ocean Nutrition Canada Limited, a company that makes and distributes omega-3 food and dietary supplement ingredients, announced that the O Trois line of chocolate bars and "fingers" from Les Truffes au Chocolat, would henceforth contain omega-3 fatty acids. Who can ask for anything more?

the fat and cholesterol content of animal foods by trimming visible fat. True, some animal foods are rich in special unsaturated fats called omega-3s that actually reduce everybody's risk of heart disease. But generally, a diet designed to lower your cholesterol emphasizes foods from plants.

- **Plant protein:** Getting your protein from plant foods is a more complicated task than getting your protein from animal foods. Blame it on the amino acids (those "building blocks" of protein). Proteins from animals are labeled *complete,* meaning that they contain all the amino acids human beings need to thrive. Proteins from plant foods are often characterized as *limited,* meaning that they lack sufficient amounts of one amino acid or another. It takes a little work to mix and match plants to get the proper protein balance, but with no cholesterol and practically no saturated fatty acids, plant proteins are worth the effort, don't ya think? At least once in a while.

Linking fatty acids and dietary fat

All fats are combinations of fatty acids. Nutritionists characterize a dietary fat or oil as saturated, monounsaturated, or polyunsaturated depending on which fatty acids make up the largest portion of the fat or oil:

✔ Foods such as butter, which are high in saturated fatty acids, are solid at room temperature and get harder when chilled.

✔ Foods such as olive oil, which are high in monounsaturated fatty acids, are liquid at room temperature; they get thicker when chilled.

✔ Foods such as corn oil, which are high in polyunsaturated fatty acids, are liquid at room temperature and stay liquid when chilled.

So how come margarine, which is composed primarily of unsaturated fatty acids, is solid? Because its fatty acids have been artificially saturated with extra hydrogen atoms. This process, called *hydrogenation,* turns an oil, such as corn oil, into a solid fat — margarine.

Hydrogenated fats are sometimes called *trans fatty acids,* but no matter what you call them, these fatty acids raise — rather than lower — cholesterol levels. As a result, these days most margarines boast "no trans fats" right on the label. I know your mother told you not to toot your own horn, but these guys have earned the right. So when you're shopping, pick them.

Table 5-1 shows the fatty acid composition of several common fats and oils. You're right: Some of the totals below don't add up to 100 percent. That's because these fats and oils also contain very small amounts of other kinds of fatty acids that don't affect the basic character of the fat. The last column, Fat Category, tells you which fatty acids are predominant in the mix.

Table 5-1	Naming Fats and Oils		
Oil/Fat	**Fatty Acid Content**		**Fat Category**
	Saturated	**Mono- unsaturated**	**Poly- unsaturated**	
Vegetable oils	7%	53%	22%	Monounsaturated
Canola oil	7%	53%	22%	Monounsaturated
Coconut oil	92%	6%	2%	Saturated
Cottonseed oil	18%	29%	48%	Polyunsaturated
Corn oil	13%	24%	59%	Polyunsaturated
Olive oil	14%	74%	9%	Monounsaturated
Palm oil	52%	38%	10%	Saturated
Peanut oil	17%	46%	32%	Monounsaturated
Safflower oil	9%	12%	74%	Polyunsaturated
Soybean oil	15%	23%	51%	Polyunsaturated

(continued)

Table 5-1 (continued)

Oil/Fat	Fatty Acid Content			Fat Category
	Saturated	Mono-unsaturated	Poly-unsaturated	
Sunflower oil	12%	19%	69%	Polyunsaturated
Butter	62%	30%	5%	Saturated
Beef tallow	46%	47%	3%	Saturated*
Lard	39%	45%	11%	Saturated*

*Because more than ⅓ of their fatty acids are saturated, beef tallow and lard are characterized as saturated fats.

Source: Institute of Shortening and Edible Oils; Nutritive Value of Foods (U.S. Department of Agriculture, 1991); Food and Life (American Council on Science and Health, 1990).

Factoring in the Fiber

Carbohydrate foods form the base for a healthful, low cholesterol diet. In 2000, the U.S. Department of Agriculture and the U.S. Department of Health and Human Services recommended that approximately 55 to 60 percent of your daily calories should come from foods such as grains (particularly whole grains) and fruits and vegetables that are high in complex carbohydrates (a term that I discuss in just a minute).

Table 5-2 does the math to show you what 55 to 60 percent of calories from carbs equals for a 1,600-calorie, 2000-calorie, 2,600-calorie, and 3,100-calorie daily diet, the range of calories for active healthy adults.

Table 5-2   Recommended Dietary Carb Intake

Calories per Day	Calories from Carbohydrates	Calories from Carbohydrates
	60%	55%
1,600	960	880
2,000	1,200	1,100
2,600	1,560	1,430
3,100	1,860	1,705

Demystifying saturation

Molecules are groups of atoms hooked together with chemical bonds (electrical charges that attract and hold atoms firmly in place). Different atoms form different numbers of bonds. For example, a carbon atom can form four bonds, an oxygen atom can form two bonds, and a hydrogen atom — poor thing! — can only form one bond.

Fatty acid molecules are long chains of carbon atoms (always an even number) with hydrogen and oxygen atoms attached to the carbons. The chain begins with a carbon atom attached to three hydrogen atoms. Imagine it looking like a cheese ball (the carbon atom) with one toothpick (a chemical bond) stuck into the top, one on the left, one on the bottom, and one on the right. And, oh, yes, an olive (a hydrogen atom) stuck onto the toothpick on top, on the left, and on the bottom. No, it doesn't matter whether it's a black olive or a stuffed green one.

A layperson sees this:

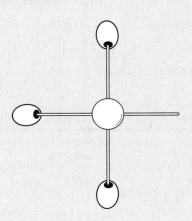

A chemist sees this:

$$
\begin{array}{c}
\text{H} \\
| \\
\text{H}-\text{C}- \\
| \\
\text{H}
\end{array}
$$

Chemists call this one-carbon, three-hydrogen unit a *methyl group* — the first piece in any fatty acid. To build the rest of the fatty acid, you add carbon atoms to the right side of the first carbon atom (on the toothpick without an olive). Then you add hydrogen atoms to the top and bottom of the carbon atoms. In the end, you have a chain that looks something like this:

$$
\begin{array}{c}
\quad\text{H}\quad\text{H}\quad\text{H}\quad\text{H} \\
\quad|\quad\ \ |\quad\ \ |\quad\ \ | \\
\text{H}-\text{C}-\text{C}-\text{C}-\text{C}-\text{etc.} \\
\quad|\quad\ \ |\quad\ \ |\quad\ \ | \\
\quad\text{H}\quad\text{H}\quad\text{H}\quad\text{H}
\end{array}
$$

See? Every carbon atom has four bonds; every hydrogen atom has just one. In real life, the chain of atoms is three-dimensional and bouncing around in space. I can't draw that here, so you'll have to take my word for it.

Meanwhile, back at the fatty acids, the last carbon in the chain is part of an *acid group,* a special unit made of one carbon atom, two oxygen atoms, and one hydrogen atom that makes a fatty acid a fatty acid. The carbon atom in the acid group still has four bonds, but two of the bonds go to one oxygen atom. The two-bond connection is called a *double bond.* This time I'll forgo the cheese, toothpicks, and olives, and just draw the thing as you can find it in a chemistry textbook:

$$
\begin{array}{c}
O \\
\parallel \\
-C-O-H
\end{array}
$$

Thank heavens that's done. Now, how do you tell the saturated fatty acid from the unsaturated one? Count the bonds between the carbons.

Saturated fatty acid

In a saturated fatty acid, all the carbons have four single bonds except for the last carbon in the chain, which has a double bond to the oxygen atom in the acid group.

$$
\begin{array}{c}
H\ H\ H\ H\ H\ H\ H\ H\ H\ H\ H\ H\ H\ H\ H\ H\ H\ H\ O \\
|\ \ |\ \ |\ \ |\ \ |\ \ |\ \ |\ \ |\ \ |\ \ |\ \ |\ \ |\ \ |\ \ |\ \ |\ \ |\ \ |\ \ |\ \ \parallel \\
H-C-C-C-C-C-C-C-C-C-C-C-C-C-C-C-C-C-C-C-O-H \\
|\ \ |\ \ |\ \ |\ \ |\ \ |\ \ |\ \ |\ \ |\ \ |\ \ |\ \ |\ \ |\ \ |\ \ |\ \ |\ \ |\ \ | \\
H\ H\ H\ H\ H\ H\ H\ H\ H\ H\ H\ H\ H\ H\ H\ H\ H
\end{array}
$$

Monounsaturated fatty acid

The following is a diagram of *oleic acid,* a monounsaturated fatty acid in olive oil. Notice that this fatty acid has one place where the carbon doesn't have four single bonds, the definition of a saturated carbon. It has two single bonds (one to the carbon on the left and one to a hydrogen) and a double bond to the next carbon atom in line. Because this fatty acid has only one instance of a double bond between carbons, it's called a monounsaturated fatty acid (*mono* = one).

$$
\begin{array}{c}
H\ H\ H\ H\ H\ H\ H\ HH\ H\ H\ H\ H\ H\ H\ O \\
|\ \ |\ \ |\ \ |\ \ |\ \ |\ \ |\ \ ||\ \ |\ \ |\ \ |\ \ |\ \ |\ \ |\ \ \parallel \\
H-C-C-C-C-C-C-C-C=C-C-C-C-C-C-C-C-C-O-H \\
|\ \ |\ \ |\ \ |\ \ |\ \ |\ \ |\ \ |\ \ ||\ \ |\ \ |\ \ |\ \ |\ \ |\ \ | \\
H\ H\ H\ H\ H\ H\ H\ H\ HH\ H\ H\ H\ H\ H\ H
\end{array}
$$

A polyunsaturated fatty acid

A polyunsaturated (*poly* = many) fatty acid has two or more carbons with two single bonds and one double bond to the next carbon in line. This diagram is a polyunsaturated fatty acid.

$$
\begin{array}{c}
H\ H\ H\ H\ H\ H\ HHH\ H\ H\ H\ H\ O \\
|\ \ |\ \ |\ \ |\ \ |\ \ |\ \ |||\ \ |\ \ |\ \ |\ \ |\ \ \parallel \\
H-C-C-C-C-C-C-C-C=C-C-C=C-C-C-C-C-C-C-O-H \\
|\ \ |\ \ |\ \ |\ \ |\ \ |\ \ |\ \ ||\ \ ||\ \ |\ \ |\ \ |\ \ |\ \ | \\
H\ H\ H\ H\ H\ H\ H\ H\ H\ H\ H\ H\ H\ H\ H
\end{array}
$$

Carbohydrates are nutrient molecules built of units of sugar. As the sidebar, "Sweet talk: Simple versus complex," explains, the more sugar units a carbohydrate molecule contains, the more complex the carbohydrate is.

When it comes to controlling your cholesterol, the most important complex carbohydrate (and the most important carbohydrate, period) is dietary fiber.

Sweet talk: Simple versus complex

Just as proteins are combinations of amino acids, and fats are combinations of fatty acids, carbohydrates are combinations of sugar units described either as simple or complex, depending on the number of sugar units in the molecule:

✔ **Monosaccharides** (*mono* = one; *saccharide* = sugar) are carbohydrates with only one sugar unit. Fructose (the sugar in fruit), glucose (the sugar you use for energy), and galactose (the sugar derived from digesting lactose, also known as milk sugar) are monosaccharides. Monosaccharides are simple carbohydrates.

✔ **Disaccharides** (*di* = two) are carbohydrates with two sugar units, Sucrose (table sugar) is a disaccharide made of one unit of fructose and one unit of glucose. Like monosaccharides, disaccharides are simple carbohydrates.

✔ **Polysaccharides** are carbohydrates with more than two sugar units. Starch, a complex carbohydrate in potatoes, pasta, and rice, is definitely a polysaccharide — it's made up of many, many sugar units (actually, many units of glucose). Dietary fiber is also made of many, many sugar units. Polysaccharides are complex carbohydrates.

Refraining from eating your shirt: Dietary fiber

The word *dietary* is stuck in front of *fiber* to make sure you understand that this fiber, which comes from food, is different from the natural and synthetic fibers, such as silk, cotton, wool, or nylon, used in fabrics.

Dietary fiber is a complex carbohydrate, but it isn't just any old complex carb like, oh, starch. Your body can digest starch, but it can't digest dietary fiber because the human gut doesn't have digestive enzymes strong enough to dissolve the chemical bonds holding the fiber molecule's sugar units together. As a result, you don't get any calories or other nutrients from dietary fiber. But that doesn't mean it's worthless. *Au contraire* — on the contrary, as they like to say in France — dietary fiber is *very* useful in helping to control cholesterol.

Foods contain two kinds of dietary fiber — insoluble dietary fiber and soluble dietary fiber. Both are important to a healthful diet, but only one helps control cholesterol.

Insoluble dietary fiber

Insoluble dietary fiber such as the cellulose, hemicellulose, and lignin in whole grains, fruit and veggie skins, and the teensy, little hard thingees in pears bulks up stool and makes it softer, reducing your risk of developing hemorrhoids and lessening the discomfort if you already have them.

Sweeping away a fiber myth

For more than 30 years, nutrition studies and experts said that consuming insoluble dietary fiber might also protect against colon cancer. But then in 1999 — wham! — new data from the *Nurses' Health Study* at Harvard University, Brigham and Women's Hospital, and Dana Farber Cancer Institute in Boston said, "Ooops!" According to the *Nurses'* numbers, no relationship — zip, zero, zilch — exists between a high-fiber diet and the risk of colon cancer.

In fact, among the 88,757 women in the 16-year study, the incidence of colon cancer was the same whether the women ate a lot of fiber or practically none. In fact, some women who

ate a lot of fruit and veggies were actually at higher risk.

These conclusions were confirmed in 2005 when a team of 29 researchers from 21 institutions in 7 different countries toted up the results of 13 separate studies. The project — called the Pooling Project of Prospective Studies of Diet and Cancer — produced exactly the same results: Eating a lot of high-fiber foods didn't reduce the risk of colorectal cancer.

On the other hand, you know these science folks. Yesterday's "yes" sometimes becomes today's "no" — or vice versa. As for tomorrow, who knows?

In the memorable words of the *New England Journal of Medicine,* insoluble dietary fiber acts like a "colonic broom," stimulating intestinal contractions that move solid waste through your digestive tract. By moving food quickly through your intestines, insoluble dietary fiber may help prevent or relieve digestive disorders such as constipation or *diverticulosis* (infection caused by food getting stuck in small pouches in the wall of your colon).

Insoluble dietary fiber has no effect on your cholesterol. To bring cholesterol into the picture, you have to turn to the second kind of dietary fiber, the soluble variety.

Soluble dietary fiber

Pectins and *gums* are soluble dietary fiber. Both dissolve in your stomach forming gels that look like the stuff made from packages of fruit gelatin. This gel is believed to sop up cholesterol and slide it out of your body, thus reducing the amount of cholesterol particles that are left to wander around your blood vessels and make trouble.

You find pectins in the fruit-part of fruits (apples are a particularly good source). Gums are most plentiful in legumes (beans and peas) and grains such as oatmeal and barley.

Fiber in animal foods

Gotcha! There's no dietary fiber in any food from animals. No fiber in meat. No fiber in fish. No fiber in chicken. No fiber in milk. No fiber in eggs. See why plant foods are so important in a cholesterol-lowering diet?

Getting it just right

Remember Goldilocks, the gal who found three bowls of porridge, one too hot, one too cold, and one just right? Well, dietary fiber is something like that.

The U.S. Department of Agriculture says that the average American woman gets about 12 grams of fiber a day from food; the average American man gets about 17 grams. These amounts are well below the current recommendations of 25 grams a day for a woman and 38 grams a day for a man.

But if you decide to stuff yourself with dietary fiber to make up for years and years of low-fiber noshing, the result may be gastric distress — an unmistakable body protest in the form of intestinal gas or diarrhea. In extreme cases, loading up on dietary fiber but failing to drink sufficient amounts of liquid to swish the fiber through your gut can lead to an intestinal obstruction. Yipes!

So remember the Golden, I mean, the Goldilocks Rule: Not too little. Not too much. Just right. And build up your fiber intake gradually, please. Your tummy, as well as your cholesterol, will thank you.

A gentle reminder

At the start of this chapter, I said that if you take care of the fat and fiber, the calories will take care of themselves. Remember? If not, that's okay — I just said it again.

Fat is high in calories; carbohydrate foods are relatively low in fat and thus relatively low in calories. Dietary fiber has no calories at all. If you limit your fats and increase your dietary fiber and complex carbs, you automatically cut calories and lose weight. Check out Table 5-3 for the breakdown.

Table 5-3	Calorie Counts
Nutrient	*Calories per Gram*
Fat	9
Carbohydrates	4
Protein	4
Dietary fiber	0

Fiber factoid

Raw food almost always has more fiber per ounce (or gram) than cooked food because cooking generally adds water, which adds weight and spreads out the fiber content. For example, a 3.5-ounce portion of dried prunes has more prunes (and thus more dietary fiber) than a 3.5-ounce portion of stewed prunes, which serves up water as well as prunes.

You Know the Deal: Everything in Moderation

Nutrition gurus like to say that there's no such thing as a bad food, only a less effective food plan. However — and it's a big *however* — some foods are more effective than others when it comes to lowering your cholesterol.

To point you in the right direction, Chapter 6 lays out a list of specific foods that help reduce cholesterol levels and the risk of heart attack. It also lists foods that can increase your cholesterol and your risk.

Okay, you've started your game plan and read about the necessary elements of said plan. Now put this cholesterol-lowering puppy together.

Building a nutritional pyramid

You're probably familiar with the old USDA/HHS Food Guide Pyramid, shown in Figure 5-1. This pyramid was used for a long time, but now there's a new kid on the block.

The food pyramid in the *Dietary Guidelines for Americans 2005* is a more elastic structure than previous versions. Instead of building block on block, this pyramid, shown in Figure 5-2, is made of triangular sections you can expand or shrink depending on your nutritional needs. And instead of being called the USDA Food Guide Pyramid, which is kind of cold, it's now known as My Pyramid. As in, warm and fuzzy, get it?

This pyramid is available online at www.mypyramid.gov/pyramid/index. html. The site provides multitudinous facts about how to stretch the pyramid one way or the other to accommodate your particular preferences. No computer access? Move on to the next section.

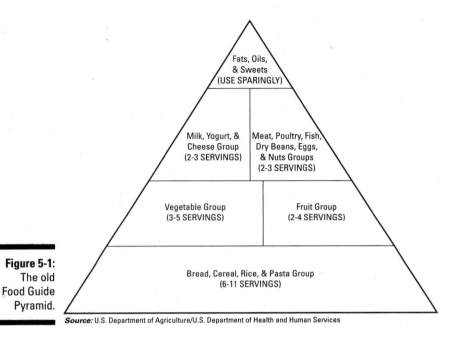

Figure 5-1:
The old
Food Guide
Pyramid.

Source: U.S. Department of Agriculture/U.S. Department of Health and Human Services

In this new pyramid, the sections stand for, from left to right:

✔ Grains

✔ Vegetables

✔ Fruit

✔ Oils

✔ Milk

✔ Meat and beans

Also, the guy climbing up the side represents (what else?) physical activity.

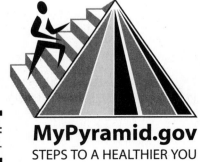

Figure 5-2:
My Pyramid.

MyPyramid.gov
STEPS TO A HEALTHIER YOU

Filling out the pyramid with daily servings

The trick to using the pyramid is to count food portions, otherwise known as *servings*. Table 5-4 and Table 5-5 show you two ways to assemble your very own diet pyramid based on the number of servings suggested by either one of two authoritative food plans, each designed to provide the nutrients required for a daily diet that delivers 1,600 calories, 2,000 calories, 2,600 calories, or 3,100 calories. Each plan is outlined as follows:

- Plan #1 is the basic USDA Food Guide, a standard healthful eating plan for healthy adult men and women.

- Plan #2 is the DASH (Dietary Approaches to Stop Hypertension) diet, a similarly healthful eating plan designed to lower blood pressure based on principles drawn from research at the National Institutes of Health.

Note for purists: The order in which the food groups are listed differs slightly on these two food plans in Tables 5-4 and 5-5.

For example, grains are Numero Uno on the DASH plan but third on the USDA design. To make it easier for you to compare the plans, I have juggled things a bit to put the food groups in the same order on both Tables 5-4 and 5-5. Whew!

Table 5-4	Daily Servings Based on the USDA Food Guide			
Food Group	**1,600 Calories/Day**	**2,000 Calories/Day**	**2,600 Calories/Day**	**3,000 Calories/Day**
Whole grains	3 servings	3 servings	4.5 servings	5 servings
Other grains	2 servings	3 servings	4.5 servings	5 servings
Fruit	3 servings	4 servings	4 servings	5 servings
Vegetables	4 servings	5 servings	5 servings	XXXXX
Dark green vegetables	4/week	6/week	6/week	6/week
Orange vegetables	3/week	4/week	5/week	5/week
Legumes	5/week	6/week	7/week	7/week
Starchy vegetables	5/week	6/week	18/week	18/week
Other vegetables	9/week	13/week	20/week	20/week

Food Group	1,600 Calories/Day	2,000 Calories/Day	2,600 Calories/Day	3,000 Calories/Day
Milk*	3 servings	3 servings	3 servings	3 servings
Lean meat and beans	5 ounces	5 ounces	7 ounces	7 ounces
Oils#	22 grams	27 grams	36 grams	44 grams
Discretionary calories	132	267	410	512

*Requirements higher for women who are pregnant or nursing.
#Represents the amount of fat added to food when it is processed, cooked, or served.
Source: *Dietary Guidelines for Americans 2005.*

Table 5-5	Daily Servings on the DASH Eating Plan			
Food Group	1,600 Calories/Day	2,000 Calories/Day	2,600 Calories/Day	3,100 Calories/Day
Grains	6 servings	6–8 servings	10–11 servings	12–13 servings
Fruit	4 servings	4–5 servings	5–6 servings	6 servings
Vegetables	3–4 servings	4–5 servings	5-6 servings	6 servings
Fat-free or low-fat milk and milk products	2–3 servings	2–3 servings	3 servings	3–4 servings
Lean meats, poultry, and fish	3–4 servings	6 or fewer servings	6 servings	6–9 servings
Fat and oils	2 servings	2–3 servings	3 servings	4 servings
Sweets	0 servings	5 or fewer servings/week	2 or fewer	2 or fewer

Source: *Dietary Guidelines for Americans 2005.*

Hey, Ma. What's a serving?

Figuring out the number of servings you need is the easy part. The hard part is figuring out what constitutes a serving. Not to worry: We do it for you. All you have to do is run your finger down Table 5-6.

Table 5-6	Dishing Up the Pyramid
Food Group	**Serving**
Grains	1 slice bread
	1 ounce ready-to-eat cereal
	½ cup cooked cereal
	½ cup cooked rice or pasta
	5–6 small crackers
Vegetables	1 cup raw, leafy vegetable
	½ cup chopped, raw vegetable
	½ cup chopped, cooked vegetable
	¾ cup vegetable juice
Fruits	1 medium piece fresh fruit
	½ cup cooked or canned chopped fruit
	¾ cup fruit juice
Dairy	1 cup milk
	1 cup yogurt
	1½ ounces natural cheese
	2 ounces processed cheese
Meat, poultry, fish, dry beans, eggs, nuts, seeds	2–3 ounces cooked lean meat
	2–3 ounces cooked lean poultry
	2–3 ounces cooked fish
	½ cup cooked dry beans
	1 egg
	2 tablespoons peanut butter
	⅓ cup nuts or seeds
Fats, oils, sweets	No specific amount; very little

Source: International Food Information Council Foundation; U.S. Department of Agriculture/U.S Department of Health and Human Services Food Guide Pyramid; Food Marketing Institute.

Notice something about these portions? Yes, indeedy, although some of the servings seem to fit the norm — a cup of milk, a slice of bread, a medium piece of fruit — other pyramid servings — especially servings of high-fat, high-cholesterol animal foods such as meat — are much smaller than the portions usually found on American plates.

(For more tips on visualizing exactly what individual servings look like, check out the "Dishing up servings" sidebar in this chapter.)

In France, where everyone eats all the high-fat foods that terrify Americans, people used to stay slim with a risk of heart disease much lower than in the U.S. But in recent years, as the portions have expanded, the risks have grown.

Do your friends in France a favor: After you memorize this part of this chapter, lend them your book. After they've got the portion sizes down pat, it's back to Vive la France! Vive la pâté de foie gras, Camembert cheese, tart tatin . . . all in USDA-acceptable serving sizes, of course.

Checking out the nutrient chart

For those of you who enjoy the challenge of totaling up grams and milligrams, heeeeeeeeeere's the ticket: Flip to the appendix where the USDA Nutrient Database is described. The Web site given lists more than 6,000 — yes, 6,000 — different foods and servings sizes. Browse to your heart's content at www.nal. usda.gov/fnic/cgi-bin/nut_search.pl.

Ending with a word for the nutrition-curious reader

This chapter explains why fats and dietary fiber figure so prominently in a cholesterol-lowering diet. But I would be remiss if I didn't tell you that there's more — much more — to discover about proteins, fats, and carbohydrates.

To find out what you're missing here, check out *Nutrition For Dummies,* 4th Edition (Wiley). In the interest of full disclosure, I have to tell you that I wrote it. More important, the book has an entire chapter devoted to each important nutrient. I wanted to include those chapters here, but my editors said that would make this book more than 500 pages long. I tried to convince them that lifting a 100-pound book three or four times a day counts as exercise, which — as you can plainly see in Chapter 8 — helps lower cholesterol. But I couldn't get them to budge on this one. So get a copy of *Nutrition For Dummies,* 4th Edition, too.

Dishing up servings

To use the serving system from the Food Guide Pyramid, it may help to get some hands-on (and eyes-on) experience with the individual portions. That way, you can store real-life versions of the recommended servings in your memory banks. So grab an 8-ounce measuring cup and a kitchen scale and head for the kitchen to play with your food and follow these steps:

✔ Broil a small steak, roast a chicken breast, or grill up a burger. When the grub is done, use your kitchen scale to weigh out a 3-ounce portion. It should be about the size of a deck of cards (okay, a small calculator). That's a meat serving.

✔ Boil some rice. Fill your measuring cup to the halfway mark with the cooked rice. Take the rice out of the cup and mush it into a ball. That's a grains or cereal serving.

✔ Tear up some greens. Fill the measuring cup to the 8-ounce mark. Dump the greens onto a salad plate. That's one serving.

✔ Open one can of veggies or fruit. Fill the measuring cup to the half mark with one or the other. Spoon the food into a small bowl. That's one serving.

✔ Pop open a can of soda. Pour it into the measuring cup right up to the 8-ounce mark. Pour that into a glass. Add some ice. It's probably more soda than you get in an upscale restaurant but less than the burger barn serves. No matter: It's still one certified USDA serving.

Chapter 6

Pinning Down the "How-To's" for a Cholesterol-Lowering Diet

In This Chapter

▶ Evaluating foods to avoid

▶ Exploring healthy plant-produced foods

▶ Trimming the fat during food preparation

C hapters 4 and 5 give you plenty of information on good food and bad food for your cholesterol. This chapter tells you ex-act-ly how to put that information to use in Real Life.

The info here is definitely hands-on, the tips you need to start changing your diet (though be sure to consult with your doctor before making any big diet changes). Naturally, the chapter is designed to be easy to follow, enabling you to turn these bits and pieces of nutrition advice into a healthful habit.

The experts call this a Good Food Plan. Go for it!

Avoiding Certain Foods (Or At Least Eating Them in Very Small Portions)

Yes, the foods listed in this section are high in fat, saturated fat, or cholesterol (or all three), but that doesn't mean they're gone from your table forever. The solution is portion control.

No, you can't have butter morning, noon, and night.

Yes, a smidgen on your baked potato now and then is okey-dokey. So is an occasional schmear of chopped liver on a canapé cracker.

And a 1-inch cube of cheddar with a fresh, crisp apple once in a while isn't all bad.

In other words, enjoy. But in moderation, please.

Butter

Butter is pure butterfat, the natural fat in milk. Just about the only redeeming virtue of butter (other than the heavenly flavor) is the fact that it's a concentrated form of energy. If you lived like your cave-person ancestors, toiling all day at manual labor, or if you lived in a very, very cold climate, you could make good use of that energy. But you don't. So you won't. And that's it for the good news.

The bad news is exactly what you expect. Butterfat is very high in saturated fat. One measly tablespoon of butter has a whopping 11 grams (g) of fat, 7.1 g of which are saturated fats. Butter only contains 3.7 g of "good" fats — 3.3 g are monounsaturated fatty acids and a miniscule 0.4 g are polyunsaturated fatty acids.

Do the math (divide 7.1 by 11), and you can see that butter is 64.5 — oh heck, call it 65 — percent saturated fat, a real heart buster. And did I mention that one tablespoon has 31 milligrams (mg) of cholesterol, 10 percent of your total daily allowance according to the diet rules I describe in Chapter 4 and Chapter 5? Now I did.

So your vote goes to margarine, right? Well, yes. As long as it's the right margarine. As you can plainly see in the section "Margarine with Trans Fatty Acids" a bit later on in this chapter.

Coconut

Nuts have been winning praise lately for their unsaturated fats, not to mention their dietary fiber. (I tell you about really good nuts later in this chapter.) But not the coconut. This big, bulky nut is a special — some may say "notorious" — case.

Yes, trying to knock open a fresh coconut uses up calories. Yes, coconut meat is high in dietary fiber, and like other nuts, it's a good source of B vitamins. Yes, a single 2-inch-square piece of fresh coconut meat has 1.09 mg of iron (7.3 percent of the recommended daily allowance for a woman of child-bearing age), and 0.49 mg of zinc (3.3 percent of the recommended daily allowance for a man, 4 percent of the recommended daily allowance for a woman). And of course, the coconut, being a plant, has no cholesterol.

Can you sense a "but" coming here? Right you are. But that same 2-inch-square piece of coconut contains 15 g of coconut oil, the fat that accounts for 85 percent of the calories in coconut meat.

Coconut oil is 89 percent saturated fatty acids, which makes it an even more highly saturated fat than butter (see the "Butter" section earlier in this chapter). Oops.

Eggs

Confused about eggs? No wonder.

For years, nutritionists insisted that eating eggs raised the risk of heart disease. Then new data from the long-running *Nurses' Health Study* (women) and the equally long-running *Physicians' Health Study* (men) turned up, showing no significant difference in risk between those who consume an average of one egg daily versus those who eat less than one egg a week.

And new laboratory analyses say that a yolk from one large egg contains only 213 to 220 mg of cholesterol, about 50 to 60 mg less than originally believed. What's a body to do? Sit tight.

The American Heart Association has upped its allowances on egg consumption to one-a-day, just like that famous brand of vitamins, so long as you figure the egg's 200+ mg of cholesterol into your daily total. In other words, if you're pigging out on red meat, don't toss a whole egg on top.

The key word there is *whole*. All the fat, including cholesterol and artery-clogging saturated fats, is in the yolk. The high protein white has none, but it does give you some minerals and some B vitamins, notably riboflavin (vitamin B2), a "visible vitamin" that may lend a faint green or yellow cast to the white.

So here's the eggs-act solution: Eat the white part of the egg and toss the yellow. Or, if you make an omelet, make do with one whole egg plus two extra whites.

By the way, no-fat, no-cholesterol egg substitutes are made of vitamin- and mineral-fortified, pasteurized egg whites containing artificial or natural colors and flavors, plus texturizers, such as gums, to make the liquid look, taste, and cook a lot like whole eggs.

Big egg

In the United States, the eggs you buy at your local food store, bazaar or emporium, come in six basic sizes, based on the minimum weight for one dozen eggs. Starting at the top, these sizes are jumbo (30 oz per dozen), extra large (27 oz), large (24 oz), medium (21 oz), small (18 oz) and peewee (15 oz).

Useful, to be sure (the most popular are the large), but none of them even holds a candle to the beauty the California Egg Commission named the largest single chicken egg ever recorded: One full pound, with a double yolk and a double shell. Sorry, I don't have any nutrition stats for this scenario.

Frankfurters

Modern hot dogs and other meat sausages are made from muscle meat similar to the fresh ground beef or pork sold at the supermarket. Like all meat products, they provide complete proteins with adequate amounts of all the essential amino acids, plus B vitamins and heme iron, the organic form of iron found in foods from animals. That's good. Unfortunately, regular franks, like other sausages, are traditionally loaded with saturated fats and cholesterol.

But notice the word *regular*. The frank, remember, is an American success story, so the same know-how that gave the world no-fat ice cream and trans fat-free margarine has come up with skinny meat and poultry franks, not to mention fairly good soybean-based veggie versions.

As you can see in Table 6-1, the new breeds of dogs are acceptable at practically anybody's table. The stats in this table come from three versions of one national brand of hot dogs. Others may vary, so check the label. Woof.

Table 6-1	Slimmed-Down Dogs (One All-Beef Hot Dog)		
Fat Content	*Regular*	*Reduced Fat*	*97% Fat Free*
Total fat	14.0 g	10.0 g	1.5 g
Saturated fat	6.0 g	4.5 g	1.0 g
Cholesterol	30.0 mg	26.0 mg	15.0 mg

Lamb

Mary's little lamb may be adorable on the hoof, but on your plate, it's the red meat with the highest proportion of saturated fat per ounce.

A 4-ounce serving of lean beef has 6 g of fat, 2.3 of them saturated. A 4-ounce serving of lamb has 23 g of fat, 9.9 of them saturated. Lean pork is somewhere in between, with 9 g of total fat, 3 of them saturated, in a 4-ounce portion. Who knew?

Liver

If you hated liver as a kid and still can't stand to see it on your plate, this is your moment to call your mom and say, "Nyah, nyah, I told you so."

Like all foods from animals, liver is rich in high-quality proteins. It's also the single best natural source of retinol ("true vitamin A"), one of the few natural sources of vitamin D, a gold mine of B vitamins (including vitamin B12), and an excellent source of heme iron (the form of iron most easily absorbed by your body).

But like other organ meats, such as brains and sweetbreads (pancreas), liver has much more cholesterol than even well-marbled red meat. For example, a 3-ounce serving of lean roast beef has 69 mg of cholesterol, but a 3-ounce serving of braised beef liver has — hold onto your hat — 330 mg of cholesterol, 30 mg more than you're supposed to have in an entire day. Just thinking about what happens if you chop up chicken liver with chicken fat makes my head ache! (For an explanation of what all that cholesterol is doing in the brains, check out Chapter 2.)

Heart and tongue aren't as high in cholesterol. They're mainly muscle, not fat, so they clock in at about the same fat and cholesterol levels as other red meat. A 3-ounce serving of heart has 164 mg of cholesterol. A similar serving of beef tongue has 91 mg of cholesterol. I guess it proves you gotta have heart, not brains. Oooooooh boy, that's lame!

Wieners

The frankfurter is a German culinary import, but stuffing the long skinny sausage into a matching bun was pure New World genius. Brooklyn butcher Charles Feltman opened the first sausage-on-a-roll stand in Coney Island in 1871. Thirty years later, cartoonist T.A. "Tad" Dorgan sketched baseball park vendors hawking the long skinny pups on buns and captioned the picture "hot dog" because he couldn't spell "dachshund."

Needless to say, the hot dog is still a favorite at baseball parks where, according to the National Hot Dog and Sausage Council, Americans gobble 7 billion total franks each summer. That's enough dogs to stretch a chain from Dodger Stadium in Los Angeles, California, to the Baseball Hall of Fame in Cooperstown, New York.

Margarine with trans fatty acids

You may think that switching to margarine eliminates the risks associated with using butter on your bread. Well, as we native New Yorkers say, fuggeddaboudit!

The problem is that all margarines aren't created equal. Some types are still made with the form of hydrogenated fat called trans fat, the fats New York City's mayor and city council banned from use by chefs in the city's restaurants in 2007.

As Chapter 5 explains, while *trans fats* aren't necessarily saturated fats, they act just like saturated fats in your body. They raise rather than lower your blood levels of cholesterol.

The word *trans* refers to the placement of atoms on molecules. No, no, don't roll your eyes. This stuff is interesting. Two molecules may contain the exact-same atoms but be totally different because of a small difference in the placement of the atoms. This small difference in atom placement makes a big difference in the way a molecule behaves.

In other words, trans fatty acids are fats behaving badly. So the margarine you want is one with the words "No Trans Fats" on the label. At least this week.

Poultry skin and dark meat

What? Poultry is bad for a heart-healthy diet? It depends on the poultry. And sometimes the part.

Ounce for ounce, skinless poultry has about the same amount of cholesterol and fat as lean red meat, but generally, poultry fat is proportionately lower in saturated fats and higher in unsaturated fats than the fat in red meats.

Decency almost prevented me from attempting to count the fat grams in crispy, crunchy chicken or duck skin, a total I feared may approach the level of the nutritionally obscene. But I figured you may want to know, so here goes:

- For chicken, serving the meat with the skin just about doubles the fat content.
- For duck, a 4-ounce serving of skin-free meat has 14 g of fat, already a pretty healthy (healthy?) helping. With the skin, a 4-ounce serving has 31.8 g of fat, 14.6 of them saturated.

Yipes!

Table 6-2 compares the fat, saturated fat, and cholesterol content of white- and dark-meat poultries with lean beef. Notice that the lean beef beats dark-meat poultry every time. My, isn't that in-ter-esting!

Table 6-2	Fat Facts: Skinless Poultry versus Lean Beef		
Four-Ounce Serving	*Total Fat*	*Saturated Fat*	*Cholesterol*
Chicken (white meat)	5.8 g	1.4 g	95.0 mg
Chicken (dark meat)	11.2 g	2.97 g	104.0 mg
Duck	14.0 g	5.3 g	112.0 mg
Goose	12.7 g	5.1 g	108.0 mg
Turkey (white meat)	4.0 g	1.2 g	78.0 mg
Turkey (dark meat)	8.0 g	2.7 g	96.0 mg
Lean beef	6.0 g	2.3 g	78.0 mg

Unfiltered coffee

In 1994, researchers at the Agricultural University in Wageningen (the Netherlands) identified two chemicals in coffee that may raise cholesterol levels.

The chemicals are *diterpenes,* substances found in the oils of the coffee bean that give coffee its wonderful flavor and aroma. The amount of diterpenes in your coffee cup varies with the brewing method.

Drip-brewed coffee, instant coffee, and percolated coffee contain only minimal amounts of diterpenes. But boiled coffees — Greek coffee, Turkish coffee, espresso, and the coffee brewed in French "press" coffee makers — may have 6 to 12 mg of diterpenes per 5-ounce cup.

This amount is significant, and the Dutch researchers estimate that continually drinking five cups of press-brewed coffee or 15 espressos a day may raise cholesterol levels 8 to 10 points.

(There are no statistics right now defining the risk for people who gobble up chocolate-covered coffee beans, but you can practically bet that some smart researcher somewhere is working on it.)

Drinking coffee may also increase homocysteine levels in your blood. *Homo-cysteine* is an amino acid produced in your body when you digest proteins. As I explain in Chapter 2, the American Heart Association has identified high levels of homocysteine as an independent risk factor for heart disease.

A 1997 study at Norway's University of Bergen found that even moderate coffee consumption (five or fewer cups a day) is linked to higher blood levels of homocysteine. This may explain the results of a 1995 study at Boston University School of Public Health in Brookline (Massachusetts) showing the risk of heart attack was 2.5 times higher among women who drank ten cups of coffee a day than among those who averaged less than one cup.

Whole-milk products

Ice cream, cheese, yogurt, cream, sour cream, half-and-half, whipped cream, milk — what do all these things have in common?

Unless the label says "low-fat," "reduced fat," "skim," or some variation thereof, every one of them contains whole milk — milk with 3.5 percent butterfat, which is how it comes from the cow.

An 8-ounce glass of whole milk has 8 g of fat, with 5.1 g of saturated fat. Compare that to an 8-ounce glass of 1 percent milk, which has only 3 g of fat, 1.6 of them saturated. Skim milk has less than 1 g of fat, with 0.3 g of satu-rated fat. The best part? All versions deliver about 300 mg of calcium, 8 g of protein, and 300 mg of vitamin D.

Playing with butterfat produces similar magic in other dairy products. Table 6-3 shows the value of reducing the fat in several kinds of milk treats.

Table 6-3	More Milk-Fat Facts		
Product	*Total Fat*	*Saturated Fat*	*Cholesterol*
Milk (8 oz)			
Whole	8.0 g	5.1 g	33.0 mg
1%	3.0 g	1.6 g	10.0 mg
Skim	<1.0 g	0.3 g	4.0 mg
Yogurt (8 oz)			
Whole milk	7.0 g	4.8 g	29.0 mg
Low-fat	4.0 g	2.3 g	14.0 mg
Fat-free	<1.0 g	0.3 g	4.0 mg

Product	Total Fat	Saturated Fat	Cholesterol
Ice cream (½ cup)			
Vanilla	7.5 g	4.5 g	58.0 mg
Ice milk (½ cup)			
Fat-free vanilla	3.0 g	1.8 g	9.0 mg

Plant-Produced Foods That Help Control Cholesterol

Chapter 5 goes on for pages and pages — well, at least lines and lines — about all the foods that can help you control your cholesterol. Literally thousands of plant foods exist that you can use on a diet designed to help control your cholesterol levels.

However, the ones listed in this section are right at the top of the list, fruit- and veggie-wise. If you don't like the foods in this section, hopefully my explanations here will encourage you to have second thoughts and start adding them to your grocery list. These are the best of the best!

Apples

Like most fruit, every variety of apples has plenty of dietary fiber: insoluble *cellulose* and *lignin* in the peel and soluble *pectins* in the flesh. As Chapter 5 explains, the former keeps things moving through your intestinal tract, and the latter sops up cholesterol and other fats, preventing them from exiting from your intestinal tract into your body and blood vessels.

The U.S. Apple Association (www.usapple.org) wants you to know another fact: When scientists at the Université Paul Sabatier in Toulouse, France, fed apples to hamsters specially bred to develop high levels of cholesterol, the hamsters' low-density lipoproteins (LDLs — the "bad" fat particles) went down and their high-density lipoproteins (HDLs — the "good" particles that carry cholesterol out of the body) went up.

The theory is that soluble pectins form a gel in your stomach that sops up fats and ferries them out of your body as waste. An added bonus: Pectins also help solidify stool, which justifies the reputation of raw apple shavings as a home remedy for diarrhea. (Purified pectin is the active ingredient in many over-the-counter, anti-diarrheal products.)

Finally, apples are rich in *flavonoids,* the naturally occurring antioxidant plant compounds that make green tea and red grapes serious players in the war against heart disease, stroke, and cancer. Sure seems to justify the time-honored adage, "An apple a day keeps the doctor away."

Avocados

For years, dieters and folks concerned about heart health avoided avocados because the luscious green fruit (yes, the avocado is a fruit, not a veggie) is high in fat. A 1-ounce serving — 1 tablespoon or 2 to 3 thin slices — has about 4.5 grams fat, which may be one reason why some people call the avocado a "butter pear."

But only a measly 0.5 gram of that fat is saturated. The rest is primarily cholesterol-lowering monounsaturated fatty acids plus polyunsaturated fatty acids (fats that don't raise cholesterol levels), including the omega-3s the American Heart Association recommends substituting for saturated fats.

The avocado also serves up about 20 vitamins and minerals, including vitamin E, vitamin C, the B vitamin folate, iron, and potassium. In addition, the avocado delivers protective *phytonutrients* (*phyto* = plant, *nutrients* = well, nutrients), such as *phytosterols* — plant compounds that look like cholesterol but actually keep the body from absorbing the cholesterol in other foods.

Chapter 14 includes a delicious recipe for Creamy Avocado Dip; try it with veggies!

Beans

Beans are little treasure chests of soluble *gums* and *pectins,* two varieties of the soluble dietary fiber that grab and hold fats in your digestive tract. Because you digest beans very slowly, unlike other high-carb foods, such as pasta and potatoes, your insulin secretion doesn't spike.

This news is good for people with diabetes. In fact, one well-known study at the University of Kentucky showed that eating a lot of beans may enable people with Type 1 diabetes (whose bodies produce practically no insulin) to reduce their daily insulin requirements by nearly 40 percent. Patients with Type 2 diabetes, whose bodies produce some insulin, may be able to cut insulin intake by 98 percent. This news is also good for people watching their cholesterol because a sudden rise in insulin has now been added to the list of risks.

But good as they are, beans aren't perfect. The human gut can't digest dietary fiber and some complex carbs, such as the sugars in beans. As a result, these guys sit in your intestines as fodder for resident friendly bacteria that munch on the carbs and then release carbon dioxide and (ugh) methane, a smelly gas.

Which leaves you with one of those conundrums that make life so interesting: Heart disease (and diabetes) or smelly gas? Smelly gas or heart disease (and diabetes)? Decisions. Decisions.

Brown rice

Score one for the original vegetarian foodies, the guys who were eating whole grains — especially brown rice — way back in the Nutritional Dark Ages before anyone even knew what cholesterol was.

Boy, were they smart cookies. All rice is low-cal, low-fat, and cholesterol-free. But when it comes to controlling your cholesterol levels, the rice to rave about is brown.

Brown rice gets its color and its nutty flavor from the *germ* (the fatty inner part of the seed) and the *bran* (the nutrient-rich outer hull).

Like oat bran, rice bran is a food worthy of respect in its own right. Oat bran gets the publicity, but as long ago as 1989, a U.S. Department of Agriculture (www.usda.gov) study showed that feeding rice bran to hamsters can reduce the animals' cholesterol levels as effectively as the better-known oat stuff.

By the way, the USA Rice Federation (www.usarice.com) says that the average American consumes about 25 pounds of rice a year. Right now, most of that consumption is white rice, without the bran. By increasing your consumption of brown rice versus white rice, you can strike a blow for low cholesterol.

Chocolate

No list of healthful foods can be considered complete if it doesn't include chocolate — the treat that says, "Hey, I've been watching my cholesterol like crazy, and I deserve a reward!"

Contrary to popular wisdom, plain dark chocolate isn't an empty-calorie food. Chocolate comes from the cocoa bean, which — like other beans — is packed with proteins, B vitamins, and vital minerals, such as iron, magnesium, and copper.

As a plant food, chocolate has no cholesterol at all. True, cocoa butter (the fat in cocoa beans) is a saturated fat, but some sweets companies have done a swell job creating chocolate products without cocoa butter, thanks to modern technology.

Wait! There's more. The cocoa bean also has small amounts of caffeine (an average of 18 milligrams (mg) per cup of cocoa, versus 130 mg per 5-ounce cup of drip-brewed coffee), *phenylethylalanine* (PEA, a mood elevator sometimes called "the love chemical"), and *theobromine* (a muscle stimulant). Zip-pi-dee-doo-dah.

And chocolate contains loads of *flavonoids* and *catechins,* the naturally occurring chemicals credited with making grapes, wine, and tea heart-healthy. In the spring of 2007, researchers reported to the annual meeting of the American Association for the Advancement of Science that consuming the flavonols in chocolate increases blood flow to the brain.

And a German study published in the June 2007 issue of the *International Journal of Medical Science* announced that cocoa consumption among the Kuna people, islanders living near Panama, reduces the risk of cancer, stroke, heart failure, and diabetes.

Is it any wonder that the Hershey Company has added Hershey's Natural Flavonol Antioxidant Milk Chocolate, Hershey's Whole Bean Chocolate, and Hershey's All Natural Extra Dark Pure Dark Chocolate to its "goodness chocolate portfolio" of antioxidant-rich chocolate bars and bits with labels prominently touring the high levels of flavonols in the bar? Surely you jest.

Grapes

Grapes are great. A single serving of 20 green Thompson seedless or deep red Tokay or Emperor grapes has 70 to 80 calories, 12 to 16 percent of the recommended dietary allowance (RDA) for vitamin C, and up to 84 percent of the potassium found in ½ cup of orange juice.

Omega chocolates

On July 3, 2007, just in time to make every nutrition-conscious American chocoholic's July 4th celebration even more celebratory, Ocean Nutrition of Canada issued a press release to announce that Canadian chocolate maker Les Truffes au Chocolat would be adding a dash of Ocean Nutrition's omega-3 fatty acids to the recipe for its O Trois chocolate bars and chocolate "fingers."

The Calgary confectioners plan to distribute these special chocolates first in western Canada, then across Canada, and finally down into the United States. Can't wait for these treats to make it to your town? Check out the Les Truffes Web site (www.lestruffes.com) for mail-order goodies.

Mae West, the Madonna of a past time, used to invite her admirers to "Come up and peel me a grape sometime." But your goal is to lower your cholesterol, so that advice isn't for you.

Grape skins and pulp contain *resveratrol,* the flavonoid some folks credit with lowering cholesterol, reducing the risk of heart attack, and maybe even protecting against some forms of cancer.

Ounce for ounce, you get more resveratrol from grape juice than from plain grapes. The darker the juice, the higher the resveratrol. Purple grape juice has more resveratrol than red grape juice, which has more than white grape juice. As for individual grape varieties, in 1998, a team of food scientists from the USDA Agricultural Research Service identified a native American grape, the muscadine, as an unusually potent source of resveratrol. So aren't you glad that about half of all muscadines grown in the U.S. are used to make grape juice?

Prefer your grape juice in the form of wine? Read all about that in Chapter 10.

Certain margarines

At the start of the margarine revolution, around the time when television sets broadcast only in black and white, margarine was a white paste in a plastic bag with a small button on top that you squeezed to release a yellow coloring to knead through the white stuff. Its only virtue was its price: lower than butter's.

A few years later, with the discovery that butter was high in cholesterol and that cholesterol caused heart attacks, margarine was transformed into health food, the non-butter that can protect your heart. Until, that is, nutrition scientists linked hydrogenated fats — the stuff that made it possible to mold the original soft margarine paste into butter-like bars — to an increased risk of heart attack.

Today, some really healthful margarines are made with *plant sterols,* natural compounds found in grains, fruits, and vegetables, and *stanols,* compounds created by adding hydrogen atoms from wood pulp and other plant sources to sterols.

Both sterols and stanols, which are from plants, thus qualifying these margarines for inclusion in this list of plant foods that protect your heart, work like little sponges, sopping up cholesterol in your intestines before it can make its way into your bloodstream. Because of this sponge-like action, your total cholesterol levels and your levels of *low-density lipoproteins* (also known as LDLs or "bad" cholesterol) fall.

The studies show that one to two 1-tablespoon servings of stanol or sterol margarines a day can lower LDLs by 10 to 17 percent with results showing up in as little as two weeks.

Some eagle-eyed readers may take out their magnifying glasses and actually read the ingredient list on the product labels, a commendable act that helps you separate nutritious food from the not-so-hot possibilities. The problem is that those who do will find the words "hydrogenated fats." The reaction may be, "Ugh! Don't hydrogenated fats clog your arteries?" The simple answer is yes. But these margarines are specially formulated to carry fats (including hydrogenated fats) out of your body. The amount of hydrogenated fats in the margarines is less than the amount of fats the margarines remove. In other words, the net impact is good for everybody. Whew!

Nuts

Pass up the pretzels. Skip the chips. At snack time, reach for the nuts. At least the almonds and walnuts.

Although nuts are technically a high-fat food, the nutrition gurus at California's Loma Linda University say that adding moderate amounts of nuts to a cholesterol-lowering diet or substituting nuts for other high-fat foods, such as meats, may cut normal to moderately high levels of total cholesterol and LDL as much as 12 percent.

These guys should know. Over the past several years, they've made headlines with nutty studies:

- ✔ In one, volunteers were told to follow one of two diets, both based on National Cholesterol Education Program (NCEP) recommendations. Diet #1 got 20 percent of its calories from fats in oils and fatty foods such as meat; Diet #2 got 20 percent of its calories from high-fat nuts (like walnuts) instead. Both diets appeared to lower cholesterol levels.

- ✔ In a second study, the Loma Lindans compared the standard NCEP diet with two almond diets, the first deriving 10 percent of its calories from nuts, the second, 20 percent. Like the walnut diet, both almond diets lowered cholesterol, lowered blood pressure, and so on.

The conclusions, dutifully reported in scientific journals such as the *American Journal of Clinical Nutrition,* are that nuts provide fatty acids and other substances that reduce the risk of blood clots, amino acids (such as arginine) that the body uses to build other clot-blocking compounds, and dietary fiber that ferries cholesterol out of your body.

In other words, it pays to be nuts about nuts (see Chapter 14's recipe for Cinnamon and Spice Almonds).

Oatmeal

For more than 30 years, scientists have known that eating foods high in *soluble* dietary fiber (more about that in Chapter 5) can lower your cholesterol. Then along came oatmeal, a gee-whiz wonder food whose primary soluble dietary fiber — *beta glucan* — is a more super-effective cholesterol buster than other types of soluble dietary fiber, such as the pectin in apples (see the section "Apples" earlier in this chapter).

But guess what? Not every oatmeal gets the job done. The Right Stuff is oatmeal with oat bran, the brown outer covering of the oatmeal grain that's often removed to make oatmeal cereal (especially the quick-cook kind).

Researchers at the University of Kentucky reported back in 1990, practically the Dark Ages for anti-cholesterol foodies, that people who add ½ cup dry oat bran (*not* oatmeal) to their regular diets may be able to lower their levels of LDL by as much as 25 percent.

Not to be outdone, scientists at Northwestern University's Feinberg School of Medicine performed a study funded by Quaker Oats. The scientists found that 208 healthy volunteers whose normal cholesterol readings averaged about 200 mg/dL were able to reduce their total cholesterol levels by an average of 9.3 percent with a low-fat, low-cholesterol diet supplemented by 2 ounces of oats or oat bran every day.

Most of the volunteers in the Northwestern study were eating oatmeal, not oat bran, so look carefully at the difference in the numbers. At the University of Kentucky, the drop in cholesterol was 25 percent. At Northwestern, it was 9.3 percent. Even more interesting, the Northwestern folks said that only about one-third of the cholesterol reduction was due to the oats.

The cereal makers rounded the Northwestern number up to 10 percent. The risk of heart attack drops two percentage points for every one point drop in cholesterol, so the National Research Council called that a potential 20 percent drop in the risk of a heart attack, but how well eating oatmeal works for you really depends on how high your cholesterol is to start.

Suppose your cholesterol clocks in higher than 250 mg/dL. Lowering it 10 percent takes you down to 225 mg/dL. Now you're within shooting distance of a safe level (under 200 mg/dL). Now assume your cholesterol level is already a safe 199 mg/dL or lower. A low-fat, low-cholesterol diet *plus* oats may drop it to 180 mg/dL, but the oats account for only 6 points of your loss. The rest is due to — get this — your low-fat, low-cholesterol diet.

In other words, at the lower cholesterol levels, what really matters is an overall low-fat, low-cholesterol diet. Adding oats makes so little difference that if you hate the stuff, it's okay to pass it by and get your soluble fiber from other foods, like brown rice (see more on that previously in this chapter).

Pomegranate

When is an apple not an apple? When it's a pomegranate, of course. Historians suspect that the pomegranate was the "apple" Eve picked in the Garden of Eden. They know for sure it was such a favorite in ancient Egypt that Moses added it to the list of goodies waiting in the Promised Land. (Check it out in Deuteronomy 8:8.)

Also, this fruit figures big in Greek mythology as well: The goddess Persephone became a semi-permanent resident of the Underworld because she couldn't resist the luscious seeds of an Underworld pomegranate.

The good part of the pomegranate (*pome* = apple, *granate* = seeds/grains) is the jelly-like red pulp in "juice sacs" surrounding the seeds. To get at it, slice through the stem end of the pomegranate, and pull off the top, taking care to avoid splashing red pomegranate juice all over you. Then slice the pomegranate into wedges and pull the wedges apart and bite into them.

Your reward as you crush the jelly around the seeds is a liquid rich in polyphenols, the antioxidant compounds that help lower "bad" cholesterol.

Nutrition researchers at Technion Faculty of Medicine and Rambam Medical Center in Haifa, Israel, rate pomegranate juice higher in polyphenols than all the current favorites, such as red wine, blueberry juice, cranberry juice, green tea, black tea, and orange juice.

Another team of Technion scientists says that the juice and the oil extracted from pomegranate seeds kill breast cancer cells in test tubes and may eventually point the way to a new drug in the fight against breast cancer.

Maybe Eve and Persephone knew what they were doing when one picked and the other one enjoyed that funny apple.

Slicing the Cholesterol from Your Dinner Plate

Reducing the amount of cholesterol lurking on your dinner plate is simply a matter of knowing which foods have what fats, and wielding your knife — or fork or spoon — accordingly.

This section is chock-full of low- or no-cholesterol alternatives and stratagems. For illustration only, I use some well-known, brand-name products as examples of low- or no-cholesterol alternatives. Feel free to substitute your own favorites. Just be sure to read the label first.

Finally, all the nutrient numbers used in this chapter come from the United States Department of Agriculture (USDA) Nutrient Database. For more on how to use this incredibly valuable tool, see the appendix.

Choosing low-fat or no-fat dairy products

Milk may not be quite the perfect food your grandmother thought it was, but modern good-food-people know that dairy products such as milk and cheese are the best natural sources of the calcium that keeps bones strong.

The problem is that these foods may be high in cholesterol and saturated fat. The solution is to opt for the low- or no-fat milk products stacked a mile high in every supermarket dairy case.

How much lower can you go? Well, one 5-ounce cup of whole milk has 33 mg cholesterol and 5 grams saturated fat. But lookie-here: one 5-ounce cup of skim (fat-free) milk has only 4.4 mg cholesterol and 0.3 grams saturated fat. If you absolutely have to have a smidgen of creaminess in your milk, one 5-ounce cup of 1-percent-fat milk has 9.8 mg cholesterol and 1.6 grams saturated fat.

One regular Kraft American Cheese slice has 20 mg cholesterol and 3 grams saturated fat; one slice of Kraft Free American cheese has no cholesterol and no fat. And here's a bonus: the regular cheese has 70 calories per slice; the fat-free cheese has only 30 calories. Yum.

Serving stew instead of steak

No matter how you slice it, red meat is red meat, cholesterol, saturated fat, and all. To compensate, start by trimming all the visible fat — yes, that white stuff on the sides. Then stew your beef or lamb, rather than broiling or roasting it. (You can do this with pork, too.)

After the cooking's done, stash your stew in the fridge for a couple of hours until a layer of white stuff — yes, more fat from the interior of the meat — hardens on top. Lift off the fat layer and away goes a whole lot of cholesterol and saturated fat.

How much? Hard to tell exactly, but clearly you've done a good-nutrition, weight-control deed for the day. You not only reduce the cholesterol and saturated fat content of the dish, but also lift away 100 calories with every tablespoon of fat.

Just thinking about that makes those tight jeans feel looser.

Washing the chopped meat

No kidding. Put a teapot of water on to boil. Put the chopped meat in a pan, breaking it into small pieces, and cook until the meat browns. Put the meat into a strainer and let the liquid fat run off, and then pour a cup of boiling water over the meat in the strainer.

Repeat the hot water bath twice. Once again, every tablespoon of fat that drains away saves you 100 calories, plus cholesterol and saturated fat.

Use the de-fatted meat in spaghetti sauce or to stuff a nutritious green pepper of cabbage leaf. Yum.

Peeling the poultry

Most of the fat and therefore most of the cholesterol in poultry is in the skin. For example, 3.5 ounces of raw chicken breast with skin has 64 mg cholesterol and 2.7 grams saturated fat. Take off the skin, and that same 3.5 ounces of chicken breast serves up 58 mg cholesterol and a miniscule 0.3 grams saturated fat.

Obviously, the way you cook the chicken may affect the fat and cholesterol levels. According to the USDA Nutrient Database, a chicken breast with skin fried in batter has nearly 30 percent more cholesterol (85 mg) and 30 percent more saturated fat (3.5 grams) than the raw stuff.

Fry the skinless chicken breast, and the saturated fat goes up 300 percent to 1.2 grams per serving — but that's still less than the fat you get from fried chicken with skin.

Got the picture? Good.

Spritzing the fish

Naturally oily fish like salmon and mackerel are rich in omega-3 fatty acids that protect your heart. Don't change the equation by drowning them in creamy, high-cholesterol, high-fat, high-calorie sauces when a spritz of lemon and some green seasonings (think dill) can do the trick.

Next.

Sparing the bread spread

Now that everybody knows vegetable oils are lower in saturated fats than butter, restaurants from pizza parlors to the fanciest white tablecloth establishments cater to their patrons' sense of sophistication by substituting a small bowl of olive oil for the standard plate of butter pats.

Before you reach for the oil, though, consider this: Vegetable oils, including the ubiquitous olive oil, aren't an unmitigated blessing. Yes, the oils have less saturated fat than butter. True, they're cholesterol-free. But the bad news is that all dietary fats — butter, margarine, oils — have about the same number of calories per serving, 100 to 125 calories per tablespoon. These unnecessary calories can pile pounds onto parts of your body and that may raise your cholesterol levels. Try the bread as is. You might like it.

By the way, don't assume that your bread is low-fat just because you didn't butter or oil it. Some breads, such as foccacia, popovers, and muffins, come pre-buttered or oiled. To test the fat content of your bread, pick up a piece and put it on your napkin. Hand sticky? Oil spots on the napkin? You know what that means.

Keeping the veggies basic

Once upon a time, when vegetables were new to the Western table and people who were used to gnawing on a haunch of beef considered them suspect at best, the accepted cooking method was to boil the plant into a no-color-no-texture-no-flavor lump.

Next came butter, cheese, and cream sauces, often broiled to a tasty, brown, fat-and-cholesterol crust. Today, the smart way to cook vegetables is as quickly and simply as possible. Steaming over bouillon works; so does broiling veggie kebobs.

Low-fat, cholesterol-free baking tip

Bake your own bread? Cake? Muffins? To reduce the fat content, don't grease the pan. Instead, bake with parchment paper. Every tablespoon of butter you don't use cuts 31 mg cholesterol and 7.3 grams saturated fat from the final product. And eliminating one tablespoon of any fat reduces the calorie count by 100 big ones.

As for flavorings, what could be better than those other plant foods: Herbs and spices. A pinch of thyme here, a sprinkle of oregano there, a dash of dill, some chives — terrific. For those of you who simply can't give up thickened sauces, the solution may be a "reduction" (boiled-down bouillon) or a cream sauce made with trans-fat-free margarine and fat-free powdered milk instead of butter and cream. Purists may wince, but try it. You may like it — and so will your arteries.

Speaking the language

No matter how dedicated the dieter, good intentions tend to fade when eating out, especially when the menu hints at exotic foreign delicacies. Not to worry, Table 6-4 lists the good and bad in six, count 'em six, popular ethnic cuisines.

Table 6-4	Choosing Low Cholesterol Ethnic Dishes	
Ethnic Food	*Low Saturated Fat/Cholesterol*	*High Saturated Fat/Cholesterol*
Chinese	Bean curd (not fried)	Batter-fried (including sweet and sour dishes)
	Moo shu chicken/pork	
	Fresh noodles	Crisp noodles (including "bird's nest")
	Steamed dumplings	Eggrolls and fried dumplings
	Sliced roast pork[1]	Spare ribs
	Vegetarian dishes, including bean curd (steamed)	Vegetarian dishes, including bean curd (fried)
	Velvet sauce (egg whites)	Shrimp and lobster sauce (egg yolks)
French	Au vapeur (steamed)	A la crème (creamed)
	En brochette (broiled)	A la mode (with ice cream)
	Grille (grilled)	Au gratin (with cheese)
		En croûte (in pastry crust)
		Remoulade (with mayonnaise)
Indian	Chutney	Batter-fried
	Dal (lentils)	Coconut milk (creamy sauces)
	Masala (curry)	Ghee (clarified butter)

Ethnic Food	Low Saturated Fat/Cholesterol	High Saturated Fat/Cholesterol
	Matta (peas)	Poori (deep-fried bread)
	Pilau (rice)	Samosas (fried turnovers)
	Raita (yogurt and cucumbers)	
Italian	Pasta (plain)	Alfredo sauce (cream, cheese)
	Picata (lemon/wine sauce)	Alla panna (with cream)
	Tomato sauces (no cream)	Carbonara (with butter, eggs, bacon)
	White clam sauce[2]	Fritto (fried)
	Wine sauces	Parmigiana (with cheese)
Japanese	Clear broth	Agemono (fried)
	Miso soup or dressing	Katsu (fried pork)
	Mushimono (steamed)	Sukiyaki (beef)
	Nimono (simmered)	Tempura (batter fried)
	Sashimi	
	Sushi (raw fish)	
	Udon (fresh noodles)	
	Yaki (broiled)	
	Yakimono (grilled)	
Mexican	Black beans and black bean soup	Refried beans[3]
	Ceviche (marinated seafood)	Tortilla shells (fried)
	Enchiladas, burritos, fajitas (minus cheese and/or sour cream)	
	Gazpacho	
	Rice and beans	

(1) Trim all visible fat
(2) The fat is olive oil
(3) While refried beans served in restaurants may be high in fat, some canned refried beans qualify as a low-fat dish. Check the label. Who knew?

Don't punish your partner

Your cholesterol may be problematic but that doesn't mean everyone else at the table is in the same situation. A considerate host or dinner partner makes accommodations. Table 6-5 shows how to adapt your controlled-cholesterol, low-fat diet for someone who doesn't have to watch the fats.

Table 6-5	Alternative Food Pairings	
Food	*Yours*	*Theirs*
Pasta	Tomato sauce	Tomato sauce plus a meatball and Parmesan cheese
Vegetables	Plain veggies	Veggies with butter or sauce
	Bean soup	Bean soup with chopped ham or sausage added
Fruit	Fresh, canned, or frozen	Fresh, canned, or frozen with cream
Poultry	Skinless	With skin
	White meat	White and dark meat
Dessert	Fat-free frozen yogurt	Ice cream
	Fat-free chocolate sauce	Hot fudge sauce
Coffee	Espresso	Cappuccino

Choosing low-fat desserts

No human being should have to give up dessert just to maintain a healthy diet. And that goes double for chocolate.

According to the Haagen Dazs Web site, one half-cup serving of Haagen Dazs chocolate ice cream has 115 mg cholesterol and (gulp!) 11 grams saturated fat. But one half-cup serving of Haagen Dazs low-fat sorbet has no, repeat no, cholesterol or saturated fat.

You can assume that similar differences apply to other varieties of frozen desserts, and take it from an expert (me), substituting the second for the first is no deprivation, particularly if you toss some fruit on the cold chocolate stuff and maybe add some Hershey's Syrup. It says right here on the bottle I just took out of my refrigerator that the chocolate syrup has zero cholesterol and fat.

Part III
Leading a Cholesterol-Lowering Lifestyle

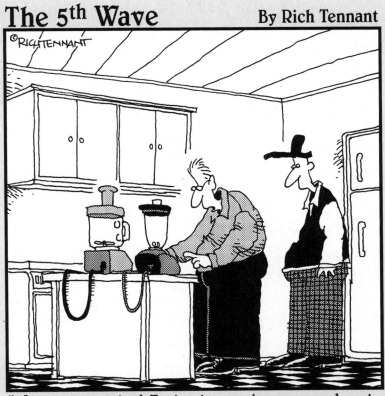

The 5th Wave — By Rich Tennant

"Mona suggested I start running every day to control my cholesterol. So far I've run the air conditioner and the lawn sprinkler. Now I'm moving on to the kitchen appliances."

In this part . . .

How you live definitely influences your cholesterol levels. Managing your weight, working your muscles, avoiding tobacco, and enjoying alcohol beverages in moderation — each of these lifestyle issues impacts your ability to keep your cholesterol within healthy bounds. The good part is that lifestyle choices are — surprise! — choices. Choose right and you win. Pretty good deal, huh? Here's an even better deal: This part provides you with some insider lifestyle information to tip the scales in your favor so that you're no longer the underdog in the "you versus cholesterol" contest.

Chapter 7

Weighing Weight's Weight on Cholesterol

*S*ome Americans worry about global warming. Others suspect that the real threat to North America isn't the rising temperature but the rising poundage of several hundred million well-padded citizens. If the trend continues, they say, the whole darned continent may soon sink. Okay, maybe that's an exaggeration, but according to *Health, United States 2006,* the 30th edition of an annual Centers for Disease Control and Prevention report on trends in health stats:

✔ Compared to 1960/1962, the percentage of overweight American adults ages 20 to 74 remained pretty much the same in 2003/2004, but the percentage of obese adults rose from 13 percent to 34 percent.

✔ The percentage of overweight children ages 6 to 11 more than doubled between 1976/1980 and 2003/2004, rising from 7 percent to 19 percent. Among adolescents ages 12 to 19, the percentage of those who were overweight more than tripled, rising from 5 percent to 17 percent.

In Canada, where the percentage of obese adults nearly doubled between 1978/1979 and 2004, things are pretty much the same. Check out these factoids from Statistics Canada's *1996/1997 to 2004/2005 National Population Health Survey*:

✔ From 1996/1997 to 2004/2005, Canadian adults, men as well as women, grew steadily heavier. Every two years, younger adults ages 18 to 33 gained more weight than did adults ages 34 to 49. Adults ages 50 to 54 also gained, but they gained less than the younger folks.

✔ The average weight gain among adult men rose from 10 pounds in 1996/1997 to 11 pounds by 2004/2005. Among women, the average gain rose from 9.9 pounds to 10.5 pounds.

While all this extra weight may not tilt the planet, it may certainly be a predictor of health problems, especially for people who work to control their cholesterol, which, come to think of it, is pretty much the title of the book you hold in your hands.

Presenting the Health Risks Posed by Extra Pounds

Many people want to lose weight to look better. Others want to gain weight for the same reason. But reaching a healthful weight — and staying there — is more than a matter of vanity. It's also about being healthy. Years and years of scientific studies and surveys have produced irrefutable evidence that excess pounds often equal higher risk of *morbidity,* doctor-speak for illness, and *mortality,* doctor-speak for you-know-what — the big D (d-e-a-t-h).

To be precise, the message from your good friends at the American Heart Association (AHA) is that being overweight raises your risk of five of the top-ten leading causes of death in the United States, Canada, and Europe:

✔ Cancer (some types)

✔ Diabetes

✔ High blood pressure

✔ Stroke

Wait! That list shows only four kinds of big trouble. The missing fifth item is, you guessed it, *coronary heart disease,* which you may know by its alias, *heart attack.* Table 7-1 lists several other weight-related problems that, although not in the big five, can certainly make you extremely uncomfortable.

Table 7-1	More Weight-Related Health Conditions
Condition	*Weight-Related Problem*
Gallbladder disease	Being overweight and/or losing weight very fast leads to the formation of gallstones.
Gout (form of arthritis that occurs primarily in men)	Being overweight is linked to high blood levels of urates, irritating byproducts of protein digestion linked to attacks of gout.

Condition	Weight-Related Problem
Incontinence	Being overweight weakens pelvic muscles, which leads to urine leakage.
Osteoarthritis	Being overweight stresses joints.
Sleep apnea	Being overweight weakens the muscles at the back of the throat that hold the airway open causing momentary cessation of breathing and frequent awakening during the night.

Connecting cholesterol with weight

You don't have to be enormously overweight to experience a connection between your higher weight and a higher risk of heart disease. Being as little as 20 percent over your suggested healthy weight — which I get to in a minute — raises your total cholesterol and your "bad" LDLs while lowering your "good" HDLs. (To brush up on this coronary alphabet soup, check out LDLs and HDLs in Chapter 2 and Chapter 3.)

But don't despair. Losing weight reverses the equation. Diet and exercise away those extra pounds, and your not-so-hot LDLs will start to fall while your hot-stuff HDLs begin to rise.

Gaining is the same as losing in this arena

Toting around too many pounds is hard on your heart and blood vessels, but gaining weight is worse because it forces your body to adapt to new, stressful conditions. Think about it. When you gain weight, you make more tissue. The tissue needs oxygen, so you have to make more blood, which carries oxygen. The extra blood stretches the chambers of your heart, which must work harder to push the blood out into your body where the extra volume of blood stresses your blood vessels. Anyone hear a diagnosis of high blood pressure in the near future?

As a result, the AHA, which ♥'s your heart, wants you to know that simply preventing weight gain is *the most important factor* in preventing your cholesterol level from rising as you grow older. Imagine! As you grow older, not gaining weight keeps your cholesterol level in check more effectively than a low-fat diet, cholesterol-lowering drugs, or exercise. And you don't have to go on a crash diet to see the benefits. According to the AHA, even a modest weight loss — say 5 to 10 percent of your total weight — lowers total cholesterol. Pretty encouraging stuff, huh?

By the way, several similar studies show that gaining weight also increases levels of *triglycerides* (check out Chapter 2), another risk factor for heart attacks. Hey, a two-for-one special: Controlling weight controls both your cholesterol and your triglycerides. What a bargain.

Figuring Out Who's Fat

Up to this point in this chapter, I have used the word *overweight* seven times, but I haven't defined it. So let me do that right now.

One way to decide whether someone's overweight is to see what he or she looks like. Right? Wrong.

Actress Lillian Russell, the femme fatale during the late 19th and early 20th centuries, weighed in at a hefty 230 pounds. One hundred years later, Nicole Richie or Eva Longoria tips the scales at, oh, maybe, 98 pounds. Your great-grandparents would have rushed these skinny merinks (great-granny's word for v-e-r-y thin) to the doctor for a weight-gain tonic. Today, it may be Russell whom people would want to ship off to the doctor.

Clearly, judging whether an individual is overweight or thin by appearance is subjective. It depends on who's doing the lookin' and the cultural standards that person applies. Conclusion: The eyeball test isn't a reliable method for determining healthful weight. You need something a tad more scientific.

Luckily, modern nutrition offers some reasonably rational options to decide who's overweight. These options include

- Body shape
- Weight charts
- Body composition

Evaluating body shape

All healthy adults have some body fat. Women generally have proportionately more body fat than men who, in turn, have proportionately more muscle tissue than women. Where a person stores the fat tissue he or she accumulates is gender-related. Men are most likely to pile excess fat around the middle (abdomen). The result is a body type called an "apple." Women usually store excess fat around their hips, buttocks, and upper thighs, a pattern called a "pear."

A more scientific name for the apple/pear shape descriptions is the *waist/hip ratio,* a measurement of the relative size of the waist and hips. To find your ratio, follow these steps:

1. **Run a tape measure around your waist.**

2. **Run a tape measure around your hips.**

3. **Divide the measurement of your waist by the measurement of your hips.**

    For example: waist (29 inches) ÷ hips (39 inches) = a waist/hip ratio of 0.74

A woman whose waist/hip ratio is higher than 0.8 or a man whose waist/hip ratio is higher than 0.95 — both apple shape numbers — may be at higher risk of weight-related health problems, including heart attacks.

However, it's only fair to point out that the BMI-plus-waist circumference described below is considered far more reliable than the apple/pear waist-to-hip ratio alone.

Charting a healthful weight

In 1990, the U.S. Department of Agriculture and Department of Health and Human Services included a weight chart in that year's edition of the *Dietary Guidelines for Americans:*

✔ The new chart numbers were *weight goals,* not *ideal weights.*

✔ The weight goals were based on the entire population of the United States.

✔ The weight charts were unisex with a single set of weight goals for men and women of the same height.

✔ Best of all, the new weight goals were divided into two age groups — one set for people ages 19 to 34 and the other for people ages 35 and older.

Table 7-2 shows the 1990 *Dietary Guidelines for Americans* weight charts for adult men and women. People with small, lighter bones and proportionately more fat tissue than muscle tissue (fat weighs less than muscle) are likely to weigh in at the low end. People with large, heavier bones and proportionately more muscle than fat, are likely to weigh in at the high end. As a general (but by no means invariable) rule, women have smaller frames and less muscle than men, so they weigh less than men of the same height and age.

Table 7-2	Weight Goals for Men and Women	
	Weight	*Weight*
Height	*Age 19 to 34*	*Age 35 and Older*
5'0"	97–128 lbs	108–138 lbs
5'1"	101–132 lbs	111–143 lbs
5'2"	104–137 lbs	115–148 lbs
5'3"	107–141 lbs	122–157 lbs
5'4"	111–146 lbs	122–157 lbs
5'5"	114–150 lbs	126–152 lbs
5'6"	118–155 lbs	130–167 lbs
5'7"	121–160 lbs	134–172 lbs
5'8"	125–164 lbs	138–178 lbs
5'9"	129–169 lbs	142–183 lbs
5'10"	132–174 lbs	146–188 lbs
5'11"	136–179 lbs	151–194 lbs
6'0"	140–184 lbs	155–199 lbs
6'1"	144–189 lbs	159–205 lbs
6'2"	148–195 lbs	164–210 lbs
6'3"	152–200 lbs	168–216 lbs
6'4"	156–205 lbs	173–222 lbs
6'5"	160–211 lbs	177–228 lbs
6'6"	164–216 lbs	182–234 lbs

Source: Nutrition and Your Health: Dietary Guidelines for Americans, 3rd ed. (U.S Department of Agriculture, U.S. Department of Health and Human Services, 1990).

For ten years, weight charts remained fairly friendly and forgiving. Then boom! The *Dietary Guidelines for Americans 2000* tossed out the higher weights for older people. As of the new millennium, the healthy weights for everyone, young or old, woman or man, were the weights for people between the ages of 19 and 34 from the 1990 *Dietary Guidelines for Americans,* which you can still find in Table 7-2. Pretty skinny thinking, if you ask me.

Then boom! — again. The *Dietary Guidelines for Americans 2005* tossed out all weight tables in favor of the body mass index chart.

Indexing your mass

In 1990, just as the *Dietary Guidelines for Americans* published its pleasantly elastic two-tier weight chart, the National Heart, Lung, and Blood Institute introduced the first federal guidelines on how to identify, evaluate, and treat people with excess poundage.

The most interesting section was the introduction of a new weight measurement: *body mass index* (BMI). BMI is a unisex measure of weight relative to height, a number — such as 24 — that serves as a predictor of your risk for weight-related illnesses, such as diabetes, high blood pressure, heart disease, stroke, gallbladder disease, and arthritic pain. The higher your number, the higher your risk. So, what's your number? Keep reading.

Calculating your BMI

The original equation used to calculate BMI was set up in kilograms for weight (W) and meters for height (H): $BMI = W \div H^2$. But if you're partial to pounds and inches, you can calculate BMI in pounds and inches as long as you add one extra step. The equation looks like this:

$$BMI = W \div H^2 \times 705$$

To get your own BMI, plug your numbers into the BMI equation. For example, if you're 5'3" tall and weigh 138 pounds, the equation for your BMI looks like this:

$$BMI = W \div H^2 \times 705$$
$$[138 \div (63 \times 63)] \times 705$$
$$(138 \div 3969) \times 705$$
$$24.5$$

Hate math? Eyes glazing over? Just run your finger down Table 7-3, which does the math for men and women from 4'11" to 6'4" tall, starting with a weight of 91 pounds. To use the table, find your appropriate height in the column labeled Height. Move across to your weight. The number at the top of the table is the BMI at your height and weight.

Table 7-3　Body Mass Index Chart

Height	Body Weight (Pounds)																
	19	20	21	22	23	24	25	26	27	28	29	30	31	32	33	34	35
58"	91	96	100	105	110	115	119	124	129	134	138	143	148	153	158	162	167
59"	94	99	104	109	114	119	124	128	133	138	143	148	153	158	163	168	173
60"	97	102	107	112	118	123	128	133	138	143	148	153	158	163	168	174	179
61"	100	106	111	116	122	127	132	137	143	148	153	158	164	169	175	180	185
62"	104	109	115	120	126	131	136	142	147	153	158	164	169	175	180	186	191
63"	107	113	118	124	130	135	141	146	152	158	163	169	175	180	186	191	197
64"	110	116	122	128	134	140	145	151	157	163	169	174	180	186	192	197	204
65"	114	120	126	132	138	144	150	156	162	168	174	180	186	192	198	204	210
66"	118	124	130	136	142	148	155	161	167	173	179	185	192	198	204	210	216
67"	121	127	134	140	146	153	159	166	172	178	185	191	198	204	211	217	223

Height	Body Weight (Pounds)																
	19	**20**	**21**	**22**	**23**	**24**	**25**	**26**	**27**	**28**	**29**	**30**	**31**	**32**	**33**	**34**	**35**
68"	125	131	138	144	151	158	164	171	177	184	190	197	203	210	216	223	230
69"	128	135	142	149	155	162	169	176	182	189	196	203	209	216	223	230	236
70"	132	139	146	153	160	167	174	181	188	195	202	209	216	222	229	236	243
71"	136	143	150	157	165	172	179	186	193	200	208	215	222	229	236	243	250
72"	140	147	154	162	169	177	184	191	199	206	213	221	228	235	242	250	258
73"	144	151	159	166	174	182	189	197	204	212	219	227	235	242	250	257	265
74"	148	155	163	171	179	186	194	202	210	218	225	233	241	249	256	264	272
75"	152	160	168	176	184	192	200	208	216	224	232	240	248	256	264	272	279
76"	156	164	172	180	189	197	205	213	221	230	238	246	254	263	271	279	287

Source: The National Heart, Lung, and Blood Institute.

Using BMI to predict health

Based on health statistics and death rates provided by the World Health Organization, the Centers for Disease Control and Prevention's National Center for Health Statistics characterize the various categories of BMI as follows:

- **Underweight:** BMI lower than 18.5.

- **Normal:** BMI of 18.5 to 24.9. (A minimal risk of weight-related health problems.)

- **Overweight:** BMI of 25 to 29.9. (A moderate risk of weight-related health problems. For reference, BMI of 25 is about 10 percent over ideal body weight.)

- **Obese:** BMI of 30 to 39.9. (High risk of weight-related health problems.)

- **Extremely obese:** BMI over 40. (The highest risk of weight-related health problems.)

BMI is a valuable health predictor for most men and women between the ages of 19 and 70, but it's not for everyone. BMI isn't a reliable guide for the following:

- Women who are pregnant or nursing. Weight gain is temporary and does not reflect a true weight/height relationship.

- People who are very tall or very short.

- Professional athletes or weight trainers. Very muscular people, such as boxer Laila Ali or the great gang of guys at the World Wrestling Federation, can have a high BMI but not be fat.

Making Lifestyle Changes

The rules of the weight-loss road are fairly simple and entirely sensible. After you decide that you really do need to lose a little weight, the following list of do's and don'ts can make life bearable — and less weighty.

Waist not

The size of your waist may affect the riskiness (or lack thereof) of your BMI. To get the relevant number, measure your waist circumference (the distance around your natural waist just above the navel). If your BMI is higher than 25, a waist circumference equal to or higher than 35 inches for a woman or 40 inches for a man puts you into a "high risk" — that is, overweight — category.

Counting those dreaded calories

Repeat after me: A healthful weight-loss regimen isn't a starvation diet. Keep these calorie requirements in mind when you're working to lose weight:

✔ Women require a food plan that provides at least 1,200 calories a day. Top limit for weight loss: 1,500 calories.

✔ Men require a food plan that provides at least 1,500 calories a day. Top limit for weight loss: 1,800 calories.

You probably noticed that I describe a totally unfair fact of life: Men and women — even when they're exactly the same weight and height — require different amounts of calories to stay healthy. A man's body has proportionately more muscle tissue than a woman's body. Muscle tissue is "active" tissue that burns calories. Therefore, men need about 10 percent more calories each day, even when they're losing weight.

Ingesting your daily vitamins and minerals

Your weight-loss food plan (have you noticed that I'm subtly substituting "food plan" for "diet?") should provide all the essential nutrients. Exactly what nutrients you need and how much of them are spelled out in excruciating detail in your copy of *Nutrition For Dummies,* 4th Edition (Wiley). (Don't have one? Get one. I wrote it. It's goooooood.)

Another good guide to vitamins and minerals is the ingredients label on any reputable brand of one-pill-a-day supplements. Or you can bookmark this page, turn to Chapter 16, and check out one of the totally excellent nutritional Web sites you find there.

Are you back? Good. I want to spend a minute covering why you should avoid fad diets, or as I like to label 'em, funny food plans. You know the ones I mean. These diets often base their recommendations on, oh, maybe one study, and it's often a dubious one. Seventeen overweight hamsters in Ohio lost weight after three months on a diet of nothing but apricots, peaches, and clam juice. Here are a few ways to spot fad diets:

✔ These diets are never endorsed by reputable organizations such as the American Heart Association or the American Dietetic Association. Instead, they use testimonials from people who may mean well but have no real nutrition expertise (like the Northeastern Ohio Hamster Owners Association).

✔ The diet plans go against generally accepted nutritional advice. (I'm no hamster expert, but I'm guessing that these furry creatures need nutrients other than those supplied by apricots, peaches, and clam juice.)

30 + 30 = ??

The perfect example of a silly food plan is the one that promises to take off 30 pounds in 30 days, a formula chosen presumably because some months do have 30 days and the numbers sound good together.

According to the American Society of Bariatric Physicians (weight loss experts), this promise is an empty one because:

✔ To lose 1 pound of body weight, you must cut out 3,500 calories.

✔ To lose 30 pounds in 30 days, you must cut out 105,000 calories (30 × 3,500 calories = 105,000 calories).

✔ If you normally get 2,800 calories a day — more than most American women and some men eat every day — you only take in 84,000 calories in 30 days.

✔ If you were to stop eating entirely for 30 days, you would still need to get rid of another 21,000 calories to reach the 105,000 mark.

Any volunteers?

Forget the pound a day business. A slow but steady loss of 5 pounds in that same 30-day period means cutting just 17,500 calories (5 × 3,500 calories = 17,500 calories). Divide 17,500 by 30, and you come up with 580 calories a day, a reduction most serious weight-loss programs can handle.

Now can I see a show of hands from volunteers?

Do yourself a favor. Fight fad diets. Who wants to eat 50 grapefruits a day anyway? You should be eating a variety of healthy, tasty foods while you're eating less.

Making the menu marvelous

A healthful food plan, even one designed to take off pounds, includes many different foods. Yes, broccoli is packed with anti-cancer *phytochemicals* (compounds found naturally in plants), plus vitamin A, vitamin C, the heart-healthy B vitamin folate, carbohydrates, and dietary fiber. But man (and woman) can't live by green florets alone.

Food variety is important to weight loss. Food is meant to be enjoyed — yes, even low-calorie food. When your weight-loss menu is interesting and tastes good, sticking to it is less of a chore. Besides, human beings are omnivores, which means they have digestive tracts equipped to handle foods from plants and animals. Although vegetarianism certainly can be a healthful choice, maybe even a moral one for folks who don't want to consume animals, your body has the ability to metabolize and use all kinds of food: meat, dairy, grains, fruits, and veggies. Why not go for it?

Living happily ever after

Here's one from the depressing-but-true file: Most people who take off weight put it back on again within three years. The only way to succeed at losing weight — which means taking it off and keeping it off — is to change your mind along with your menu. The goal isn't a quick 10 pounds off your hips. The goal is a lifelong healthful weight.

To reach this goal, organizations such as the American Heart Association, the American Diabetes Association, and the American Dietetic Association, their international counterparts, and all the relevant governmental agencies across the globe offer pretty much the same prescription: Eat less, eat a variety of foods, get the nutrients you need, step up your exercise time, and take the time you need to lose pounds safely.

Boring? Yup. Sensible? Yup. A way to succeed? Without a doubt.

Tossing Out the Scales

Now that I've spent an entire chapter talking about weight and how weight gain may adversely affect your cholesterol levels and, by implication, your risk of heart disease, I'm slamming on the breaks. I'm going to reverse engines and back-peddle a bit to mention those special times when weight doesn't seem to matter at all. The truth is that most people pick up pounds as they grow older, and many manage to stay healthy anyway.

One way to explain this seemingly odd situation among an older population is to suggest that people who've experienced weight-related illnesses have already gone to their reward. The ones left standing (or sitting) are older folks whose general health is so good that weight is irrelevant. A second possibility is that individual human beings really are individuals with unique bundles of genes and possibilities. Trying to make these unique individuals fit into strict, predictable categories is like trying to map the stars in the sky. It works, but only up to a point.

For example, the experts who invented BMI admit that its value in predicting weight-related health risks depends to some extent on age. In your 30s, a lower BMI is clearly linked to better health. In your 70s (and later), no convincing evidence supports the idea that BMI and/or weight itself makes a difference. In fact, some recent studies suggest that a higher BMI (below the obesity mark, of course) is protective for women of a certain age. In between, the relationship between BMI — or weight — and health is, well, in between — more important early on, less important later in life.

The inescapable conclusion? Human beings are more diverse and complicated than any weight and health charts. Case closed.

Chapter 8

Exercising Options to Control Your Cholesterol

Regular exercise is such an important part of a heart-healthy lifestyle that the authors of the *Dietary Guidelines for Americans 2005* (U.S. Departments of Agriculture and Health and Human Services) put "Physical Activity" right before the info on every single type of food a healthy diet is likely to include.

According to the American Heart Association, exercise can alter your cholesterol levels, pushing up your HDLs (the "good" cholesterol) and pushing down the LDLs (the "bad" cholesterol). In other words, moving your bod is good for your heart.

This chapter presents tips on how to use exercise to help with controlling your cholesterol. Hey, isn't that the title of this book? You bet.

Sweating the Definition: Exercise

Do you know what exercise is? That isn't a trick question — really. When many people hear the word *exercise,* they think of things such as professional-level sports, a 10-mile run, or a hop-'til-you-drop celebrity workout. But in reality, *exercise* is nothing more than simple movement.

If you're not training for the Olympics, your favorite sport — golf, tennis, or even ping-pong — is good exercise. No, dusting the house is not good exercise, but if you get down on your knees and really scrub the floor or, as the American Heart Association (AHA) suggests, "vacuum vigorously," that counts. (You can even clean to music to get a good rhythm going.)

Walking is also good exercise. No, let me revise that: Walking is a *great* exercise that moves virtually every part of your body. (Swing those arms! Shift those eyes from right to left! Turn that head!)

Of course, you may prefer riding a stationary bike in front of the TV, jogging a mile before or after work, dancing, mowing the lawn, or raking leaves — all of which come with the AHA seal of approval (as long as your doctor gives the green light).

You can estimate how effective an exercise is in two ways:

- ✔ By counting the calories you use up
- ✔ By counting your heartbeats while you're doing the exercise

Counting calories

The more calories an exercise consumes, the harder you're working. Table 8-1 classifies very light, light, moderate, and heavy activity by calorie count. Table 8-2 tells you approximately how many calories you burn by engaging in some specific activities for either 15 minutes or one hour.

The numbers in the first chart come from the U.S. Department of Agriculture. I found the numbers in the second chart in *Fitness For Dummies*, 3rd Edition, by Suzanne Schlosberg and Liz Neporent (Wiley), a terrific book for recovering couch potatoes who can't tell a rowing machine from a washing machine.

Table 8-1	Estimated Calorie Use per Activity Level	
Activity Level	**Calories Used per Hour**	**Examples of Activities**
Very light	80–100	Painting pictures, driving, typing, sewing, ironing, cooking, playing cards, playing a musical instrument
Light	110–160	Walking on a level surface at 2.5 to 3.0 mph, house cleaning, child care, golf

Activity Level	Calories Used per Hour	Examples of Activities
Moderate	170–240	Walking 3.5 to 4.0 mph, weeding, bicycling, dancing
Heavy	250–350	Carrying packages uphill, heavy digging, basketball, climbing, football, soccer

Source: U.S. Department of Agriculture, "Food and Your Weight," Home and Garden Bulletin, 74.

Table 8-2	Estimated Calorie Use per Exercise	
Exercise	*Calories Used (15 Minutes)*	*Calories Used (1 Hour)*
Aerobic dance	171	684
Bicycling (12 mph)	142	566
Downhill skiing	105	420
Golf (carrying clubs)	87	348
Jumping rope (60–80 skips/minute)	143	572
Rowing machine	104	415
Running (10-minute mile)	183	731
Swimming (freestyle, 35 yards/minute)	124	497
Tennis (singles)	116	464
Tennis (doubles)	43	170
Walking (20-minute mile, flat ground)	60	240
Walking (20-minute mile, hills)	81	324
Water aerobics	70	280

Source: Suzanne Schlosberg and Liz Neporent, Fitness For Dummies, 3rd Edition (Wiley Publishing, Inc.).

Counting heartbeats

Aerobic, as in "aerobic exercise," means "with air." An aerobic exercise is an exercise that forces you to use oxygen, challenging your heart to beat faster and your lungs to breathe more deeply.

Exercises that use your big muscles — the ones in your legs, back, and chest — are the ones most likely to be aerobic. Walking, running, swimming, bicycling, and climbing up (not down) stairs are all aerobic exercises. When you do these exercises, your heartbeat begins to speed up. That's good.

How fast should your heart be beating during exercise? Grab a piece of paper and a pencil and follow these three steps to find your "target range" for how fast your heart should beat while you're exercising:

1. **Subtract your age from 220.**

   The number you get is your estimated *maximum heart rate.* For example, Ellen is 27 years old. 220 – 27 = 193 (which means 193 beats per minute).

2. **Divide that number by 2.**

   The number you get is the low point for your "target range." In Ellen's case, 193÷2 = 96.5. Oh, call it 97. The low point for Ellen's target range is 97 beats per minute. If her heart is thumping out 97 beats per minute, she knows she's not exerting herself to her fullest potential.

3. **Multiply the original number by 0.85.**

   The number you get is the top boundary for your "target rate." In Ellen's case, 193 × 0.85 = 165. If her heartbeat hits 165 beats per minute while she's working out, man, she knows she's working out! If it goes higher than 165, she needs to slow it down.

To burn fat and receive heart-healthy benefits from exercising, you must reach — and hold — your personal target heartbeat range for at least 30 minutes, at least three times a week. (But only after checking in with your doctor.)

Pairing Exercise and . . .

Everybody knows that exercise makes your heart healthy. But here's a fact to make it beat a bit faster: Regular exercise — even as little as a brisk 30-minute walk several times a week — also improves your cholesterol profile.

How about that? The same exercise regimen that strengthens your heart will

✔ Lower your total cholesterol

✔ Lower your low-density lipoproteins (LDLs) — the "bad" fat-and-protein particles that ferry cholesterol into your arteries

✔ Raise your high-density lipoproteins (HDLs) — the "good" fat-and-protein particles that carry cholesterol out of your body

How does exercise do all this good stuff? Nobody knows for sure. It may have something to do with exercise enabling your heart to pump extra oxygen-toting blood out into your body. Or it may not.

Either way, why look a gift horse — carrying lower total cholesterol, lower LDLs, and higher HDLs — in the mouth? Especially when he's packing even more good stuff in his saddlebags (and getting rid of yours), such as the possibility that exercise may change your arteries so that they're less susceptible to cholesterol damage.

CRP

C-reactive protein (CRP) — discussed in detail in Chapter 3 — is a compound in your blood that medical folks regard as an indicator of otherwise-invisible arterial inflammation.

Inflamed arteries have rough interior surfaces with many little nooks and crannies that may snag cholesterol particles as they float by. If that happens, the snagged cholesterol attracts other particles, eventually building the kind of plaque that blocks the artery and leads to a heart attack.

In 2002, data from a six-year study of 128 males in Finland ages 50 to 60 showed that those who engaged in even mild exercise, such as walking, reduced their CRP levels by 16 percent, suggesting that their arteries were healthier than before they began exercising.

By the way, the change even occurred in men who have a gene that increases their risk of blood clots.

Blood pressure

Blood pressure is the term used to describe the force exerted by your heart when it pushes blood out into your arteries. If your arteries are narrowed in any way, your heart must work harder to get blood out.

Exercise relaxes and dilates your blood vessels, lowering your risk of high blood pressure. Some research has suggested that exercise also widens blood vessels enough to allow a stray piece of cholesterol gunk to float on through rather than block the artery. Only a suggestion, but sure sounds good!

Triglycerides

Triglycerides are the most common fats found in food and the most common fats circulating through your blood. Having high triglyceride levels raises your risk of heart attack. Exercise lowers triglycerides, thus lowering your risk of heart attack. To find out more about triglycerides, check out Chapter 2.

Weight control

If you're overweight, losing weight makes you look and feel better. It also lowers your total cholesterol and raises your HDLs.

Regular exercise is such an efficient weight loss technique that the American Society of Bariatric Physicians (the group of fine folks who treat weight disorders) considers a regular exercise plan the number one predictor for long-term weight stability.

In other words, you can lose weight by cutting calories, but according to the bariatric docs, you'll lose pounds faster and keep them off longer if you exercise.

Exercise can also change your body shape — and not just by making your muscles bulge. For example, exercise can transform a person's "fruit" shape from the round-in-the middle "apple" shape known to carry a higher risk of heart attack to a slimmer, trimmer . . . banana? Carrot? No, wait. That's a vegetable. Well, you get the idea.

Your body

If you need a refresher course on the whole-body health benefits of exercise, stick around for the next few paragraphs. The short version is

- ✔ Exercise builds muscle.
- ✔ Your heart is a muscle.
- ✔ Exercise strengthens your heart.

When you exercise, your heart pumps out more blood. More blood means more oxygen to every part of your body. More oxygen means healthier body tissues. Keep exercising. Your heart is only one of the organs and systems that benefits from regular exercise.

Exercise also strengthens bones, revs up your brain, keeps your digestive system moving along, sharpens your immune system, and improves your mood.

To save time (yours) and space (the publisher's), I've put all this good stuff into Table 8-3, which lists the various ways in which a regular exercise program tunes up your body and mind.

Table 8-3	Tuning Up Your Body and Mind
Organ/System	*Exercise Benefits*
Blood fats	Lowers total cholesterol, lowers LDLs, raises HDLs, lowers triglycerides
Blood vessels	Increases blood flow, relaxes blood vessels (reducing risk of high blood pressure), reduces risk of cholesterol damage
Bones	Strengthens muscles that support bones; slows, stops, or even reverses age-related bone loss (reducing the risk of osteoporosis)
Brain	Increases flow of oxygenated blood to brain tissue, quickens and clarifies thinking, increases production of *endorphins* (natural chemicals that calm mood and reduce pain), improves sleep patterns
Digestive tract	Reduces risk of cancer (reason unknown), reduces incidence of constipation
Fatty tissue	Reduces amount, lowers weight
Heart	Strengthens muscle, improves function
Immune system	Improves immune response (mechanism not yet identified)
Lungs	Improves breathing
Muscles	Strengthens and enlarges (providing support for bones)
Miscellaneous	Quickens metabolism, uses calories, raises body temperature

---

Burning the midnight bulb

Does thinking about an exercise program use up energy? Yes, but not as much as you may imagine. To solve a crossword puzzle — or write a chapter of this book — the average brain uses about one calorie every four minutes. That's only one-third of the amount of energy needed to keep a 60-watt bulb burning for the same length of time.

Does that mean that even really smart people are pretty dim bulbs? Sorry, I couldn't resist that one.

Riding the Stationary Bike into the Sunset

Did you wake up this morning and decide it's time to exercise? Well, don't just do something. Sit there! Yes, you heard me right. Untie your running shoes. Unzip your warm-up jacket. Brew yourself a cup of tea, coffee, or whatever, and relax in your favorite armchair while you carefully consider how to put together an exercise program that fits your individual needs.

Just keep in mind that you want to choose an exercise (or exercises) that works your muscles. Yoga, for example, is a wonderful relaxation technique, but — sorry about this — it won't jump-start your heart or raise your HDLs.

The Web is totally jam-packed with special sites that offer balanced advice on exercise and its billions of benefits — well maybe not *that* many — for your body. To save you hours of surfing time, expand your universe by typing **exercise sites** into the search box of any search engine. Doing this often brings up one site with links to many other sites. How handy!

Table 8-4 shows several useful exercise and health sites. Wait! Did I mention you should always check with your own doctor before starting an exercise program? I think I did, but now I'm sure. It never hurts to be sure.

Table 8-4	Surfing for Exercise and Health
Organization	*Internet Address*
American Alliance for Health, Physical Education, Recreation, and Dance	www.aahperd.org
American College of Sports Medicine	www.acsm.org

Organization	Internet Address
American Council on Exercise	www.acefitness.org
American Heart Association	www.americanheart.org
The President's Council on Physical Fitness	www.fitness.gov

Checking with your medical mechanic

You wouldn't take your car out for a 3,000-mile trip without a tune-up would you? For your body, starting a new exercise program is the equivalent of that multi-mile trip.

The first step on the way to a healthful exercise regimen should be an appointment with your doctor so he can run a basic body check. He may even want to do a stress test.

This caution clearly applies to anyone who's already had a heart attack. But it's also recommended for people who've never had even the slightest hint of heart trouble. Even if you are (or think you are) a healthy young person, this is one time when it's definitely better to be safe than sorry.

Exercise is hard work, and you want to be sure your body can handle it without folding on you. Call your doctor first. No exceptions!

If you skipped this all-important step and headed straight for a health club or gym, turn right around and walk out of any facility that lets you sign up for an exercise program without first checking your vital signs.

Setting yourself up for success

An exercise program should make you feel good about the program and about yourself. If you choose a regimen that's too strenuous, you're apt to quit in the middle. Bummer.

Your exercise goal is to rev up your body and lower your cholesterol, not wear yourself to a frazzle in an unsuccessful attempt to qualify for the Olympic couch-potato-turned-pro-athlete team.

In other words, it's A-okay to settle for the warm and fuzzy sense of well-being you get by stretching your muscles while walking a mile, riding a stationary bike, or once in a while picking up the pace to jog (if you really want to that is).

Here are a few helpful hints:

- ✔ **Have realistic expectations.** Rome wasn't built in a day, and that new, fabulously healthy, lower-cholesterol body of yours won't be either.

  - • **Start small:** If you've been sedentary for the last 15 years, you shouldn't expect to sprint 3 miles a day out of the gate. Walk first and work up to a run; start with 1 mile and work your way up to the 3-mile plan.

  - • **Give yourself time:** Positive changes in your body won't pop up overnight. Give yourself at least six months of effort to see noticeable change.

- ✔ **Exercise some days, not every day.** You intend to wake up every morning at 5 a.m. and jog? Who — I mean whom — are you kidding? Set a more realistic goal of a jog every other day, and you're more likely to stick to the schedule. By the way, the three-times-a-week rule comes from the American Heart Association. For the AHA — and you — three times can be the charm.

- ✔ **Reward yourself.** But not with a huge stack of pancakes drizzled in syrup when you get back from your morning run. Try other rewards like a new article of clothing, a plant, or a CD. If you prefer to indulge in food rewards, do so less often.

Choosing something you like

As the AHA puts it, choose "activities that are fun, not exhausting." If you hate football, loathe jogging, despise aerobics, and can't stand to get your hair wet in a pool, you won't make it past the first week with an exercise regimen that includes these activities.

In other words, your aim is to find some kind of movement you actually enjoy — or at least one that fits into your normal daily routine. No one can tell you exactly what that exercise is — you know what you enjoy. What I can share with you is the assurance that anything that moves your muscles benefits your body.

If everything else fails to pass your "I like that" test, there's always walking (briskly, that is).

Here are a few ideas to set the wheels in motion:

- ✔ Biking (streets, parks, hills, or flats)

- ✔ Hiking (meadows or mountains, doesn't matter)

- ✔ Working out along with a TV fitness guru — start slow, work up

Sticking to a schedule

To get the most from your exercise, follow a consistent regimen of moderately intense movement for at least 30 minutes a day five days a week, if possible. Okay, okay, three days a week. As I said before, the AHA says three days is okay, and even a recovering couch potato can remember Monday, Wednesday, and Friday. Try it: Monday — Wednesday — Friday. See?

Did you know that you don't have to do all your exercise at once? You can break it up into two or three sessions during the day. For example, suppose you drive to work or take public transportation. Instead of driving all the way to the front door, park your car 15 minutes away from work and walk. Or get off the bus or train at a stop 15 minutes before your final destination and, yes, walk. Doing that twice a day equals (can you believe it?) 30 minutes of moderate-intensity exercise.

Don't ya just love it when things work out the way they're supposed to?

No pain, no gain? No way

"No pain, no gain" is an out-of-date, never-was-right slogan that deserves a decent burial once and for all. Pain means injury. Injury is bad for the body. Yes, the pros play with problems — after all, they're playing for millions (dollars, not fans) — but that's why so many of them end up hobbling around at a really tender age.

Avoid anything that requires you to twist yourself into a pretzel or perform activities that feel uncomfortable. True, stretching muscles that haven't moved in heaven knows how long can leave you with *some* soreness, but if your exercise leaves you hobbling, you're doing something wrong. This book is *Controlling Cholesterol For Dummies,* not *Fitness For Dummies,* so my best advice is that you seek guidance from a professional trainer or check out *Fitness For Dummies,* 3rd Edition, by Suzanne Schlosberg and Liz Neporent (Wiley), which also lays out rules for finding a trainer. Think of it as a two-fer bargain — and safe, sane, and sensible besides.

Rating an exercise program or gym

How can you tell if a fitness program or plan or video is right for you? That's easy. The program fits your needs, which means

- It fits into your schedule (rather than forcing you to shift your life around to accommodate *it*).

- ✔ You're comfortable with the exercise expertise required.
- ✔ The price is right.

Here are some examples of what can work for you:

- ✔ Group programs, such as an exercise class at the local YMCA/YWCA, are great for people with no talent as self-starters. They're not so great for people who hate to play follow the leader.
- ✔ Individual trainers are great for folks who hate to leave the house (and can afford the trainer). They're not so great for people who enjoy working out in the company of others.
- ✔ Videotapes are a delight! You get to sit and watch someone else work up a sweat on TV. No, wait, that's not how it's supposed to work. If that's what you're doing, join a group or get a trainer. Of course, using a tape properly gives you the freedom to exercise at your own speed and on your own schedule.

If you go the videotape route, remember that being a TV sitcom star may not be the best training in the world for handling other people's bodies. Any videotape you choose should have guides to exercise and skill levels printed on the box. A credit for an expert adviser is also good.

As for gyms and health clubs: No matter what type of program you choose, be sure to check out the instructor by taking in the diplomas on the wall. Preferably, your exercise guru should have a four-year college degree in exercise science or a related field.

Certification from a recognized group for fitness professionals such as these is also a really, really good recommendation:

- ✔ American Council on Exercise (ACE)
- ✔ American College of Sports Medicine (ACSM)
- ✔ National Academy of Sports Medicine (NASM)
- ✔ National Strength and Conditioning Association (NSCA)

Then, after you have your ducks in a row, start your engines. You may be mixing metaphors, but you'll also be benefiting your heart — and optimizing your cholesterol. Pretty good, all around.

Chapter 9

Weeding Out Tobacco's Role in High Cholesterol

In This Chapter

▶ Explaining how smoking affects cholesterol levels

▶ Noting the connections between smoking and cholesterol

▶ Identifying the typical smoker

▶ Finding ways to break the habit

Consider this chapter, in fact, this entire book, a nonsmoking area. In fact, close your eyes and visualize little signs up all over the virtual walls explaining what's wrong with tolerating tobacco, how tobacco interacts with cholesterol, and showing how to quit, right now. Then think about how this will make your healthful life style even more so.

Enumerating Smoking's Health Hazards

Puffing on a lit tobacco stick, that is, inhaling smoke from burning, dead leaves produces the following reactions in your body:

✔ Raises the level of carbon monoxide in your blood, which reduces the amount of life-giving oxygen

✔ Injures the lining of your blood vessels

✔ Constricts arteries that may already be narrowed by cholesterol plaque

✔ Heightens your risk of high blood pressure

✔ Reduces the amount of blood carrying oxygen to your body tissues

✔ Makes it more likely that your blood will clot

✔ Increases your risk of *sudden cardiac death,* a genuinely catastrophic moment when, without warning, your heart may stop beating forever

Not to mention, smoking increases your risk of these forms of cancer:

- ✔ Bladder
- ✔ Esophagus (throat)
- ✔ Lungs
- ✔ Pancreas

And, if that's not enough to get to you thinking, how about this: Smoking also destroys your good looks by promoting facial wrinkles.

But did you notice that this list of bad stuff smoking can do to your body is incomplete? Look carefully. Something is missing. What can it be? Surely you jest. It's smoking's ability to upset your cholesterol — specifically your "bad" cholesterol.

Burning up the cholesterol charts

The relationship between smoking and cholesterol is straightforward. Over time, lighting up and inhaling all those deep, "flavorful" breaths will

- ✔ Increase your total cholesterol levels.
- ✔ Decrease the level of your *high-density lipoproteins* (HDLs), the "good" cholesterol described in detail in Chapters 2 and 3 of this book.
- ✔ Hasten the buildup of cholesterol plaque on damaged blood-vessel walls.
- ✔ Constrict your blood vessels, increasing the risk that a passing clump of cholesterol may block blood flow.
- ✔ Increase the level of *triglycerides* in your blood, another risk factor for heart attacks (check out Chapter 2).
- ✔ **Double your risk of heart attack, regardless of your cholesterol level.**

That last point deserves serious attention, so I've asked my editor to print it in boldface type, and doggone if she didn't do it!

Although many studies demonstrate a relationship between smoking and heart disease, many smokers are convinced that having a low cholesterol level reduces their risk of smoking-related heart disease. They're wrong. Low cholesterol levels don't protect smokers from heart disease. I can say this with impunity because I've read the results of the *Korea Medical Insurance Company Study,* the first effort to pin down a relationship between smoking, cholesterol levels, and the risk of heart attack. (Check out the "East Asia's heart disease" sidebar in this chapter.) Do I do my homework, or what?

East Asia's heart disease

East Asia is a part of the world that's best known for gorgeous scenery and scrumptious food. But it's also known for having a large population of smokers and a rate of heart disease that's now among the highest in the world. The confusing part of this equation has been that East Asians have a high risk of heart attack even though they generally have low cholesterol levels. A good guess to clear up this confusion may be that their love of smoking is an independent risk factor against which low cholesterol offers no protection. And by golly, that's exactly what turned up in data from the 10-year, 106,745-man *Korea Medical Insurance Corporation Study,* named for the volunteers who were all Korean men with insurance policies from the Korea Medical Insurance Corporation.

Based on the number of men who were either hospitalized or died from heart attack or stroke during the study, the researchers found that smoking significantly increased the risk of heart attack and stroke. Even among men with very low cholesterol levels, smokers had a risk of heart attack and stroke that was 330 percent higher than that of nonsmokers.

Conclusion? As reported in the *Journal of the American Medical Association,* "This study demonstrates that . . . a low cholesterol level confers no protective benefit against smoking-related atherosclerotic cardiovascular disease." Translation: Low cholesterol levels provide no protection for smokers against heart disease caused by smoking.

Getting a bad deal on secondhand smoke

As if your own smoking weren't bad enough for your body, somebody else's smoking can also be hazardous to your health.

Secondhand smoke, also known as *environmental tobacco smoke,* isn't something you buy in a secondhand store. It's the smoke you inhale from other people's cigarettes, pipes, or cigars and from the air that people breathe out while they're smoking.

Like all tobacco smoke, this recycled version contains at least 250 toxic chemicals including at least 50 known carcinogens, which is why, in 2006, the Centers for Disease Control and Prevention (CDC) issued yet another warning on secondhand smoke. For the umpteenth time, the CDC repeated that exposure to secondhand smoke increases the risk of heart disease by 25 to 30 percent in adult nonsmokers and increases their risk of lung cancer by 20 to 30 percent.

As for the effect on kids, don't ask. No, do ask.

Kids and secondhand smoke

If you smoke, children in the room smoke, too. No, they don't actually light up, but they do breathe the same air you do, so if you exhale smoke into the air, they breathe it into their lungs. In fact, the American Heart Association states that 43 percent of all American kids between the ages of 2 months and 11 years are exposed to secondhand smoke at home.

While their lungs are still developing, smoke from other people's burning tobacco may slow the normal rate of lung development in children and increase a child's risk of

- ✔ Eye, nose, and throat irritations
- ✔ Middle ear infections
- ✔ Reduced lung functions
- ✔ Respiratory irritations (cough, phlegm, and wheezing)
- ✔ Respiratory tract infections (pneumonia and bronchitis)
- ✔ Worsened asthma (or new cases)

Clearing the air

Is the word getting out? You bet.

No-smoking-in-public-spaces laws to ban smoking in offices, hotels, restaurants, and other indoor spaces are now commonplace in the United States. And by summer 2007, American cities had passed at least 1,124 laws banning smoking outdoors in places such as amusement parks, zoos (including the National Zoo in Washington D.C.), beaches (no more burying your butts in the sand), golf courses, and — get this one — cemeteries.

Across the Atlantic, in 2004, Ireland became the first European country to ban smoking in all workplaces, including the legendary Irish pubs. Sweden and Italy soon followed suit, and then came the big one: France.

In 2007, the French banned smoking in public practically everywhere: airports, railway stations, hospitals, schools, shops, offices, and so on. Today, in Paris, where people practically invented serious, sexy smoking, many restaurants and most cafes still permit your pampered pooch to dine along with you, but may now ban *les cigarettes,* which is French for *small cigars* — cigarettes.

Sacre bleu! But no smoke-blue air.

Identifying the Smokers

Despite all the terrible things that are known about smoking, including its effects on cholesterol levels and the consequent risk of heart disease, many people continue to puff away.

You may wonder who these smokers are. Well, wonder no more: The hard-working statisticians at the Centers for Disease Control and Prevention (CDC) and the National Center for Health Statistics (NCHS) have crunched the numbers and come up with figures to identify U.S. smokers by age, gender, ethnicity, and level of education. It's a hard job, but somebody had to do it.

Gender and ethnicity

The percentage of American men who smoke is slightly higher than the percentage of American women who smoke, perhaps because some women still cling to the discredited idea that women are at lower risk of tobacco-related lung cancer. Silly girls.

When it comes to ethnicity, there are distinct differences among Americans. Table 9-1 shows who is more likely to light up.

Table 9-1	U.S. Smokers by Ethnicity
Population (age 18 and up)	*Percentage Who Smoke*
All American adults	20.9
Non-Hispanic Whites	21.9
Non-Hispanic Blacks	21.5
Hispanics	16.2
Asians	13.3
Native Americans/Alaskan Natives	32.0

Source: Centers for Disease Control, Fact Sheet, Adult Cigarette Smoking in the United States: Current Estimates, updated November 2006.

Getting older, getting smarter

When you count smokers, age matters. So do educational levels. According to the CDC, more than 2,000 new smokers younger than the age of 18 light up every day for the first time. That's the bad news.

The good news is that as Americans get older, they're less likely to smoke. Higher levels of education also seem to reduce the likelihood that people will smoke. Maybe the message of Table 9-2 is that as Americans get older (and smarter), they really do get wiser. At least when it comes to smoking.

Table 9-2	American Cigarette Smokers: By Age and Education
Population	*Percentage Who Smoke*
18–24 year olds	24.4
25–44 year olds	24.1
45–64 year olds	21.9
65+ year olds	8.6
Middle school students	8
High school students	23
High school graduates	43.2
College graduates	10.7
Graduate degree (master's or doctorate)	7.1

Source: Centers for Disease Control, Fact Sheet, Adult Cigarette Smoking in the United States: Current Estimates, updated November 2006. Fact Sheet, Youth and Tobaccos Use: Current Estimates, updated December 2006.

Mapping the smokers

Okay. You've made it past gender, ethnicity, age, and education. How else do researchers classify American smokers? Geography!

Poison control

Because smoking delivers relatively small amounts of nicotine to the body, cases of nicotine poisoning are rare, if not unknown, among smokers. But eating one cigarette, three cigarette butts, one pinch of chewing tobacco, or any tobacco-replacement medication, such as that found in nicotine gums or patches, is hazardous for an infant, small child, or pet.

Nicotine poisoning is a medical emergency that requires *immediate* medical assistance! Check with your local poison control center before administering any therapy. The possibility of your tobacco use harming another person in this way is just one more reason to seriously consider the information contained in the "Breaking the Habit" section in this chapter.

Where you live in the United States says a lot about whether you're likely to be a smoker. According to the CDC:

- ✔ In 2005, the percentage of adults who smoke ranged from a high of 28.7 percent in Kentucky and 27.3 percent in Indiana all the way down to a low of 11.5 percent in Utah.

- ✔ For men, the states with the highest percentages of smokers were Kentucky (30.6 percent), Indiana (29.7 percent), and Alabama (28.5 percent). Lowest? Utah, again, at 13.7 percent.

- ✔ More women smoke in Kentucky (26.9 percent), West Virginia (26 percent), and Indiana (25.1 percent). Fewer light up in good old Utah (9.3 percent).

What makes the difference? Must be something in the air.

For those of you who prefer pictures, Figure 9-1 shows the CDC smoking map of the United States in 2005 with the states ranked according to the percentage of adults who are smokers (defined here as people who smoke every day).

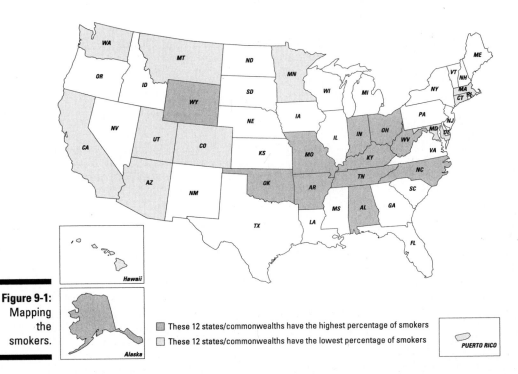

Figure 9-1:
Mapping
the
smokers.

■ These 12 states/commonwealths have the highest percentage of smokers
□ These 12 states/commonwealths have the lowest percentage of smokers

PUERTO RICO

Breaking the Habit

A smoker's risk of coronary artery disease (CAD) rises in direct relationship to the number of cigarettes he or she smokes each day:

- ✔ Smokers who quit have only half the CAD risk of people who keep smoking.

- ✔ People who quit after having coronary artery bypass surgery or a heart attack, fairly good signals that it's time to quit, lower their risk of early death.

- ✔ Quitting decreases the likelihood of illness and the risk of death for people with *atherosclerosis* (cholesterol buildup) in arteries other than those that supply the heart and brain.

Ending your relationship with tobacco isn't a Sunday walk in the park. Nicotine is such a rewarding drug that leaving it behind takes time and effort — a lot of time and effort in many cases. People often feel guilty when their first attempt at breaking the habit isn't totally successful. That's nonsense!

Not quitting forever the first time you try to stop smoking is neither a crime nor a moral failure. In fact, not making it the first ten or twenty times isn't the end of the world. Every time you stop smoking, you keep your body free of tobacco smoke for hours, days, or weeks. Consider that an accomplishment to celebrate. In the end, the only important thing is the end of smoking. Eventually, you'll get there.

But from the moment you stop (for as long as you stop), your body benefits. Table 9-3 shows exactly how.

Table 9-3   The Surgeon General's Ex-Smoker's Timetable to Health

Time Since Quitting	Effect on Your Body
20 minutes	Heart rate drops
12 hours	Carbon monoxide level in your blood falls to normal
2 weeks to 3 months	Circulation improves and lung function improves
1 to 9 months	Coughing and shortness of breath decrease; lungs regain normal ability and clear mucus cleans the lungs, reducing the risk of infection

Smoking with the enemy

Nicotine is a naturally-occurring *phytochemical* (*phyto* = plant) named for Jean Nicot, a 16th-century French ambassador to Portugal who sent a gift of tobacco seeds to Catherine de' Medici, queen mother of France, along with a glowing description of the plant's ability to cure practically every illness. Eventually, the tobacco plant was christened with the genus *Nicotiana* in his honor.

In small doses, nicotine is a stimulant that revs up the *autonomic nervous system* — nerves that control involuntary body functions, such as heartbeat, breathing, and the expansion of blood vessels. Cigarette smokers who inhale tobacco smoke into their lungs get a virtually instantaneous nicotine hit. Within ten seconds after puffing, they feel the effects of nicotine in their brains. (Cigar and pipe smokers rarely inhale, so the nicotine they get is absorbed relatively slowly through the mucous membrane lining of the mouth.)

In the brain, nicotine activates natural chemicals called *neurotransmitters* that enable brain cells to fire pleasure messages back and forth among themselves. Alas, the effect fades in a few minutes. To maintain the high, a smoker must take a second puff, and then a third, and so on throughout the day. Pretty soon, another three-pack-a-day habit is born.

But addiction isn't nicotine's only hazard to your health. In large doses, nicotine is a poison that can overload and shut down vital body systems, producing symptoms such as

- Confusion, agitation, and depression
- Convulsions, coma, and death
- Elevated blood pressure
- Gastrointestinal upset
- Muscle spasms and weakness
- Rapid heartbeat
- Respiratory problems

Is this really something that you want to welcome into your life?

Time Since Quitting	Effect on Your Body
1 year	Risk of coronary heart disease drops to half that of a smoker
5 years	Risk of stroke drops to that of a person who never smoked
10 years	Incidence of lung cancer death falls to half that of a smoker; risk of cancers of the mouth, throat, esophagus, bladder, cervix, and pancreas decreases
15 years	Risk of coronary heart disease is that of a nonsmoker

Choosing How to Quit

When you decide to quit — right now would be a really good time — you have four basic ways to go:

- You can just quit.
- You can quit with the help of medication.
- You can quit with the help of a behavior-modification program.
- You can try one method from column A, one from column B, and one from column C — in other words, you can take the smorgasbord approach.

The good points and bad points of each of these methods are described in the following sections.

Quitting cold turkey

I decided to stop smoking when my habit reached three packs a day and everything — my apartment, my clothes, my hair — smelled like dead cigarettes.

As a highly competitive, Type A person, I couldn't stand the thought of being beaten by a paper tube filled with crumbled leaves. Naturally, when I decided to quit, I took the cold-turkey route. The first six weeks weren't pleasant. I really, really wanted a cigarette, and it was really, really hard not to give in to my craving. Worse yet, I was so used to lighting up when I typed that I couldn't write a coherent sentence for weeks. Luckily, my editors understood and supported my desire to quit. To make the situation bearable, I made some concessions to reality. You may also find them useful.

Concession #1: Stop smoking, but don't throw out the cigarettes

An about-to-be-ex-smoker's worst nightmare is waking up at 4 a.m. without a cig in the house. At that point, resolve dissolves during a frantic search through every possible drawer and coat pocket in the house. Without the comforting thought that a cigarette is close at hand, should it be necessary, the willpower-challenged sort of ex-smoker may succumb to panic and rush to the corner gas station to buy — you guessed it — cigarettes!

To keep my own panic in check, I kept a pack of cigarettes in my purse for about two years, and I kept a pack in the back of my desk drawer for what turned out to be seven years. When I found the withered cigarettes by accident, seven years after I had stopped smoking, I was able toss them in the trash without a second's hesitation.

Concession #2: Don't promise more than you can deliver

When coworkers stopped at my office door to say, "Hey, I hear you've stopped smoking," I would grin like a Cheshire cat and purr, "Well, at least for this morning," or "this afternoon," or whatever.

A lot of people consider this weak-willed. I call it telling the truth. I knew, for example, that I could make it through an hour, and then four hours, and then a morning, and then an afternoon, and then a day. But I really didn't know what would happen after these increasingly longer periods of smoke-free time. By not saying "Never!" to the possibility of smoking again, I avoided setting myself up for a fall.

Concession #3: Don't be a nag

Ex-smokers can be very annoying. It's not their business if someone else wants to muck up his lungs or stink up her clothes. After you decide to stop smoking, let other people come to the same conclusion on their own. And don't give up your smoking friends. The funny thing is that smokers may smell bad, but they're often looser and more fun than nonsmokers.

Concession #4: Don't sweat the small, guilty pleasures

Once in a while, when we're out walking, my husband and I get a whiff of a pipe or a cigar. Our eyes sparkle. Our step quickens. And we follow that smoker for a couple of blocks, remembering. But we've never lit up — so far (see Concession #2).

Letting loose

After I stopped smoking, it was only a matter of time until my husband gave into my nagging. (I didn't mean you shouldn't nag your loved ones; just leave strangers alone.) Several years later, we received an assignment to write about a weekend at a honeymoon hotel. In the dining room, the seating plan was tables for eight. On the first night, the only open seats were at a smoking table. We agreed to sit there, and we had such a great time that we kept going back to sit with the smokers. (No, we didn't smoke.)

The last morning, there were no open seats at our regular table, so we sat with the ex-smokers. What pills! They kept grabbing the butter and wouldn't let us have it. Frankly, a discreet smoker's cough would've been more welcome.

Applying effective medicines

For some people, the path to a smoke-free nirvana runs through a prescription, either for the antidepressant medication bupropion (formerly known as Wellbutrin; now known as Zyban) or the new nicotine-blocker varenicline (Chantix).

Anti-smoking medicine #1: Buproprion

In several well-controlled studies, buproprion (Zyban) alone, with no counseling or other therapy, helped nearly 50 percent of the people who took it stay smoke free for seven weeks and aided roughly 23 percent of people in avoiding cigarettes for at least a year. These figures may not sound all that impressive, until you hear that only 4 to 7 percent of smokers who try to quit on their own are able to make it for a full year without cigarettes. As a result, in 1997, the Food and Drug Administration (FDA) approved buproprion as a stop-smoking aid.

Buproprion does have some potential adverse effects: upset stomach, headache, insomnia, irritability, and seizures in people with a history of seizure disorders. But the medicine also has an interesting benefit in addition to its ability to diminish cravings for a smoke. Smokers who kick the habit often gain weight in the process, but buproprion actually produces a slight weight loss. No smoking, no weight gain, and it's covered by insurance? Glory, glory!

Anti-smoking medicine #2: Varenicline

When you smoke, the nicotine in your tobacco hooks onto receptors in your brain that tell the brain to release dopamine, a natural mood elevator. The newest anti-smoking med, varenicline (Chantix), approved by the FDA in the spring of 2006, is a chemical that clicks into place on these brain receptors, blocking nicotine so that smoking fails to produce its usual "high." In double-blind studies (studies in which neither the researchers nor the subjects know what they are getting), varenicline enabled 44 percent of people who had been smokers for as long as 24 years to quit smoking after 12 weeks.

The most common side effects of varenicline are gastric upset (nausea, vomiting, intestinal gas, and constipation) and sleep disturbance (frequent waking and vivid dreams). The drug has not been approved for women who are pregnant, plan to be pregnant, or are nursing. In addition, this medicine may interact with anticoagulants ("blood thinners"), asthma medication, and insulin.

Get your nicotine here!

Smoking is both a chemical addiction and a psychological habit. By stopping smoking, you immediately break the psychological habit of putting a cigarette in your mouth. Nicotine replacement therapy (NRT) products help deal with the chemical addiction by delivering small doses of nicotine to your bloodstream to make up for what you give up when you quit cigarettes. They also help reduce your cig cravings by lessening common withdrawal symptoms such as irritability, headache, sleep disturbances, and fatigue.

Most cigarettes sold in the United States contain 10 milligrams (mg) of nicotine each, delivering about 1 to 2 mg of nicotine per smoked cigarette — yes, you lose some nicotine because the cigarette burns down between puffs. The best way to use all nicotine replacements is to start at a dose equivalent to the number of cigarettes you smoke a day, and over each subsequent month, reduce the amount you use daily by either going to a lower concentration or fewer ingestions of nicotine. NRTs are often most successful when taken along with buproprion.

To get the best results from a NRT, start using your preferred method as soon as you quit smoking. You shouldn't use any NRT for longer than three months. Some people find these products incredibly effective when used on their own; others may need the extra help that can come from counseling or participating in a smoking-cessation program with other people. And always check with your doctor before starting to use these products. Like all medicines, they (the NRTs) do have potential side effects and interactions.

Nicotine chewing gums

You don't need a prescription to buy nicotine-replacement chewing gum, but you do need to be 18 or older. The manufacturers' directions usually tell you to start with one tablet per hour. If you smoked fewer than 24 cigarettes a day, the 2-mg gum should be fine; people who smoked more may need the 4-mg dose. To get the most bang from your gum, avoid food and beverages for 15 minutes before chewing. (Some foods and beverages reduce the gum's effect.)

If necessary, you can take an additional piece to tamp down a sudden craving, but you shouldn't use more than 30 pieces of gum a day. And do remember to follow the directions when chewing the gum. You stick the wad between your lip and gum so that the nicotine makes its way into your system. If you forget to do that, the gum may make you queasy.

Transdermal patches

The nicotine patch is a medical device that delivers a constant amount of nicotine through your skin. Nicotine patches come in two versions: a 16-hour patch that you wear while you're awake and a 24-hour patch for people who wake up craving a cigarette. The patch, which started life as a prescription drug, is now available over the counter.

But it's always a good idea to check with your doctor before using it because, as the American Lung Association notes, potential side effects may include

- Headache, dizziness, and blurred vision
- Itchy or burning skin
- Sleep disturbance (vivid dreams)
- Upset stomach and diarrhea

When you remove your nicotine patch, dispose of it carefully and as directed. (The package comes with storage space for used patches.) **Remember:** Nicotine is a poison. The amount of nicotine in your discarded patches may be lethal for pets and small children.

Inhalers

The nicotine inhaler is a plastic cylinder that looks like a cigarette, but instead of tobacco, it contains a pressurized cartridge filled with nicotine mist. When you puff on the inhaler, the nicotine mist is absorbed through the mucous membrane lining your mouth and throat.

The inhaler is a prescription product, with a maximum dose of six cartridges a day. Ask your doctor about the inhaler's risks and benefits, and be absolutely sure to read the instructions carefully before using this device.

Nasal sprays

You can take two spritzes from this pump bottle, one in each nostril, up to five times an hour. The spray delivers nicotine straight to the mucous membrane lining your nose, which lets the nicotine zip into your bloodstream faster than it does with gums, patches, or inhalers.

Like the inhaler, the spray is a prescription product. And, as with all nicotine-replacement therapies, you should read the patient insert to check out the possible side effects and drug interactions.

Comparing the alternatives

Table 9-4 briefly reviews the different types of nicotine-replacement products. All are available as generics and as brand-name meds. As with most drugs, you can count on the generics being equally effective at a lower price.

Table 9-4	Nicotine Replacement Therapy Products	
Product Type	*OTC/Prescription*	*Nicotine Per Dose*
Chewing gum	OTC	2 mg, 4 mg
Inhaler	Prescription	10 mg
Nasal spray	Prescription	10 mg
Transdermal patch	OTC	16-hour (5 mg, 10 mg, 15 mg)
		24-hour (7 mg, 11 mg, 14 mg, 21 mg)

Source: *James J. Rybacki, The Essential Guide to Prescription Drugs 2006 (New York: Collins, 2006).*

Modifying your behavior

When you decide to quit smoking, behavior modification programs can be a valuable tool in teaching you how to avoid or ignore the emotional and physical triggers, such as anxiety or nicotine cravings, that tell you to light up.

Here are some suggestions:

✔ You can get your behavior-modification advice from a stop-smoking clinic or a stop-smoking book. As with every other step associated with quitting smoking, the best solution is the one that works for you.

For information about behavior-modification programs to help you quit smoking — and even good books on how to toss the tobacco — visit the American Lung Association (ALA) Web site at www.lungusa.org. The ALA has a ton of information to help you declare freedom from smoking.

✔ Don't want to go through ALA? No problem. You can also call your local hospital, YMCA, or YWCA. At least one of these organizations is almost guaranteed to have a low-cost or maybe even free smoking-cessation program.

Hypnosis and acupuncture

Think of hypnosis and acupuncture therapies as effortless behavior modification. Someone else does the work — waving a magic hypnosis wand or sticking skinny needles in various parts of your body — and you reap the benefits.

Many hospitals have trained professional hypnotists and acupuncturists on staff, so one path to a reliable practitioner is through your doctor or local hospital.

Although no evidence shows that either hypnosis or acupuncture is any more effective at ending your smoking habit than the other stop-smoking therapies, both approaches do turn some smokers into ex-smokers. If you're one of those people, hooray! If not, just pack up your bags and move on to another method. Just remember — no quitting on your quitting. Okay?

Future perfect

Today's stop-smoking techniques aren't perfect, so smarties around the world are always on the lookout for better ways to break the habit. This section covers two interesting works-in-progress.

Eating your way out of the cigarette pack

Believe it or not, in 2007, scientists at Duke University's Nicotine Research Program in Durham, North Carolina, the very heart of tobacco-growing country, reported that drinking milk and water or eating fruits and veggies seems to make tobacco taste yucky, while alcohol beverages, coffee, and meat have just the opposite effect.

Is this the way to a stop-smoking diet? Couldn't hurt, according to program director Jed E. Rose, who recommends diet modification along with any standard stop-smoking stratagem you prefer.

Anticipating the quit-smoking vaccine

Wouldn't it be nifty if you could just zip off to the doctor for an anti-smoking shot? Take heart: Dr. Dorothy Hatsukami and her colleagues at the University of Minnesota Medical School are working on it.

Their solution, reported in the November 2005 issue of the medical journal *Clinical Pharmacology and Therapeutics,* is a vaccine that enables your body to produce nicotine antibodies — teensy molecules that hook on to nicotine molecules to prevent them from making their way into your brain.

Volunteers given the experimental vaccine four times in one 26-week period were more likely to be able to stay away from cigarettes for 30 days without nasty withdrawal symptoms than those given a placebo (look-alike) injection. Both those who received the vaccine and those who received the placebo reported a similar incidence of mild or moderate side effects (headache, cough, or upper respiratory tract infection).

Hatsukami's research is a work in progress. Keep your eyes peeled for more info.

Movie babes and butts

Many smokers lit up their first cigarettes because some movie star looked so darned cool smoking. Unfortunately, some of the greatest stars, such as John Wayne and Bogie, went to their untimely reward courtesy of that cool cig. Nonetheless, smoking is still a prominent silver-screen fixture. In *Basic Instinct,* Sharon Stone uttered this really great line: "What are they going to do, arrest me for smoking?" These days, in a lot of American cities, the answer is, "We could if we wanted to."

Take the following quiz and match the star with the movie in which she lit up. And by the way, if you still think that smoking is sexy, imagine the poor hero who had to kiss the glamorous woman with the awful tobacco breath.

Movie	*Smoker*
1. *Now Voyager*	a. Audrey Hepburn
2. *In The Bedroom*	b. Everyone on screen
3. *My Best Friend's Wedding*	c. Demi Moore
4. *Basic Instinct*	d. Bette Davis
5. *St. Elmo's Fire*	e. Sissy Spacek
6. *Breakfast at Tiffany's*	f. Cameron Diaz
7. *Grease*	g. Julia Roberts
8. *Vanilla Sky*	h. Sharon Stone
9. *The Fabulous Baker Boys*	i. Lauren Bacall
10. *Troop Beverly Hills*	j. Michelle Pfeiffer
11. *To Have and Have Not*	k. Shelley Long

Answers: 1. d, 2. e, 3. g, 4. h, 5. c, 6. a, 7. b, 8. f, 9. j, 10. k, 11. i.

Chapter 10

The Grape, the Grains, and Your Cholesterol

*A*lcohol beverages are among mankind's oldest home remedies and simple pleasures. The ancient Greeks and Romans called wine a gift from the gods — now that's holding it in pretty high regard. As for distilled spirits, the Gaels (early inhabitants of Ireland) called them *uisgebeatha* (whis-key-ba). The French came up with *eau de vie* (o-duh-vee). And the Scandinavians dubbed the hard stuff *aquavit* (ah-kwa-veet). Take your pick — they all mean "water of life."

The funny thing is that this translation may turn out to be a scientifically accurate description. Drinking moderate amounts of alcohol appears to benefit your heart. (No, that doesn't mean you should start drinking if you've been abstaining from drinking up to now.)

Yes, excessive drinking is hazardous to your health, and you can read about that later on in this chapter, but first, the good stuff, including alcohol's ability to lower your cholesterol.

Wait! One more thing. Throughout this chapter — and throughout this book — beer, wine, and spirits are called *alcohol beverages,* not *alcoholic beverages.* After all, who ever heard of a beverage that can drink enough to become an alcoholic?

Toasting to Your Heart

The Dietary Guidelines for Americans 2005 from the U.S. Department of Agriculture and Department of Health and Human Services is a primer for healthy eating (and drinking). So you may be interested to read that the guidelines state flat out that compared to nondrinkers, adults who consume one to two alcohol beverages a day appear to have a lower risk of coronary heart disease.

Clearly, the Guidelines' authors, sober scientific ladies and gentlemen every one, have been doing their reading. Which is to say, they've been looking at a series of recent studies showing that moderate use of alcohol beverages has the following effects:

- ✔ Lowers total cholesterol

- ✔ Raises levels of "good" cholesterol (check out these *high-density lipoproteins,* also known as HDLs, in Chapters 2 and 3)

- ✔ Lowers blood pressure

- ✔ Relaxes muscles (including the heart muscle)

Okay, you're right. Maybe that last bullet point doesn't affect your cholesterol, but it does make you feel good. Does all this sound good enough for you to take a look at the data that convinced the experts? If so, keep reading.

Studying the studies

The evidence that moderate drinking benefits the heart comes from really reliable studies from real, reliable sources, such as the American Cancer Society (ACS), the American Heart Association (AHA), and the long-running, 70,000-women *Nurses' Health Study* (NHS) from the Harvard Medical School, Harvard School of Public Health, and Brigham and Women's Hospital in Boston. Hey, it don't get more reliable than that, right?

Here are the studies of proof:

- ✔ **Really Reliable Study #1:** The ACS's *Cancer Prevention Study I* (CPS-I) followed more than 1 million Americans in 25 states for 12 years. Analyzing the lifestyles of 276,802 middle-aged men and the circumstances of those who died during the study period, the researchers concluded that men who drink moderately lower their risk of heart attack — 21 percent lower for men who have one drink a day than for men who never drink. In addition, men who have one or two drinks a day are 22 percent less likely to die of a stroke.

✔ **Really Reliable Study #2:** An analysis of the data for nearly 600,000 women in CPS-I showed that, like men, women who drink occasionally or have one drink a day are less likely to die of heart attack than women who don't drink at all.

✔ **Really Reliable Study #3:** In 2002, researchers at the NHS issued a new report on 70,891 women who were 25 to 42 years old when the study began in 1989. This time the subject was alcohol. The conclusion? Women who have one-quarter to one-half drink a day — in real life, this equals two or three drinks a week — are 15 percent less likely to develop high blood pressure than women who never drink. At the other end of the spectrum, women who have more than ten drinks a week are 30 percent more likely to have high blood pressure. The results were the same regardless of the type of drink (beer, wine, or spirits) the women preferred. Nice.

Subscribe to the NHS newsletter, which details the current progress of both the original *Nurses' Health Study* and the *Nurses' Health Study II*. Visit `www.channing.harvard.edu/nhs/newsletters/index.shtml`.

What happens as alcohol moves through your body?

How is it that alcohol beverages may benefit your heart, your blood vessels, and your cholesterol profile? First, a bit of physiology. Unlike other foods, which must be digested before your cells can absorb them, alcohol can flow directly through body membranes into your bloodstream.

For example, when you eat a burger, none of its protein, fat, carbs, vitamins, or minerals get into your bloodstream until the burger has made its way through your stomach and your small intestines.

The latest edition of *Nutrition For Dummies* (Wiley), which I also wrote, has an entire chapter on how alcohol affects your body. But for an outline of the path that the grape juice, oops, alcohol takes, check out these steps:

1. **You take a sip of a really good merlot (or my personal favorite, Chianti).**

2. **Small amounts of alcohol immediately pass through the membranes of your mouth and throat into your bloodstream.**

   This process happens so fast that the alcohol reaches your brain within seconds of your sip.

3. **Some of the alcohol goes directly from your stomach to your bloodstream.**

4. **Most of the alcohol goes from your bloodstream to all the organs (such as your heart) in your body.**

5. **Alcohol relaxes the heart muscles, reducing the force with which the muscle contracts (your heartbeat).**

6. **Your heart pumps out slightly less blood for a few minutes.**

7. **When your heartbeat slows and your heart pumps out less blood, a couple of things occur:**

   • Blood vessels all over your body relax, and your blood pressure goes down.

   • Blood *platelets* — the particles that make it possible for blood to clot — become less sticky and less likely to clump together. For a while (oh, maybe an hour or so), your risk of blood clot-related heart attack and stroke goes down.

8. **Your heart muscle's contractions soon return to normal, but as the alcohol circulates through your body, your blood vessels may remain relaxed, and your blood pressure may remain low for as long as half an hour.**

Although the immediate result of moderate drinking is beneficial, heavy drinking or alcohol abuse can raise your blood pressure over the long term.

Focusing on cholesterol

Lipoproteins, the fat-and-protein particles on which cholesterol travels, come in two varieties:

✔ **HDLs (high-density lipoproteins)** are labeled good because they carry cholesterol out of the body.

✔ **LDLs (low-density lipoproteins)** are called bad because they take cholesterol into your arteries.

But as Chapter 2 explains, when you're talking lipoproteins, size is as important as type because large LDLs are less likely than small LDLs to make their way into arteries.

The *Cardiovascular Health Study* (CHS), funded by the National Heart, Lung, and Blood Institute (NHLBI) was designed to evaluate risk factors for heart disease in men and women 65 and older. Data from the 1,850-person study, which ran from 1989 to 1999, has served as a base for more than 400 research papers and 120 follow-up studies.

In 2007, a team of researchers from Beth Israel Deaconess Medical Center (Boston), the University of Pittsburgh, the University of Vermont (Burlington) and the University of Washington (Seattle) combed through the CHS's data in search of medical gold. What they found was that men and women who consumed 7 to 13 drinks a week had the highest number of small LDLs, which have a higher chance of getting into the arteries, thus increasing their risk of blockage. Score another round for moderation — one to two drinks a day.

Identifying Alcohol's Heart-Healthy Compound

If you've read the previous pages of this chapter, you've gathered that moderate drinking has a few benefits. But what exactly is in the alcohol beverages that does the trick? I'm glad you asked.

Unfortunately, the studies that show alcohol's benefits for your heart and blood vessels don't necessarily agree on exactly which kind of alcohol beverage or which constituent in the beverage makes moderate amounts of alcohol beneficial. Is it the alcohol itself? Or something else?

Surveying the studies

On the one hand, lots of studies show similar benefits with all kinds of alcohol beverages — beer, wine, and spirits — suggesting that the active ingredient may simply be the alcohol.

On the other hand, one or two studies have shown special benefits for beer. The best you can say about this development is that it's just one or two studies; before accepting this as a medical gospel, you'd have to see — yes — more studies.

Grooving on grapes

Grape skins and pulp are rich in resveratrol, and grapes belong on a heart-healthy diet. Not only are they low in calories, they're high in nutrients and yummy as all get out. A single serving of 20 green Thompson seedless or deep-red Tokay or Emperor grapes has 70 to 80 calories, 12 to 16 percent of the recommended daily allowance of vitamin C, and up to 84 percent of the potassium in ½ cup of orange juice. And there's a teensy little bit of dietary fiber in the grape's skin, plus astringent tannins that make your mouth pucker.

Maybe that's why Mae West, your great-great-grandpa's sex symbol, whose delightfully raunchy wit is available today on DVDs from the very modern Amazon.com, used to ask her beaus to "peel me a grape." If you want to peel the grapes you toss into your fruit salad, choose American varieties such as the Catawba, Concord, Delaware, Niagara, or Scuppernong. These grapes are called "slipskins" because (surprise) the skin comes off easily. Peeling a European variety, such as an Emperor, Tokay, Malaga, Muscat, or Thompson, is more of a challenge. Here's a little Euro-grape-peeling lesson:

1. Drop the grape into boiling water for a few seconds.

2. Then fish it out with a slotted spoon (to spare your fingers).

3. Finally, plunge the little darling into cold water.

The hot water makes the water under the skin expand so the skin swells; the cold water makes it burst and peel back.

Or you can just eat your grapes with the skin on.

Note: Ounce for ounce, you get more resveratrol from grape juice than from plain grapes. The darker the juice, the higher the resveratrol. Drink up! The following minitable shows you the nutrients in grapes and grape juice, depending on the kind of grapes you ingest.

Nutrients in Grapes and Grape Juice

Nutrient	Red Grapes (20)	White Grapes (20)	Grape Juice (4 oz)
Calories	80	70	77
Carbohydrates	20 g	18 g	19 g
Dietary fiber	<1 g	<1 g	2 g
Vitamin C	12 mg	10 mg	<1 mg
Potassium	210 mg	184 mg	167 mg

Source: U.S. Department of Agriculture.

On the third hand — there're always more than two hands in this kind of discussion — the first hint of alcohol's heart benefits showed up in France, where folks eat lots and lots of high-fat food — pâté! cheese! butter! — but generally have a lower rate of heart disease than people in the United States. Researchers eventually linked this situation, sometimes called "The French Paradox," to the facts that (a) the French serve their fatty foods in very small portions, and (b) the French also drink lots and lots of wine.

Nothing in science is ever simple, is it?

Since researchers have turned their attention to the heart-healthy French, several studies have shown a correlation between low heart disease, favorable cholesterol profiles, and red wine consumption. This research leads to the interesting possibility that the important ingredient in alcohol is actually something in the skin, pulp, and seeds of grapes — the parts of the fruit more widely used in making red wines. Ladies and gentlemen, meet resveratrol.

Zeroing in on resveratrol

Resveratrol is a *flavonoid,* one of a group of plant chemicals credited with lowering cholesterol and reducing inflammation of body tissues, such as the lining of blood vessels, thus reducing your risk of heart attack.

The juice from purple grapes has more resveratrol than the juice from red grapes, which has more resveratrol than the juice from white grapes. (Get the red wine connection?) To be even more specific, in 1998, a team of food scientists from the USDA Agricultural Research Service identified a native American grape, the muscadine, as an unusually potent source of resveratrol. About half of all muscadines grown in the United States are used to make grape juice. With that in mind, nondrinkers can get their resveratrol from grapes and grape juice. Don't you love it when science serves up something for everybody?

Drinking in Moderation

So far in this chapter, we've been talking about the benefits of moderate drinking. Here's what "moderate drinking" means, from the *Dietary Guidelines for Americans:*

- ✔ One drink a day for a woman
- ✔ Two drinks a day for a man

Damaging the liver

Alcohol has to be metabolized in the liver by ADH, which is found in the *mitochondria* (the cellular powerhouses that convert nutrients into energy-yielding molecules that fuel the cells) of the liver cells. If the amount of alcohol presented to the mitochondria exceeds the amount of alcohol the enzyme can detoxify, the alcohol poisons the mitochondria and causes the liver cell to die.

The first change in the liver is seen as fat depositing in the liver cells. If excessive alcohol ingestion is continued, *alcoholic hepatitis* (an inflammation within the liver cells) occurs.

If excessive ingestion of alcohol is stopped at either of these first two stages, the liver cells may return to normal.

The liver is one of the few regenerative organs in the body. If you surgically remove half of the liver, the body will regrow the half that's removed. If, however, excessive alcohol ingestion continues, *cirrhosis*, the final stage of liver damage, occurs. Cirrhosis is a scarring of the liver cells that's an irreversible stage of liver disease and frequently leads to death.

Why does *moderate* mean different things for men and women? It's an enzyme thing. To metabolize (to get rid of, to use up) the alcohol you drink, your body calls on enzymes called *alcohol dehydrogenases* (ADH). You produce one form of ADH — *gastric alcohol dehydrogenase* (GADH) — in your stomach (where alcohol metabolism begins) and another form of ADH in your liver, the primary alcohol-metabolizing plant.

The average woman makes less GADH than the average man. As a result, more unmetabolized alcohol flows from her stomach into her bloodstream on its way to her liver. With more unmetabolized alcohol in her blood, the average woman is likely to become tipsy on smaller amounts of alcohol than is necessary to produce the same effect in the average man.

Most people (men as well as women) need a full hour to produce enough ADH to metabolize the amount of alcohol — ½ ounce — in one drink. But that's an average: Some people still have unmetabolized alcohol circulating in their blood for as long as two to three hours after they take a drink.

Which brings me to the next question: What's one drink? According to the American Heart Association, one drink equals

- 12 ounces of regular beer
- 5 ounces of wine
- 1.5 ounces of 80 proof distilled spirits
- 1 ounce of 100 proof distilled spirits

What makes these different amounts of beer, wine, and spirits equivalent? Each serves up approximately 15 grams of ethyl alcohol, the only alcohol used in alcohol beverages.

Checking Out the Risks, Too

Alcohol is a serious product. Having read this far, you know it has benefits. But you can assume that it also has risks. You're right.

The following sections focus on the risks of alcohol consumption.

Alcohol and cancer

The same studies that applaud the effects of moderate drinking on heart health are less reassuring about the relationship between alcohol and cancer:

- ✔ The American Cancer Society's *Cancer Prevention Study I* shows that people who take more than two drinks a day have a higher incidence of cancer of the mouth and throat (esophagus).

- ✔ Researchers at the University of Oklahoma say that men who drink five or more beers a day double their risk of rectal cancer.

- ✔ American Cancer Society statistics show a higher risk of breast cancer among women who have more than three drinks a week.

The reassuring note? With the exception of breast cancer, the damage appears to be linked to amounts of alcohol that exceed the moderate levels set by the *Dietary Guidelines for Americans.* For info on the moderate levels, see the "Studying the studies" section earlier in this chapter.

Alcohol and birth defects

Fetal alcohol syndrome (FAS) is a collection of birth defects including (but not limited to) low birth weight, heart defects, retardation, and facial deformities.

FAS has been documented only in babies born to women who experts describe as "chronic alcohol abusers who drink heavily during pregnancy." No evidence ties the syndrome to one or two drinks during pregnancy, or even one or two drinks a week during pregnancy.

About 7 percent of the babies born in the United States each year have a birth defect. Often the parents of these children feel guilty even though their behavior had absolutely nothing to do with the birth defect. To make the case even stronger, the U.S. federal government requires that a warning about birth defects appear on all bottles of alcohol beverages.

To date, no solid scientific medical evidence says, "Avoid all alcohol while pregnant." But human beings are complicated forms of life, and the possibility of lifelong guilt if you have a drink while pregnant and then deliver a child with birth defects isn't worth the moment's pleasure.

Alcohol and the morning after

The stories from the morning after a night of too much alcohol aren't fiction. They're a miserable physical fact.

If you ever have too much to drink one evening, the next morning you may experience many of the following symptoms:

- You're thirsty because alcohol, a diuretic, has caused you to lose a lot of water through excessive urination.

- Your stomach hurts because alcohol irritates your stomach lining.

- You're queasy because having your stomach irritated stimulates the release of extra stomach acid and *histamine,* the same immune system chemical that makes the skin around a mosquito bite red and itchy. (Who wouldn't be queasy when her stomach looks like one big bug bite?)

- Your muscles ache because processing alcohol through your liver requires an enzyme normally used to convert *lactic acid,* a byproduct of muscle activity, to compounds you can use for energy. The extra lactic acid piles up painfully in your muscles.

- You have a headache. Alcohol dilates (relaxes) blood vessels, including some in your scalp. The dilated blood vessels swell, making your head hurt.

And when you're talking headache, don't forget the Red Wine Problem. When grapes ferment, their protein molecules split into fragments. One fragment, called *tyramine,* slows your body's metabolism of alcohol, so alcohol keeps circulating through your bloodstream, causing a headache and other unpleasant sensations. Red wine has more tyramine than other kinds of alcohol.

A word to the wise

When experts talk about alcohol abuse, they don't mean warming the vodka or chilling the brandy. The foodies among us may wince, but these gourmet gaffes aren't the point. They mean allowing alcohol to interfere with your ability to enjoy a normal, productive life. If you or someone you know is drinking too much, too often, don't miss this easy opportunity to find help.

1. **Get up right now and walk over to your computer.**

2. **Turn it on.**

3. **Connect to the Internet.**

   What? You have broadband and it's *always* on? Well, skip this step and go to Step 4.

4. **Go to this site: `www.findtreatment.samhsa.gov`.**

   You're now looking at the Web site for the Substance Abuse & Mental Health Services Administration (SAMHSA), a division of the U.S. Department of Health and Human Services. This particular page enables you to find a treatment center right in your own backyard.

5. **Click on the link to the treatment facility locator.**

   You get a map of the United States.

6. **Click on your state, and a short questionnaire pops up.**

   The nice folks at SAMHSA have already filled in your state.

7. **Add your city.**

   City and state are required, but you can narrow your search by including your zip code, street address, and the radius around your home.

8. **Click** Continue **to get a map of your neighborhood with the treatment centers clearly marked.**

Try it. Your friends and loved ones will certainly cheer you on. If you don't have Internet access readily available, try calling 800-662-HELP (4357).

These results are inevitable if you drink too much. Only time heals by enabling you to metabolize alcohol and eliminate it from your body. Hangover remedies or preventives are myths. For example, some people say that you should take an aspirin while drinking to avoid the headache, but the aspirin will intensify the irritation of your stomach lining. To avoid the morning after, drink moderately the night before.

Alcohol and sulfite sensitivity

Sulfur compounds (sulfites) are preservatives widely used to protect the freshness of products such as dried fruits. Some wines also contain sulfur compounds to slow down spoilage by yeasts still active in an aging wine.

Unfortunately, some people are sensitive or allergic to these compounds and may experience potentially serious reactions if exposed to foods containing sulfites. To avoid problems, the government requires all alcohol products containing sulfites to say so on the label. Sounds sensible to me.

An allergic reaction to sulfites can be life-threatening. If you experience intense itching, hives, swelling of your body, a "tight" feeling in your throat (due to swollen tissues), or breathing problems after drinking alcohol, go directly to the closest emergency room or call 911.

Alcohol and drug interactions

If you drink alcohol, even once in a while, when your doctor hands you a prescription, hand her a request for the lowdown on how the drug may interact with alcohol. The grape and the grain make some drugs stronger and reduce the effectiveness of others.

Table 10-1 lists some of the known interactions between alcohol and a few common prescription and over-the-counter (OTC) drugs. This short list gives you an idea of some of the general alcohol-drug interactions likely to occur, but it's definitely not complete.

Always check with your doctor — or pharmacist — to be sure that your medication isn't on the alcohol no-no list.

Table 10-1	Alcohol-Drug Interactions
If You Drink Alcohol While You're Taking This Type of Drug	*This May Occur*
Acetaminophen	Increased liver toxicity
Aspirin and other anti-arthritis/ anti-inflammatory drugs (continuous use)	Increased stomach bleeding; irritation
Anticoagulants (blood thinners)	Increased bleeding
Antidepressants	Increased drowsiness/intoxication; high blood pressure (depends on type of drug; check with your doctor)
Antihistamines	Increased sedation
Diuretics	Low blood pressure
Insulin	Very low blood sugar
Sleeping pills and tranquilizers	Increased sedation

Source: James J. Rybacki, The Essential Guide to Prescription Drugs 2006 (Collins 2006).

Rating Alcohol Beverages as Food

People make alcohol beverages from virtually every sugar-containing, carbohydrate food found on the planet, but the most common choices are cereal grains, fruit, honey, and potatoes. All these foods produce alcohol when fermented, but the alcohols have slightly different flavors and colors.

Table 10-2 shows you which foods are used to produce the different kinds of alcohol beverages.

Table 10-2	Which Food Makes That Drink?
Food	*Alcohol*
Agave plant	Tequila
Apples	"Hard" cider
Barley	Beer, various distilled spirits
Corn	Bourbon, corn whiskey, beer
Grapes and other fruits	Wine
Honey	Mead
Milk	Kumiss (koumiss), kefir
Potatoes	Vodka
Rice	Sake, rice wine
Rye	Whiskey
Sugar cane	Rum
Wheat	Beer, various distilled spirits

Counting content

No alcohol beverage is 100 percent alcohol. The beverage is always alcohol plus water and, if it's a wine or beer, some residue of the foods from which it was made. You can tell how much alcohol is actually in an alcohol beverage through the following two ways:

✔ **Alcohol by volume:** *Alcohol by volume* measures the amount of alcohol as a percentage of all the liquid in the container. For example, if your container holds 10 ounces of liquid and 1 ounce of that liquid is alcohol, the product is 10 percent alcohol by volume. A simple equation: Alcohol content÷Total amount of liquid = Alcohol by volume.

The label on every bottle of wine and spirits sold in the United States must show the alcohol content as *alcohol by volume* (written as *12% alcohol by volume* or *Alc. 12% by vol.* — check out Figure 10-1). When talking to each other, people who make and market alcohol beverages sometimes use the shorthand abbreviation ABV, but this isn't permitted on beverage labels. For reasons too complicated to explain in less than, say, ten pages, using the term *alcohol by volume* or *proof* on beer bottles or cans is optional. Figure 10-1 shows you where to find the ABV on a typical wine label.

✔ **Proof:** The label may also show *proof,* an older way of measuring the alcohol in an alcohol beverage. Proof is two times the alcohol by volume. For example, an alcohol beverage that's 10 percent alcohol by volume is 20 proof. Simple equation: Alcohol by volume × 2 = Proof.

Front label

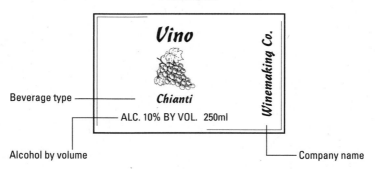

Beverage type —————

Alcohol by volume —————

————— Company name

Back label

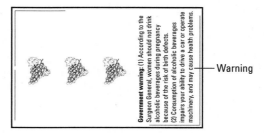

————— Warning

Figure 10-1:
A wine
label.

Counting calories

On its own, alcohol has no nutrients — zero, zilch, zip — other than energy (7 calories per gram), so distilled spirits such as whiskey have nothing to offer, nutritionally speaking, other than calories. Beer, wine, cider, and other fermented beverages contain some of the food from which they were made, so they also contain small amounts of proteins, carbohydrates, vitamins, and minerals.

Tables 10-3 and 10-4 show the nutrient content for one serving of several types of alcohol beverages. As you can imagine, the amounts listed here are averages. For example, some sweet wines may have higher amounts of carbohydrates (sugars) than this chart shows, but very dry (not sweet) wines have less. Just go with the flow.

Table 10-3	Nutrients in Alcohol Beverages			
Beverage	*Serving size*	*Calories*	*Protein*	*Carbohydrates*
Beer				
Regular	12 oz	153 g	1.6 g	12.6 g
Light	12 oz	103 g	0.9 g	5.8 g
Spirits				
86 proof/43% ABV	1.5 oz	105 g	0 g	trace
Wine				
Red table wine	5 oz	125 g	0.1 g	3.8 g
White table wine	5 oz	122 g	0.1 g	3.8 g

Source: USDA National Nutrient Database, www.nal.usda.gov/fnic/food comp/search.

Table 10-4			More Nutrients in Alcohol Beverages						
Beverage	**Thiamin (B1)**	**Riboflavin (B2)**	**Niacin (mcg)**	**Calcium**	**Phosphorus**	**Iron**	**Potassium**	**Sodium**	
Beer									
Regular	0.02 mg	0.09 mg	1.8 mcg	14 mg	50 mg	0.1 NE	96 mg	14 mg	
Light	0.02 mg	0.05 mg	1.4 mcg	14 mg	42 mg	0.1 NE	74 mg	14 mg	
Spirits									
86 proof/43% ABV	trace	trace	trace	0 mcg	2 mg	0.02 NE	1 mg	0 mcg	
Wine									
Red table wine	0 mg	0.01mg	0.2 mcg	12 mg	34 mg	0.7 NE	187 mg	6 mg	
White table wine	0 mg	0.02 mg	0.2 mcg	13 mg	26 mg	0.4 NE	104 mg	7 mg	

Source: USDA National Nutrient Database, www.nal.usda.gov/fnic/foodcomp/search.

Part IV

Cutting Cholesterol with Nutrients and Medicine

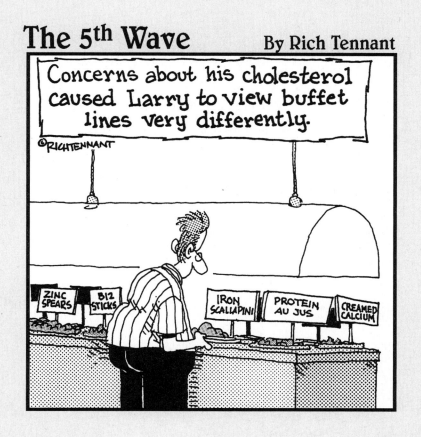

The 5th Wave   By Rich Tennant

Concerns about his cholesterol caused Larry to view buffet lines very differently.

In this part . . .

When food and lifestyle tweaks, turns, or transformations aren't sufficient to control your cholesterol levels, you and your doctor may decide to move on to that old standard: A Pill for Every Ill. But before popping a pill — no matter how beneficial — a smart health consumer does the research. This part makes research a cinch. I evaluate the virtues of nutritional supplements, cholesterol-lowering medications, and — yikes! — medical products that may be counterproductive to your quest for the Big Prize — an improved cholesterol profile.

Chapter 11

Vitamins, Minerals, and Other Good Stuff

*O*ne day, vitamins, minerals, and phytochemicals (*phyto* = plants) are the cat's meow. The next day, they're thrown out with the cat's litter. Although taking vitamin pills and other nutritional supplements is sometimes touted as one way to lower cholesterol, most studies come up a bit short of proclaiming it a certainty. Or worse: At least one study shows that taking extra vitamins may reduce the effectiveness of cholesterol-lowering medications.

As a result, the best advice on supplements may be one that's tried and true (and a bit boring): A balanced diet beats supplements hands down. In this case, I'm talking about a balanced, low-cholesterol, controlled-fat diet. A few exceptions exist to the advice I just laid on you, and I promise to discuss those exceptions in this chapter, along with all the info you need concerning cholesterol and how it relates to vitamins, minerals, fiber, and other dietary supplements.

For the lowdown on cholesterol-lowering prescription meds, check out Chapter 12; for cholesterol-lowering diets, your best bets are Chapters 4 and 5.

Identifying Supplements

Every year, Americans snap up more than $3 billion worth of nutritional supplements. Some people use them for "nutritional insurance;" others see supplements as a quick and easy way to get vitamins, minerals, and other good stuff without the pesky fat and sugars found in food.

But you're reading a book about cholesterol, so for you, the most interesting statement about supplements may be that some appear to help lower total cholesterol and *low-density lipoproteins* (LDLs) while raising *high-density lipoproteins* (HDLs), the cholesterol particles you can read more about in Chapter 2.

The U.S. government considers dietary supplements to be food products, not drugs. As a result, supplements aren't regulated as strictly as drugs, and very few serious studies exist to show how these pills affect cholesterol. Every rule, however, has an exception. Which is the point of this chapter, so read on.

Popping a Vitamin and Mineral Pill May Help Lower Cholesterol

Some nutrients play an important role in keeping your heart healthy. For example, calcium enables muscle cells, including heart muscle cells, to send messages back and forth, and selenium protects against *Keshan disease,* a disorder of the heart muscle whose symptoms include rapid heartbeat, enlarged heart, and (in severe cases) heart failure.

But when it comes to lowering cholesterol, most nutrients are no-shows. The one stellar exception is niacin. The maybes are vitamin E, vitamin C, and calcium.

How niacin helps control cholesterol

Niacin is a B vitamin considered essential for proper growth and development. It's intimately involved in the work of *enzymes,* naturally occurring compounds in your body that power various processes such as digestion.

In fact, niacin is a component of one enzyme that enables oxygen to flow into your body tissues. Like thiamin (vitamin B1), niacin helps you maintain a healthy appetite. It also participates in the digestion of sugars and fat. You get niacin directly from these foods:

- **Dairy products:** Your body converts the amino acid tryptophan found in milk and dairy foods into niacin.

- **Grains:** Grains are a source of niacin, but your body can't absorb them efficiently unless they've been treated with lime (the mineral, not the fruit — see the nearby sidebar "Limelicious").

- **Meat, fish, and poultry:** No need to explain these three, right?

The niacin you get from food helps your body function in all of these ways, and it also protects you against the niacin-deficiency disease *pellagra.* The symptoms of pellagra include diarrhea, skin lesions, confusion, and dementia. But the amount of niacin found in food is too small to affect your cholesterol. For that, you need industrial-strength niacin.

Numbering normal niacin needs

In the United States, the *r*ecommended *d*ietary *a*llowance of each nutrient is usually abbreviated as RDA, a term comparable to the Canadian RNI (*r*ecommended *n*utrient *i*ntake).

The RDA for niacin is described in terms of niacin equivalents (NE), as in milligrams of niacin equivalents (mg/NE). For example, 60 mg of tryptophan (an amino acid in milk) = 1 mg of niacin = 1 niacin equivalent (mg/NE).

The basic adult requirement for niacin is 14 mg/NE per day for women and 16 mg/NE per day for men. The amount of niacin required to lower cholesterol levels is dramatically higher.

Measuring medically-effective levels of niacin

If you take an immediate-release form of niacin, a product that sends the vitamin right into your bloodstream, the starting dose is 100 mg/NE three times a day. The starting dose for an extended-release form of niacin, a product that releases the niacin gradually into your bloodstream, is one 375-mg/NE pill once a day.

So much for the techy details. Now, on to the practical part.

Balancing the benefits and risks of medical-strength niacin

As a medication, large doses of niacin

- ✔ Lower your triglycerides (fats in your blood; see Chapter 2)
- ✔ Lower your total cholesterol up to 10 percent
- ✔ Lower your LDLs by as much as 14 percent
- ✔ Raise your HDLs by as much as 25 percent

Limelicious

Treating grain with lime is a common practice in Central American and South American countries. Lime enables the body to absorb the niacin efficiently. In these countries, lime is added to cornmeal used to make tortillas.

In the United States, breads and cereals are routinely fortified with niacin, which makes the use of lime unnecessary.

So far, everything sounds pretty good, but like most medication, a cholesterol-lowering dose of niacin has potential side effects. Like what?

- Like a *niacin flush,* a feeling of sudden warmth similar to the hot flashes some women experience at menopause, which is kind of weird if you're not yet in menopause — or if you're male

- Like making your diabetes or arthritis medication less effective

- Like skin rashes, hives, itching, muscle pain, peptic ulcers, upset stomach, nausea, diarrhea, liver damage, vision problems, dizziness, and fainting

Call 911 or go immediately to the closest emergency room if you experience any of these symptoms while taking niacin supplements.

Worse yet (can it really get worse?), if you develop any of these symptoms and decide to stop taking niacin cold turkey, your total cholesterol and your LDLs will rebound, zooming skyward, almost certainly higher than they were before you started taking niacin.

One way to avoid this state of affairs is to taper off niacin, taking a little bit less every day.

If a pill — including a vitamin pill — is powerful enough to alter your cholesterol profile, it's powerful enough to be troublesome — an example of how something natural may be helpful but not necessarily harmless.

For more info on niacin and other cholesterol-lowering medications, turn to Chapter 12.

Evaluating vitamin E and vitamin C

Vitamin E is a fat-soluble nutrient (a vitamin that dissolves in fat and can be stored in your fatty tissue). Vitamin C is water-soluble (a vitamin that dissolves in water and is eliminated when you urinate). But the two nutrients have one interesting trait in common: Both are *antioxidants.*

Antioxidants are substances that prevent fragments of molecules from hooking up to form potentially damaging compounds inside your body.

For example, many cured meats contain added vitamin C and vitamin E to prevent fragments of preservatives called nitrates and nitrites from hooking up to form carcinogens called nitrosamines.

Linking antioxidants and cholesterol

Low-density lipoproteins (LDLs) are fat-and-protein particles sometimes called "bad" cholesterol because they ferry cholesterol into arteries. Combining with oxygen makes LDLs more damaging.

So it seems reasonable to assume that anything that prevents LDLs and oxygen from mating should lower your risk of clogged arteries.

One such "anything" may be antioxidant vitamins. In fact, during the 1990s, several major scientific studies at thoroughly reputable scientific institutions suggested that antioxidant vitamins E and C could protect your heart muscle and blood vessels from cholesterol damage.

This led many respected scientists (and some nutritional theorists) to say that taking a lot of E and C would be good medicine. But they may have been off on the wrong path.

More recent studies suggest contrary conclusions: Taking antioxidant vitamins may reduce the effectiveness of cholesterol-lowering statin drugs, *and* antioxidant vitamins may actually convince your liver to churn out more cholesterol.

Subverting the statins

In August 2001, *Atherosclerosis, Thrombosis, and Vascular Biology,* a journal of the American Heart Association, published a report from a one-year study at the University of Washington School of Medicine.

The study included 153 volunteers between the ages of 33 and 74 who had arteries narrowed by cholesterol plaque and low levels of HDLs, the "good" cholesterol. Each volunteer was randomly assigned to one of the following "treatment" regimens:

- **Regimen #1:** The cholesterol-lowering drug Simvastatin (Zocor), plus niacin, and antioxidant vitamins E and C (for a rundown on Simvastatin and other "statins" see Chapter 12)
- **Regimen #2:** Simvastatin and niacin
- **Regimen #3:** Antioxidant vitamins alone
- **Regimen #4:** A placebo (pill with inactive ingredients; basically a sugar pill)

Ordinarily, both Simvastatin and niacin lower total cholesterol and LDLs while boosting HDLs, but volunteers who took Simvastatin, niacin, and antioxidants experienced a smaller increase in HDLs than volunteers who took the drugs alone, and their levels of HDL (2) — a kind of "super good" cholesterol — didn't budge a bit. Boy, did that surprise the researchers!

As a result, the editorial accompanying the report concluded that doctors should tell their patients that taking antioxidants with a statin drug, such as Simvastatin, or with niacin may not be a good idea.

But the editorial also noted that the study was so small that it couldn't be considered conclusive, especially since vitamin E — a natural anticoagulant that reduces the risk of blood clots — has been shown to lower the risk of heart disease.

Ticking off tocotrienols

Tocotrienols are phytochemicals similar to vitamin E. One measly study shows that taking tocotrienols lowers LDLs, so some companies are packing tocotrienols in pills and selling them as cholesterol-lowering supplements.

But if you take vitamin E while taking tocotrienols, the former cancels out the effects of the latter. Too complicated for me!

Then, believe it or not, results from another study, this one from Oxford University (England), showed no ill effects from combining antioxidants with a statin drug, leading the Brits to suggest that the problem may lie with the niacin.

Making the body make more cholesterol

In April 2004, a team of researchers at New York University School of Medicine's Lipid Treatment and Research Center reported that when mice were fed a diet rich in the antioxidant vitamins E, C, and beta-carotene, their livers churned more than normal amounts of VLDLs (very low-density lipoproteins).

VLDLs are one form of LDLs, the fat-and-protein particles that carry cholesterol into arteries. (For more on the various forms of lipoproteins, see Chapter 2.)

Would this also happen in human beings? The researchers couldn't say for sure; after all, mice aren't people.

However, the study — plus a raft of others casting doubt on the anti-cholesterol powers of antioxidants — may have been what led the American Heart Association to issue the following statement in 2007:

> "The American Heart Association doesn't recommend using antioxidant vitamin supplements until more complete data are available. We continue to recommend that people eat a variety of nutrient-rich foods daily from all the basic food groups."

Can calcium supplements counter cholesterol?

Remember when your mother told you to drink your milk because — all together now — "Calcium makes strong bones and teeth." Would mom say the same thing about calcium's ability to lower the level of cholesterol circulating in your older body? Maybe.

In May 2003, a team of researchers from the Department of Medicine at the University of Auckland (New Zealand) reported that when 223 postmenopausal women who weren't being treated for high cholesterol or osteoporosis were given either calcium supplements (1 g/day) or a placebo (a look-alike pill with no calcium) for 12 months, HDL levels rose about 7 percent among those taking the calcium, while LDL and total cholesterol levels went down slightly.

Conclusion? For older women, calcium supplements may protect arteries, as well as bones. Good job, mate.

Fighting Cholesterol with Dietary Fiber

As you can read in Chapter 5, there are two kinds of dietary fiber — insoluble dietary fiber (which doesn't dissolve in your intestinal tract) and soluble dietary fiber (which does dissolve in your gut).

There's absolutely no doubt that eating foods like beans, fruits, veggies, and grains, which are all high in soluble dietary fiber, lowers your cholesterol. You can read all about oatmeal and beans, the quintessential soluble-dietary-fiber factories, in Chapter 6.

But suppose you totally loathe high-fiber foods. Suppose just looking at fruits, veggies, grains, and beans makes you go, "Ugh!" Far be it from me to say, "Boy! You're missing some good stuff." No, my job here is to answer the question dancing across your lips: "Can I get my fiber from supplements?" Well . . . maybe.

Soluble dietary fiber lowers your cholesterol levels by mopping up cholesterol in your digestive tract before it gets into your bloodstream. To do this job effectively, the fiber must absorb water and form a gel.

To date, more than 50 separate scientific studies (notice the subtle, albeit compelling, alliteration) attest to the ability of some soluble-fiber supplements to lower total cholesterol and LDLs. The soluble dietary fibers most often studied in these tests are

- **Guar gum:** A sticky, soluble dietary fiber from a plant commonly cultivated in India as cattle feed. Guar gum is also known as guar flour or bentonite.
- **Pectin:** A soluble fiber found most prominently in apples.
- **Psyllium:** A sticky soluble fiber also known as plantago seed or plantain seed.

But not all supplements containing these fibers are equally effective. For a soluble-fiber supplement to lower your cholesterol, it must form a strong gel that can attract and hold cholesterol in your gut. Unfortunately, some methods of processing fiber to make supplements break up the strands of carbohydrates that form the gel, thus weakening the whole darned thing.

To be certain that a dietary-fiber supplement will actually lower cholesterol, the manufacturer has to test it, a time-consuming and expensive process. As a result, very few fiber supplements can actually prove they will lower your cholesterol. Sorry about that.

Psyllium alert! Psyllium alert! Some people are allergic to psyllium. If they eat the stuff, they may end up with hives or a rash, respiratory problems, or — worst-case scenario — the potentially lethal, whole-body reaction called *anaphylaxis.* In other words, something natural may be helpful but not necessarily harmless. If you consume some psyllium and start feeling itchy or have trouble breathing, get to the nearest emergency room or call an ambulance.

Phabulous Phytochemicals

Perhaps the most fascinating nutritional discovery of the past several years has been the identification of *phytochemicals,* naturally occurring compounds in plants. Some of these compounds actually mimic powerful medicines such as the female sex hormone estrogen and the cholesterol-lowering statin drugs. Who wouldn't be impressed with these natural wonders?

Sticking with sterols

Plants are great little pretenders. They often manufacture compounds that resemble chemicals found in animal (human) bodies but don't seem to carry the problems associated with animal (human) chemistry.

One good example is *phytosterols,* substances that resemble cholesterol so closely that your digestive tract can't tell what's a phytosterol and what's cholesterol.

If you eat phytosterols along with a meal that includes cholesterol, your body is likely to absorb phytosterols (which won't clog your arteries) in place of cholesterol (which may).

This principle has inspired the creation of special cholesterol-lowering margarines that promise to change your cholesterol profile for the better, although the exact decrease in total cholesterol and LDLs and the increase in HDLs will vary with the dose and the body. For more on the sterol margarines, see Chapter 6.

As with dietary fiber supplements, the question here is whether you can cram enough of the good stuff into a pill to let you take your sterols as a supplement rather than a food. This time, the answer is why bother? The sterol studies say you must wolf down at least 3,000 milligrams (mg) of sterols per day to produce a noticeable change in your cholesterol levels. Each tablespoon of sterol margarine provides 1,700 mg, so two tablespoons per day more than does the trick.

By comparison, the *University of California Berkeley Wellness Letter* says that the doses of sterols in supplement pills are "too small to have any effect." How small? Usually in the under-400-mg-per-pill range, which means you'd need about eight pills a day to make a difference. I say, pass up the pills, and "butter" (note the qualifying quote marks) your bread.

The *sterols* in sterol margarine or cholesterol-lowering supplements aren't the same as the *steroids* sometimes used illegally by athletes to bulk up their muscles. Do I need to add that steroids, which can really mess up your body systems, are a definite no-no? Make that, NO-NO. And go ahead and add an exclamation point, as in *never, ever* use these drugs!

Getting the goods on garlic supplements

As a food, garlic is yummy. As a cholesterol buster, it's so-so. In the mid-1970s, a number of studies suggested that phytochemicals in garlic, particularly the smelly mustard compounds such as allicin, were useful in lowering cholesterol. Later research is mixed.

Some studies say, yes, garlic and garlic supplements can lower cholesterol. Others say not in this lifetime. In 2007, Christopher Gardner, assistant professor of medicine at Stanford University, ran a trial with 192 adults — in this case, people older than 50 — whose average LDL level was 140. Six days a week for six months, the volunteers were given the equivalent of one clove of garlic (either as a pill or as plain raw garlic mixed into food) or a dummy pill. Monthly blood tests failed to show any change in cholesterol levels, but more than half the people who got garlic reported bad breath and body odor.

Conclusion: Pass this supplement by. Otherwise, people may pass you by.

Waiting for the Next Study

This section may be a good opportunity to remind you that it takes a while to shake down all the data from new medical studies and that this situation sometimes leaves doctors and patients confused.

At one recent medical convention, speakers presented the findings from four large treatment trials whose aim was to determine if taking vitamin E may help prevent heart attack. Three of the trials showed that vitamin E had no beneficial effect on the heart, and one showed that vitamin E caused more heart attacks than the placebo.

At the beginning of the presentations, the doctors in the audience were asked, "How many of you are taking vitamin E for your heart?" and about half of them raised their hands.

After the presentation of the trials, the doctors were asked, "How many of you will be taking vitamin E in the future?" and no one raised his or her hand.

Who's right? I hate to say this, but who knows? The only conclusive answers about vitamins, minerals, phytochemicals, and cholesterol will come — arrrgh! — with time.

Chapter 12

Prescribing Lower Cholesterol

*O*kay, so you've changed your diet to conform to the guidelines in Chapters 4 and 5, you've stepped up your exercise (see Chapter 8), and you've lost a couple of pounds — maybe even more than a couple of pounds. But — can it be? — your cholesterol levels are still higher than your doctor considers healthy. What to do?

You may be a candidate for cholesterol-lowering drugs. This chapter, with eight tables and one very detailed drawing of your innards, compares the effectiveness of different kinds of drugs, explains the unfamiliar words used to name these drugs, lists potential side effects, and generally gives you the facts you need to make an informed decision as to whether you're a candidate for cholesterol-busting meds. So read it.

Introducing Cholesterol-Lowering Medicines

Modern medicine has reduced the number of deaths from heart attacks, but, until recently, it hadn't substantially lowered the number of heart attacks or cases of heart disease. One possible way to accomplish this is to eliminate the cause of many heart attacks — that is, to lower the amount of cholesterol swimming around in the blood.

Doctors currently use one (or more) of four different kinds of meds to lower cholesterol, which I list here:

- ✔ Statin drugs
- ✔ Cholesterol blockers
- ✔ Bile acid sequestrants
- ✔ Triglyceride inhibitors (including the B vitamin niacin)

To explain the particulars about these meds, I have created a separate section for each starting right after the nifty picture of your insides in Figure 12-1, which shows where in your body the cholesterol-lowering drugs do their good work.

Patients with high cholesterol (particularly those who've already had a heart attack) may also be given anticoagulants (blood thinners) such as aspirin and clopidogrel (Plavix). Anticoagulants don't lower cholesterol, but they do reduce the risk of blood clots, thus reducing the risk that a blood clot gets stuck in a cholesterol-clogged artery.

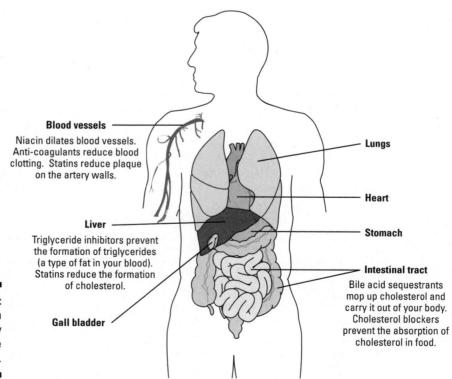

Blood vessels
Niacin dilates blood vessels. Anti-coagulants reduce blood clotting. Statins reduce plaque on the artery walls.

Lungs

Heart

Liver
Triglyceride inhibitors prevent the formation of triglycerides (a type of fat in your blood). Statins reduce the formation of cholesterol.

Stomach

Intestinal tract
Bile acid sequestrants mop up cholesterol and carry it out of your body. Cholesterol blockers prevent the absorption of cholesterol in food.

Gall bladder

Figure 12-1:
Seeing in the body where the meds work.

Cutting cholesterol off at the source: Statins

Atorvastatin (Lipitor), fluvastatin (Lescol), pravastatin (Pravachol), simvastatin (Zocor), and rosuvastatin (Crestor) are medicines known collectively as "statins." The statins reduce the body's synthesis of cholesterol, which means they are definitely heart-healthy. In fact, the usual dozens of studies cited in cases like this show that taking a statin drug can do all these good things:

✔ Lower your LDLs

✔ Raise your HDLs

✔ Reduce your *plaque* (the technical term for gunk sticking to your artery walls that may break off and form clots, which can block the flow of blood and cause a heart attack)

✔ Protect the lining of your arteries

   All arteries are lined with tissue called *endothelium*. When the endothelium doesn't function properly, the artery starts to build up plaque. Statins, as well as some other drugs, keep the endothelium healthy — another way these drugs lower your risk of heart attack or stroke.

✔ Lower your *C-reactive protein,* another risk factor for heart attack that you can check out in Chapter 3

✔ Reduce your risk of a first heart attack

✔ Reduce your risk of a second heart attack if you've already had one

✔ Reduce your risk of stroke

Statins are sold as single ingredient pills or combo pills that add a second heart-healthy drug such as one that lowers blood pressure. Table 12-1 lists the various statin products currently on your drugstore shelf or behind the counter.

Table 12-1	What's in That Statin Pill?
Single Ingredient Products	
Brand Name	*Generic Statin*
Lescol	Fluvastatin
Lipitor	Atorvastatin
Mevacor	Lovastatin
Pravachol	Pravastatin

(continued)

Table 12-1 (continued)

Single Ingredient Products	
Brand Name	**Generic Statin**
Zocor	Simvastatin
Crestor	Rosuvastatin

Combination Products		
Brand Name	**Generic Statin**	**Additional Ingredient(s)**
Advicor	Lovastatin	Niacin/nicotinic acid (extended release)*
Caduet	Atorvastatin	Amlodipine besy late (Norvasc)#
Vytorin	Simvastatin	Ezetimibe (Zetia)@

*Reduces triglycerides
#Lowers blood pressure
@Blocks absorption of cholesterol from food; the value of ezetimibe is currently under review (see sidebar, "Questioning a cholesterol buster"

Statin side effects

Because you're reading this book, I know that you're an informed medical consumer. Because you're an informed medical consumer, *you* know that even beneficial medicines may pose problems for some patients.

When statins first came on the market, manufacturers included a notice in the small print of their product information about muscle cramps, aches, pain, and weakness, but it sure looked insignificant. Yet from their introduction in the late 1980s, it was clear that statins may trigger *rhabdomyolysis,* an excessive breakdown of muscle tissue creating a flood of waste cells that tumble through the bloodstream and into the kidneys where they may clog small passages and — theoretically — cause kidney failure.

Until the summer of 2001, the word *theoretically* was very, very important. In clinical trials of more than 50,000 patients, researchers hadn't linked a single death to statin-triggered kidney failure. But cerivastatin (Baycol), a new statin introduced by Bayer A.G. in 1997, was different. The incidence of rhabdomyolysis among Baycol users was about ten times higher than among people taking other statin drugs, and the reaction was more likely to be really serious — read: fatal.

Name games

When the words on this page move from unfamiliar to incomprehensible, you know you're into the serious stuff. That's the case with *HMG-CoA reductase inhibitors,* the scientifically-correct name for statins.

The easy way to define HMG-CoA reductase inhibitors is to work backwards, starting with the last word in the name. *Inhibitor* is plain English for something that keeps something else from doing something.

Now, move back one word to *reductase.* Note the ending *-ase,* which is the scientific shorthand for *enzyme.* Now you know an HMG-CoA reductase inhibitor is a drug that interferes with (inhibits) the action of an enzyme. Hey, that's not bad for a non-scientist!

Next step: *CoA.* The initials stand for *coenzyme A.* But if you look that term up in *Stedman's Medical Dictionary,* the one most science writers use, it directs you to *HMG-CoA,* the abbreviation for — take a deep breath — *beta-hydroxy-beta-methyl-glutaryl-CoA.*

What in the world is beta-hy.... No, no, not again. I'm going to stick to the abbreviation. HMG-CoA is an important player in converting fats to lipoproteins and cholesterol.

Put it all together, filter out the science speak (well, most of it), and you get the plain-language definition of an HMG-CoA reductase inhibitor: A drug that reduces the activity of an enzyme needed to turn fats into lipoproteins and cholesterol, especially the nasty little LDLs.

Wait. Don't leave. I'm not done.

The generic names for all HMG-CoA reductase inhibitors end in *–statin* because, as the International Union of Pure and Applied Chemistry and the International Union of Biochemistry and Molecular Biology so carefully note, the suffix *–statin* stands for "factors inhibiting the release (and perhaps the synthesis) of pituitary hormones."

Now we're done. Whew.

By August 7, 2001, when Bayer took Baycol off the market, at least 31 deaths had been linked to the medication in the United States, and the Food and Drug Administration (FDA) had reports of nine more deaths abroad. The total number of deaths linked to Baycol has never been finalized, but the estimated number of cases of rhabdomyolysis eventually rose into the thousands, and according to the *Kaiser Daily Health Policy Report* of November 23, 2004, Bayer has settled nearly 3,000 lawsuits about Baycol-related injuries.

Today, the package inserts and advertising for all statin drugs include a warning about muscle pain, usually like this **in bold black type.** Forewarned, after all, is forearmed. The following list details the currently recognized side effects of statin drugs:

> ✓ **Common side effects:** Abnormal results on tests for liver enzymes (temporary), allergic rash, fatigue, headache and dizziness, low blood pressure, upset stomach (nausea, gas, diarrhea, or constipation)

> ✔ **Less common/potentially serious side effects:** Persistent abnormal results on liver function test, accompanied by hepatitis, abnormally low platelets (particles that enable blood to clot), emotional depression, memory loss, muscle pain and tenderness, muscle loss (rhabdomyolysis), protein in the urine

Naturally, because you are, as noted above, an informed medical consumer, you tell your doctor right away if you experience any of the more serious side effects. Right away. No waiting. Really.

Statin interactions with other drugs

If you take a statin along with a drug that blocks the action of liver enzymes required to eliminate statins from your body, the level of statins floating about your organs and tissues may rise high enough to cause serious muscle damage — and maybe even kidney failure — which isn't a good thing. Among the drugs known to hit those liver enzymes and trigger this reaction are the antibiotics clarithromycin (Biaxin) and erythromycin; oral fungus fighters, such as keto-conazole and other meds whose names end in –*azole;* and protease inhibitors (HIV/AIDS drugs).

Taking two or more meds at once is a balancing act, so always tell your doctor *exactly* what you're taking when she prescribes a new medicine, including a statin.

Nature's cholesterol busters: Not

Hate doctors? Don't want to spend all your money on prescription drugs? Think you can find an inexpensive over-the-counter cholesterol buster? Fuggeddabboudit.

In the late 1980s, health food stores did a nifty business selling a "natural" cholesterol buster called Cholestin. The active ingredient in Cholestin was red yeast rice (or red rice yeast) produced by fermenting a particular strain of rice with — what else? — yeast, a process that created a form of *lovastatin,* the statin drug sold under the brand name Mevacor.

Because red yeast rice was introduced as a dietary supplement, not a drug, it didn't have to go through the rigorous tests for safety and effectiveness required of lovastatin. Was it safe? Probably as safe as lovastatin. Did that mean perfectly harmless? Clearly not, as you can see for yourself by reading the side effects listed for lovastatin earlier in this chapter.

In 2000, the 10th U.S. Circuit Court of Appeals ruled that red yeast rice was a drug and therefore subject to regulation by the Food and Drug Administration (FDA). After that, the FDA went all out after any company selling red yeast rice, demanding to see proof — real scientific studies, please — demonstrating the safety and effectiveness of any product containing red yeast rice.

As an inevitable result, while products listing red yeast rice as an ingredient are still available on health food and drugstore shelves, the rice is made differently and no longer contains any statin. Other "natural" cholesterol-lowering products may contain various herbs, vitamins, dietary fiber, and plant compounds such as stanols and sterols (the anti-cholesterol ingredients in some margarines described in Chapter 6). You don't need a prescription for these products and the packages sure are pretty, but none of them will lower cholesterol as effectively as statin drugs.

Trading bile for cholesterol: Bile acid sequestrants

Right off the bat, here are a couple of those unfamiliar words I mentioned at the start of this chapter. Don't panic. Just take 'em one at a time. *Bile acids* are digestive aids stored in your gallbladder. (If your gallbladder has been removed, your body still makes bile acids but releases them into the digestive tract instead of storing them.)

Bile acids enable you to metabolize fats so that your body can absorb fatty acids (no, ice cream doesn't go straight from your lips to your hips) and convert them to useful products such as — you got it — cholesterol. *Bile acid sequestrants* are compounds that grab up bile acids in your intestines and eliminate them via your feces before the bile acids can do their job on fats.

You take bile acid sequestrants right before you eat so they're readily available when the gallbladder begins to release bile acids for digestion. As the bile acid sequestrants grab up so much bile acid that you can't efficiently digest fats, your body says, "Whoa there! I need some more of this stuff." As a result, you begin to convert some of the cholesterol in your body to bile acids to replace the ones you've mopped up and eliminated, and the amount of cholesterol and triglycerides in your blood goes down.

The different bile acid sequestrants

The most commonly used bile acid sequestrants, listed in alphabetical order by their generic names, are

- ✔ **Cholestyramine:** Available either as a powder to mix with a clear liquid, such as water or juice, or as a chewable bar. The brand names for cholestyramine are Prevalite and Questran.

- ✔ **Colesevelam:** Available in tablet form — a unique selling point. The brand name for colesevelam is Welchol.

- ✔ **Colestipol:** Available as coated tablets, flavored granules, a liquid, or in packets of powder (to be dissolved in water). The brand names for colestipol are Colestid and Lestid.

Taking low doses of bile sequestrants (8 gram/day) may knock cholesterol levels down by 10 to 15 percent. Tripling the dose may lower LDL levels by 25 percent.

Taking bile sequestrants with a second drug improves their performance. For example, in one drug trial, taking colesevelam alone cut total cholesterol by about 10 percent and LDLs by about 18 percent. Taking colesevelam plus a statin drug cut total cholesterol up to 21 percent and LDLs up to 32 percent.

The side effects of bile acid sequestrants

Bile acid sequestrants have been in use for so long that their overall long-term safety is well established. But there are some drawbacks:

- ✔ **Common side effects:** Constipation, loss of appetite, gastric upset (indigestion, gas, nausea, vomiting, diarrhea), headache and dizziness, muscle and joint pain, discolored teeth

- ✔ **Less common, more serious side effects:** Reduced absorption of calcium, leading to increased side effects; risk of osteoporosis (loss of bone density); vitamin deficiencies due to reduced absorption of vitamins A, D, E, and K, as well as the B vitamins folic acid and niacin; decreased effectiveness of painkillers, diuretics, some diabetes drugs, some antibiotics, and some antifungal drugs

To reduce the side effects of bile acid sequestrants, the FDA suggests that you

- ✔ Start with small doses.

- ✔ Drink a lot of water to prevent constipation.

- ✔ Ask your doctor about the need for nutritional supplements and the possibility of drug interactions.

Finishing off another kind of fat: Triglyceride inhibitors

Triglyceride inhibitors are medicines that reduce your liver's natural production of triglycerides, a fat that circulates in your blood. Lowering the level of triglycerides means you convert less dietary fat to lipoproteins. As a result, triglyceride inhibitors lower the production of LDLs, the "bad" cholesterol. No surprise there. But for some unknown reason, they also increase the levels of HDLs, the "good" cholesterol. Down with the bad, up with the good. Go figure.

The most commonly used triglyceride inhibitors are fibrates and the B vitamin niacin, which are covered in the following sections.

Fighting cholesterol with fibrates

Fibrates, also known as fibric acids, are a class of drugs that reduce blood levels of triglycerides and increase the levels of HDLs ("good" cholesterol). The fibrates include clofibrate (Atromid-S), fenofibrate (Tricor), and gemfibrozil (Gemcor, Lopid). Because these drugs haven't been shown to reduce the overall incidence of heart attack, they're not considered first-line treatment.

The fibrates come in capsules to be taken twice a day — 30 minutes before breakfast and 30 minutes before dinner. What? You have to get up half an hour early to take a pill? Oh, well . . .

Because taking fibrates may raise blood sugar, these drugs are rarely prescribed for people with diabetes. Following are other possible side effects of fibrates:

- **Common side effects:** Allergic, itchy, skin rashes and hives; blurred vision; fatigue; gastric upset (diarrhea, gas, nausea, vomiting); headache and dizziness; muscle aches

- **Less common, more serious side effects:** Flu-like symptoms (chills, fever, sore throat); gallstones; kidney failure; lower blood levels of potassium; lower levels of white blood cells (the cells that protect against infection); muscle weakness or loss of muscle tissue; Raynaud's syndrome (constriction of small blood vessels in hands and feet)

Nipping the numbers with niacin

The recommended dietary allowance (RDA) for niacin is 16 mg/day for a man, 14 mg/day for a woman. Taking much larger amounts of this familiar B vitamin appears to reduce triglycerides. For example, in various clinical trials, people taking doses of niacin up to 375 mg/day were able to cut their total cholesterol levels by up to 10 percent and their LDLs by up to 14 percent while raising their HDLs by as much as 25 percent.

In addition, niacin/nicotinic acid dilates blood vessels so that (theoretically) blood flows more easily through even clogged blood vessels. When niacin dilates blood vessels, it causes a feeling of warmth and flushing much like the "hot flashes" many women experience at menopause. To reduce this effect, doctors who prescribe niacin often opt for the *sustained release* or *extended release* form of the med. Instead of sending niacin zooming into your bloodstream as soon as — or pretty soon after — you take the pill, these babies release their niacin slowly, over several hours. In 2006 and 2007, several studies showed that combining niacin with a statin drug was an even more effective treatment.

Currently, niacin is available as a single ingredient drug either as a generic or under the brand names Niacor, Nicolar, Niaspan, and Slo-Niacin. Advicor is a sustained release combination drug containing niacin and lovastatin (Mevacor) in two doses: 500 mg niacin/20 mg lovastatin and 1,000 mg niacin/20 mg lovastatin.

Questioning a cholesterol buster

The scenario is familiar: You open your morning newspaper or turn on the evening news and read or hear that a prestigious pharmaceutical company has discovered a splendiferous new medicine that will solve one of your most pressing health problems like, oh, high cholesterol. The FDA has signed on, so you hotfoot it over to the doctor who prescibes the new med. And then what happens? Two weeks, two months, or two years down the road — "Oooops!" they say. "We think we missed something here."

Ezetimibe (Zetia) is the first prescription drug created specifically to lower LDLs ("bad" cholesterol) by reducing your body's absorption of the cholesterol in food. The med was introduced in 2003 as a single ingredient product (Zetia) and in 2004 as the second ingredient (along with simvastatin) in the combo pill Vytorin. When the FDA approved ezetimibe in 2003, it did so on the basis of several small trials, none of which ran longer than three months — and which hinted at trouble ahead. The people in the trial took either ezetimibe or a look-alike pill without ezetimibe, and the people in the ezetimibe group were 11 times more likely to experience serious adverse effects, most commonly liver damage. (Other possible side effects in the ezetimibe group — allergic reactions, increased risk of gallstones, and potentially serious muscle and liver damage — were described as "rare.")

In December 2007, this situation became more troublesome when non-government experts on drug safety, including researchers at the University of Washington, discovered that Merck and Schering-Plough, the companies that jointly market ezetimibe, had not published the data from a 2-year, 760-person clinical trial called "Enhance" that ended in April 2006 and was originally scheduled to be made public in 2007. The FDA said the agency had seen the unpublished studies and considered ezetimibe safe, but in January 2008, when the study was finally published, ezetimibe's rep took a tumble.

The Enhance study was designed specifically to show that ezetimibe not only lowers LDLs ("bad" cholesterol), but also — like statins — reduces the buildup of plaque inside blood vessels that can lead to heart attack and stroke. In fact, that did not happen. Patients in the trial took either simvastatin (Zocor) alone or a combination of simvastatin and ezetimibe (Vytorin). Simvastatin alone lowered LDLs by 41 percent on average; simvastatin plus ezetimibe, by 58 percent. But among patients given the combination pill, the plaque accumulated twice as fast as among those taking simvastatin alone. In short, taking ezetimibe appeared to increase the risk of both heart attack and stroke.

Many experts called this development "shocking." Others said the data required further investigation. Congress called for an inquiry into the delay in releasing the trial results. Merck and Schering-Plough announced that the results of a longer, larger study of ezetimibe would be released in a few years. Patients and doctors fumed.

As of this writing, both Zetia and Vytorin are still on the market, but stay tuned — and if you are taking either one, be sure to check with your doctor for the latest update.

The possible side effects of single-ingredient niacin are as follows:

- ✔ Reduced effectiveness of diabetes medicines
- ✔ Reduced effectiveness of drugs used to treat gout (a form of arthritis)

> ✔ Reduced effectiveness of painkillers and anti-inflammatory drugs such as ibuprofen (Advil), naproxen (Naprosyn), and naproxen sodium (Aleve and Anaprox)
>
> ✔ Liver damage (high doses)
>
> ✔ Dizziness

Check earlier in this chapter for the side effects of statin drugs.

The word *niacin* is used interchangeably for two different chemical compounds, *nicotinic acid* and *nicotinamide* (also known as *niacinamide*). Nicotinic acid reduces levels of triglycerides. Nicotinamide does not. Also, the niacin sold as a dietary supplement (vitamin) isn't a substitute for prescription niacin, **a product whose use must be monitored by your doctor.**

Comparing the Benefits of Cholesterol-Buster Drugs

Assuming that you worked your way through all the paragraphs before this, you're now definitely an expert on the virtues of the various drugs your doctor may prescribe to lower your cholesterol. What? You didn't read every single word? Twice? Not to worry. Table 12-2 pretty much sums it all up as of Winter 2008.

The doses listed in Table 12-2 are the highest prescribed in one day. They are not the doses prescribed for every patient. In fact, your doctor may achieve satisfactory results — lower LDLs — with lower doses. **Do not change your dose of any of these medicines without your doctor's approval!**

Table 12-2	Comparing Cholesterol-Lowering Drugs		
Drug Class	*Generic Name*	*Brand Name*	*Max Drop in LDLs at Highest Daily Dose of This Medicine*
Statin	Rosuvastatin	Crestor	63% (40 mg)
Statin	Atorvastatin	Lipitor	60% (80 mg)
Statin	Fluvastatin	Lescol	36% (80 mg)
Statin	Lovastatin	Mevacor	42% (80 mg)
		Altocor+	41% (60 mg)

(continued)

Table 12-2 *(continued)*

Drug Class	Generic Name	Brand Name	Max Drop in LDLs at Highest Daily Dose of This Medicine
Statin	Pravastatin	Pravachol	37% (80 mg)
Statin	Simvastatin	Zocor	47% (80 mg)
Statin combination	Lovastatin/ nicotinic acid	Advicor	40%* (1,000mg/20 mg)
Statin combination	Atorvastatin/ amlodipine besylate	Caduet	50%# (80 mg/10mg)
Bile acid sequestrant	Cholestyramine	Prevalite, Questran	N/A
Bile acid sequestrant	Colesevelam	Welchol	18% (six 625 mg tablets)
Bile acid sequestrant	Colestipol	Colestid, Lestid	23% (five 1,000 mg/1 gm packets)
Triglyceride inhibitor	Fenofibrate	Tricor	20% (200 mg)
Triglyceride inhibitor	Gemfibrozil	Lopid	20% (1,200 mg)

+ Altocor is an extended-release form of lovastatin
*Estimate based on effect of lovastatin.
#Estimate based on effect of atorvastatin.
Sources: *Drug comparisons: HMG-COA Reductase Inhibitors,*
www.drugdigest.or/DD/Comparison/New Comparison/0,10621,37-15,00,
updated July 2007; Physicians' Desk Reference 2004, 58th ed. (Montvale, New Jersey: Thomson PDR, 2004); James J. Rybacki, Essential Guide to Prescription Drugs 2006 (New York: Collins, 2006); Allan Gaw, et.al., Effects of Colestipol Alone and in Combination With Simvastatin on Apolipoprotein B Metabolism, Arteriosclerosis, Thrombosis, and Vascular Biology. 1996;16:236-249; individual product Web sites.

Picking the Perfect Pill Candidate

Should you be using a cholesterol-lowering medicine? Maybe. One way to decide is to review the recommendations of the experts at the National Heart, Lung, and Blood Institute's Web site: www.nhlbi.nih.gov. The recommendations are contained in two reports:

✔ *The Third Report of the Expert Panel on Detection, Evaluation, and Treatment of High Blood Cholesterol in Adults* (Adult Treatment Panel III)

✔ ATP III Update 2004: *Implications of Recent Clinical Trials for the ATP III Guidelines*

To save time, ink, and the lives of all the trees that would otherwise be cut down to make the paper for the extra pages required to print that entire title over and over again, I've made an important decision. From now on, I refer to these reports by their nicknames: ATP III and ATP III Update. If you're absolutely committed to reading both reports in their mind-numbing entirety, feel free to visit www.nhlbi.nih.gov/guidelines/cholesterol/index.htm.

Meanwhile, I dance through the highlights:

✔ In the context of ATP III and ATP III Update, a *major risk factor* is diabetes, high blood pressure, high levels of LDLs, high levels of triglycerides, smoking, being older than 45 (men) or 55 (women), or having a family history of early heart disease (before 55 for your dad, before 55 for your mom).

✔ To estimate your risk of suffering a heart attack in the next ten years, click the interactive National Cholesterol Education Project (NCEP) Risk Assessment Tool for Estimating Your 10-Year Risk of Having a Heart Attack at http://hp2010.nhlbihin.net/atpiii/calculator.asp.

No computer handy? Zip over to the library computer, or check with your doctor.

Categorizing risk

ATP III divided Americans into four large categories based on their risk of heart disease. The categories are

✔ **High risk:** Known coronary artery disease and/or blocked arteries in the legs or brain, plus multiple major risk factors

✔ **Intermediate risk:** No known vascular disease, at least two major risk factors, and 10 to 20 percent risk of heart attack in the next ten years

✔ **Moderate risk:** No known vascular disease, at least two major risk factors

✔ **Low risk:** One or no major risk factors, less than 10 percent risk of heart attack in the next ten years

The ATP III Update revised the risk categories as follows

- ✔ **Very high risk:** Previous heart attack or stroke, plus several major risk factors
- ✔ **High risk:** Known coronary artery disease and/or blocked arteries in the legs or brain, plus multiple major risk factors
- ✔ **Moderately high risk:** No known vascular disease, at least two major risk factors
- ✔ **Moderate risk:** No known vascular disease, at least two major risk factors
- ✔ **Low risk:** One or no major risk factors, less than 10 percent risk of heart attack in the next ten years

As a result of this update, several million more Americans were now classified as being at high risk or very high risk, necessitating — you guessed it — more meds.

Recommending treatment

The treatment recommendations in both ATP III and ATP III Update are both based on the proposition that lowering a person's level of LDLs lowers her risk of heart attack. The difference lies in the decision about who needs to be treated and how low she needs to go.

ATP III's treatment recommendations were simple:

- ✔ The first line of defense in ATP III is diet. The report recommends that a whopping 65 million Americans change what they eat in order to lower their cholesterol.
- ✔ If changing the diet doesn't do the trick, the NHLBI recommends that an almost-equally-whopping 35 million Americans with a more than 20-percent risk of heart attack in the next ten years and/or an LDL level higher than 130 mg/dL begin drug treatment to push their LDLs down to 100 mg/dL.

The treatment recommendations in the ATP III Update are dramatically different:

- ✔ For people in the very high risk and high risk categories, the recommended level of LDLs was lowered to 70 mg/dL, a level virtually impossible to reach without drugs.
- ✔ If a very high-risk or high-risk person has high levels of triglycerides, a fibrate or nicotinic acid should be given along with a cholesterol-lowering med.

✔ The best option for moderately high-risk people is to aim for LDL levels less than 100 mg/dL. Any moderately high-risk person with LDL levels of more than 130 mg/dL plus major risk factors is a candidate for cholesterol-lowering drugs.

✔ Low-risk people don't have to take cholesterol-lowering drugs.

Seems like practically everyone you know is a candidate for cholesterol-buster meds. Not surprisingly, that conclusion hasn't been universally applauded.

Many critics note (correctly) that the ATP III Update pretty much ignores the benefits of lifestyle changes such as diet and exercise, while passing over studies showing virtually no benefits in giving cholesterol-lowering meds to older people. Others are distressed by the makeup of the ATP III Update panel: Eight of the nine panel members had financial ties to companies producing cholesterol-lowering drugs. Ooops.

As the debate simmers, will the ATP III Update recommendations become the norm? Maybe. Should you check with your own doctor before diving into drugs? You bet. Case closed.

Chapter 13

Identifying Meds That Raise Cholesterol

. . . .

In This Chapter

▶ Finding the facts on hormones and HDLs

▶ Discovering how diuretics affect blood fats

▶ Protecting statins

▶ Naming the problems with vasoconstrictors

. . . .

*B*elieve it or not, several common medications, such as *diuretics* (also known as water pills), work like a dream to cure or alleviate conditions they were designed to treat, such as swelling caused by water retention, but may send your "bad" cholesterol up, your "good" cholesterol down, and your triglycerides heaven-knows-where (see the section "Lowering Fluids with Diuretics" later in this chapter).

The following sections make up a representative list of medicines that may alter your cholesterol levels, sending some kinds of cholesterol up and others down. But hey, forewarned is forearmed.

Hankering for Hormones

In the past few decades, hormone products have become part of everyday life. The female sex hormones estrogen and progesterone are used for birth control, "morning after" pills, and postmenopausal hormone replacement therapy. Some athletes skirt the law by using steroids (male hormones) to build muscles. In each case, the use of hormones, like the ones listed in this section, can have unexpected effects on cholesterol levels.

Birth control pills

The most popular oral contraceptives (OCs) are a combination of the female hormones *estrogen* and *progestin* (a synthetic form of progesterone, the second female sex hormone). The less effective and thus less frequently used "mini-pill" is plain progestin.

Estrogen seems to be the more cholesterol-friendly female hormone. Estrogen lowers total cholesterol and boosts HDLs, the "good" cholesterol. But higher doses of progestins lower HDLs. You can read all about it for yourself in this quote from the package insert that comes with all OCs sold in the United States:

> *A positive association has been observed between the amount of estrogen and progestogen [another way to say "progestin"] in oral contraceptives and the risk of vascular disease. A decline in serum high-density lipoproteins had been reported with many progestational agents. Estrogens increase HDL cholesterol. The net effect of oral contraceptives depends on a balance achieved between doses of estrogen and progestogen. Most scientists now believe that the reason women on hormone replacement therapy had a higher incidence of heart attacks is because the therapy stimulates the clotting system, and since the first event in a heart attack is a clot forming in the coronary arteries, that is the reason for the increased number of heart attacks and not the effects of cholesterol.*

Hormone replacement therapy (HRT)

Now that researchers have proven the link between HRT and a higher risk of breast cancer and disproved the assumption that taking hormones after menopause lowers a woman's risk of heart disease, fewer women are using these pills.

For those who do — or for those women who take estrogen for a few weeks or months after a surgical menopause (translation: total hysterectomy that removes both the uterus and the ovaries) — I want to point out that estrogen does increase levels of HDLs. Wait. I already said that in the preceding section.

Table 13-1 lists the words used for "estrogen" or "progestin" on the labels for birth control pills and postmenopausal hormone-therapy products.

Table 13-1	Hormones in OCs and HRTs
Estrogens	*Progestins*
Estradiol	Ethynodial
Estrogens, conjugated	Hydroxyprogesterone

Estrogens	Progestins
Estrogens, esterfied	Medroxyprogesterone
Estropipate	Megestrol
	Norethindrone
	Norgestrel

Muscle builders

The male sex hormone testosterone promotes muscle mass, which is why the average man has bigger biceps than the average woman.

In medicine, *anabolic androgenic steroids* (muscle-building, testosterone-like compounds) are used legally to treat the results of abnormally low levels of testosterone, such as delayed male puberty, some forms of impotence, and the wasting of lean muscle mass associated with certain illnesses — AIDS being one of them.

Although these meds are banned from all legitimate athletic competition, some athletes use them secretly in an attempt to enhance performance. In the long run, it's a losing game. According to the National Institute on Drug Abuse (www.nida.nih.gov), steroid abuse — using the drugs to build muscles for athletic competition — comes with a full complement of horrible side effects, including liver tumors; liver cancer; yellowish pigmentation of skin, tissues, and body fluids; high blood pressure; kidney tumors; severe acne; trembling; shrunken testicles; infertility; increased risk of prostate cancer; male pattern baldness (in men and women) . . . no, no, I can't go on. This book is called *Controlling Cholesterol For Dummies,* not *Steroids For Dummies,* so I have to stick with the main event: Taking anabolic androgenic steroids raises LDLs and lowers HDLs. No gold medal there, guys.

Lowering Fluids with Diuretics

Diuretics are drugs that make you urinate more frequently, eliminating excess fluids from your body tissues. Some ingredients, such as caffeine, in over-the-counter (OTC) products have a diuretic effect, but the most effective diuretics are the ones available only by prescription.

Common prescription diuretics

Prescription diuretics may be either *single ingredient products* or *combination products*. The active ingredient in a single ingredient prescription diuretic is most commonly either furosemide, spironolactone, or a member of the thiazide drug family. Table 13-2 lists some well-known single ingredient prescription diuretics.

Table 13-2	Single Ingredient Prescription Diuretics	
Class of Diuretic	*Generic Name*	*Brand Name*
Thiazide	Bendroflumethiazide	Naturetin
	Chlorothiazide	Diachlor, Diuril
	Hydroflumethiazide	Diucardon
	Methyclothiazide	Aquatensen
Furosemide	Furosemide	Fumide-MD, Furose
		Lasimide, Lasix
Spironolactone	Spironolactone	Aldactone

The primary active ingredient in combination diuretic products is commonly a thiazide diuretic. The second active ingredient varies according to what the drug is designed to accomplish. This is done because diuretics make most blood-pressure-lowering drugs work better. For example:

- The active ingredients in Aldochlor are a thiazide diuretic (chlorothiazide) and methyldopa, a drug that lowers blood pressure by relaxing blood vessels.

- The active ingredients in Aldactazide are a thiazide diuretic (hydrochlorothiazide) and spironolactone, a drug that reduces the amount of the mineral potassium lost when you take a diuretic and urinate a lot (yes, your body eliminates potassium through urinating).

- The active ingredients in Lopressor HCT are a thiazide diuretic (hyrochlorothiazide) and metroprolol tartrate, a drug that helps control the rapidity and force of your heartbeat.

Diuretics and cholesterol levels

Taking either a thiazide or furosemide diuretic raises total cholesterol levels and levels of triglyerides (another blood fat described in Chapter 2). The increase, however, is believed to be small enough that it doesn't increase the risk of heart disease. Because diuretics are so valuable for controlling high blood pressure, your doctor can work with you to establish a diet that helps control your cholesterol while allowing you to continue taking the water pills.

Any medicine, prescription or over-the-counter, that causes you to lose too much water can have serious effects, like causing you to collapse from dehydration. That's why you should never use diuretics without the knowledge or consent of your own personal physician.

Sabotaging Cholesterol Therapy

Your cholesterol is on the high side, so your doctor prescribes a cholesterol-lowering statin drug, such as atorvastatin (Lipitor), pravastatin (Pravachol), or simvastatin (Zocor), or a statin combo drug, such as Vytorin. You take the pills right on schedule, but when your doctor tests your blood, your cholesterol level hasn't gone down. Why? One possibility is that you're taking a second medication that makes your statin less effective. Gee. Sometimes you can't win for losing.

Considering interactions between cholesterol and meds, I thought it important to mention statin interactions. But for more on how the other meds you take can affect a statin's ability to control your cholesterol, turn back to Chapter 12, which has absolutely everything you need to know about statins and other cholesterol-lowering drugs, including these pesky drug/drug interactions.

Narrowing Your Options

Having high cholesterol is risky because cholesterol particles in your bloodstream may snag on artery walls, catch other particles floating by, and build plaque deposits that block the artery, stop the normal flow of blood to your heart, and trigger a heart attack. Given this set of facts, you can understand why medicines that further narrow the blood vessels may be problematic for someone with high cholesterol or known coronary artery disease.

Drugs that make blood vessels constrict (narrow down) are called *vasoconstrictors*. Drugs that make blood vessels dilate (open wider) are called *vasodilators*. Vasoconstrictors raise your blood pressure and vasodilators lower it.

Vasoconstrictors are used in both prescription and OTC medicines, as you can see here:

- An example of a prescription vasoconstrictor product is the Epipen, a device that enables the patient to inject a dose of epinephrine.

- An example of an OTC vasoconstrictor product is a cold remedy, cough medicine, or anti-asthma product in which the vasoconstrictor functions as a *decongestant,* an ingredient that helps shrink swollen tissues in your nose and throat. Hemorrhoid relief products may also contain vasoconstrictors, but you apply them to your skin, so they're less likely to be problematic.

By the way, if you're still smoking, you should know that nicotine is a vasoconstrictor. For more about smoking and your cholesterol, check out Chapter 9.

Right now, take a look at Table 13-3, which contains a list of common decongestant ingredients from the *Physicians' Desk Reference 2001.* All these ingredients are vasoconstrictors, so if you have high cholesterol, you want to ask your doctor before using these products.

Table 13-3	Representative Vasoconstrictor Ingredients			
Ingredient	*Product Application*			
	Nasal	*Eye*	*Oral*	*Inhaler*
Epinephrine*	X	X		X
Naphazoline		X		
Oxymetazoline	X			
Phenylephrine	X		X	
Pseudoephedrine*			X	
Tetrahydrozaline		X	X	

*Epinephrine is also used as an injectible drug. Pseudoephedrine can be used to make the street drug known as "crystal meth." As a result, products containing these vasoconstrictors are still available without a prescription, but must be sold from behind the pharmacy counter rather than simply stacked on open drugstore shelves.

Getting the Last Word

Every drug can be valuable — heck, even lifesaving — when prescribed for the condition it's intended to treat and for a patient whose body tolerates the medicine. On the other hand, every drug has side effects. And sometimes a drug that works for one person is ineffective or downright dangerous for another person.

The trick is to maximize the benefits and minimize the risks. In other words, try to knock off the illness or medical condition without harming the patient. Doing that requires you and your doctor to work together. She by doing her homework so she knows what may go wrong; you by taking your meds as directed and reporting any problems immediately. And each of you needs to listen to one another. It's a hard job, but you can do it. So do it.

Chapter 14

Mouth-Watering Morsels for Special Occasions

From *Low-Cholesterol Cookbook For Dummies* by Molly Siple, MS, RD

In This Chapter

▶ Creating healthy munchies with satisfying flavor and crunch

▶ Trying some delicious heart-healthy recipes

*W*hen your doc gives you the good news that your cholesterol is under control, you have cause to celebrate. And even when you're still working toward lowering your cholesterol, special occasions abound. Unfortunately, party foods, by definition, are full of flavor and not short on fat. But missing your son's wedding, skipping out on your best friend's birthday party, or opting not to throw your annual holiday bash isn't an option.

The good news is that many of the foods recommended for heart health are already standard party fare. Nuts to nibble, avocado in guacamole, smoked salmon with capers, and olives of all sorts are green-light foods. Making sure they're healthy is just a matter of how you prepare them.

Think of cooking as an art rather than a science. The recipes in this chapter are guidelines; don't stress if you can't find the exact ingredients or if your measurements are just a bit off. Adding a little more or less of an ingredient won't ruin anything, and you just might end up creating something you like even better. The prep time estimates I give you include the time it takes to wash fruits and veggies under cold running water and to cut, assemble, and measure all ingredients. The temperature for all recipes is in Fahrenheit. Also note that the little tomato you see on the "tabs" in front of the recipe names indicate that the recipe is vegetarian.

In this chapter, you discover heart-healthy foods with crunch that haven't been deep-fried, and satisfying nibbles high in the right sort of fats. I give an assortment of quick and easy recipes for basic party offerings, including a vegetarian pâté and marinated olives. Presentation of food is also part of the drill. Read on to find all sorts of suggestions for creating scrumptious party offerings that meet your dietary needs.

If you love this chapter, check out *Low-Cholesterol Cookbook For Dummies* by Molly Siple, MS, RD (Wiley) for more great culinary tips and tempting recipes to help get your cholesterol under control.

Little Bites a Cardiologist Would Love

The hors d'oeuvres and little nibbles that meet the nutritional requirements of a cholesterol-lowering, heart-healthy diet are so numerous they would fill a buffet table. These morsels feature raw vegetables, fresh herbs, healthy fats, chicken, and fish. In addition, these foods are eaten in very small amounts, but many are so tasty that you'll be tempted to make a meal out of them.

Adding crunch to party fare

Healthy foods, perhaps because they're never deep-fried, often lack crunch, leaving you longing for the sound of crispy food and a satisfying chew. Party favorites like potato chips and tacos are full of crunch, while healthier foods, such as grains, nut butters, and vegetables, are quiet foods. The following gives you ways to combine the best of both worlds: the cholesterol-conscious and the crispy.

Crostini

Toast is crunchy, so how about starting with that and making some crostini, which means "little toasts" in Italian. Here's how to prepare crostini:

1. **Adjust the rack of a broiler so that it's at least 4 inches from the heat source and preheat the broiler.**

2. **Cut a slim baguette of French bread (about 2 inches in diameter and sold in specialty bakeries and upscale supermarkets) into thin slices and place on a large baking sheet.**

   Cut slices of bread on the diagonal for a stylish presentation.

3. **Brush the slices on one or both sides with a little olive oil and rub one or both sides with a halved clove of garlic.**

4. **Broil the bread so that one side is lightly toasted.**

5. **Turn the bread over and broil for a minute or two, making sure that the bread doesn't toast all the way through.**

Use crostini as a platform for other foods. Here are some suggested toppings:

- ✓ A smear of tapenade, an olive paste seasoned with capers, anchovies, garlic, and lemon juice and sold in jars

- ✓ Goat cheese mixed with fresh herbs, such as basil and parsley, and topped with a sliver of sun-dried tomato

- ✓ A spoonful of garlicky, mashed cannellini beans scented with oregano

Homemade baked tortilla chips

Instead of noshing on corn chips fried in who-knows-what kind of oil and loads of salt, enjoy the crunch of home-baked tortilla chips. Start with corn tortillas or whole-wheat tortillas, both made with whole grains, far healthier than white flour tortillas. Here's the procedure:

1. **Using a pastry brush, brush each side of a corn tortilla with unrefined safflower oil or lightly spray each side, using an oil sprayer filled with unrefined oil.**

   To give the chips a southwest flavor, sprinkle the oiled tortillas with ground cumin or chili powder.

2. **Stack the tortillas and cut them into 8 wedges, as you would a pie.**

3. **Place the wedges in a single layer on an ungreased baking sheet and bake in a preheated 400-degree oven, until they just begin to become golden, 10 to 12 minutes.**

Serve tortilla chips with a bean dip for a dose of soluble fiber. Or use guacamole, which is a great source of folate, or classic tomato salsa, which is full of healthy ingredients.

Doing the crudité dip

Eating raw vegetables at parties became chic when the veggies took on the name *crudité,* which is French for "raw." They are indeed refreshing, crispy, and full of all the vitamins and minerals nature gave them. But what do you do with all the bits of vegetable after you cut them? Choose one of the following ideas to bring order to the chaos:

- ✓ Start with sticks of carrot, celery, and seeded cucumber, and maybe some blanched asparagus or blanched string beans, and give each vegetable a separate container, such as glass tumblers, colorful ceramic mugs, or small flower vases. Cluster the containers on the serving table, creating a vegetable forest.

- ✓ Arrange vegetables on a long, rectangular platter or basket lined with kale, and give each vegetable its own row.

✔ Tuck raw vegetables between the leaves of a full head of Boston lettuce, following the instructions in the recipe, Crudité with Mango Salsa and Creamy Avocado Dip.

Figure on 1 cup of dip for every 20 guests. If you're serving chunky dips, you may need a bit more.

The fat of the matter: Acceptable appetizers

One of the great pleasures of party food is that it's full of hard-to-resist assertive flavors, in part because the food is also full of fat, a flavor carrier. Taking a holiday from diet restrictions, the most careful of eaters will graciously accept the hot cheese puffs and chocolate truffles being offered. But there's no reason you can't enjoy the feel of fat, even if you're watching your cholesterol. You have options.

Nuts and olives

Nuts and olives are two classic cocktail nibbles that are perfectly acceptable heart-healthy foods. In numerous studies, both nuts and olives, the basis of the famed Mediterranean diet, have been linked to a lower risk of heart disease. In addition, the monounsaturated and polyunsaturated fats in these foods help control cholesterol.

So which nuts have the most of these healthy fats and are low in the cholesterol-raising saturated kind? Here are a few that fit the bill:

✔ Almonds

✔ Filberts

✔ Pecans

✔ Pistachios

✔ Walnuts

One way to include nuts in a party menu is to add walnuts to hummus, pureeing them along with the other ingredients. The rich, mellow flavor of walnuts blends well with the flavors of the other ingredients, and walnuts add omega-3 fatty acids, making hummus even more nutritious. Here's how to make it: In a food processor, combine 2 cups chickpeas (one 15-ounce can), ½ cup walnuts, ½ cup tahini sesame paste, ¼ cup fresh lemon juice, and 1 clove garlic, plus water or oil to reach the desired consistency. Season with cumin and salt.

Cheeses

You can save on fat by eating lowfat and nonfat cheeses or having a soy cheese look-alike, but I can't promise you great flavor or texture in all cases. For instance, I'd rather have a shaving of world-class Parmigiano-Reggiano as a garnish for slices of pear topped with a paper-thin slice of prosciutto, than a large wedge of rubbery, nonfat mozzarella any day. But do sample some lowfat cheese and see what you think. For instance, lowfat ricotta can be very satisfying. If you want to cut back on fat intake and still eat cheese, modified products let you keep these creamy-tasting foods in your diet.

When shopping for cheese, be sure to read the label for content of total fat and saturated fat as well as cholesterol. The amounts present vary among producers. Cheeses such as Camembert, Brie, Roquefort, cheddar, and American processed cheese can contain more than 25 percent of your daily quota of saturated fat and about 10 percent of a day's worth of cholesterol. And these amounts are in just 1 ounce, which isn't very much, especially for a devoted cheese eater. Best to stay away from these unless you can stop after one nibble. Feta and mozzarella, the full-fat kind, are lower in fat and cholesterol and are better choices.

For the feel of fat on the tongue, use lowfat yogurt and lowfat sour cream, both very palatable, in your hors d'oeuvres.

Caviar

If any food says "special occasion," it's caviar. Caviar is salted fish eggs, so, just like chicken eggs, it's a whole food and a balanced source of nutrition. In addition, although fat contributes 61 percent of the calories, caviar, like fish, contains mostly the healthy monounsaturated and polyunsaturated kinds. Admittedly, caviar is high in sodium (containing 240 mg per tablespoon) and in cholesterol (containing 31.3 mg per teaspoon), but you're not likely to be eating a bowlful of caviar anyway.

I give you two ways of serving caviar that give you a smidgeon of this glamorous stuff. On a budget, use black lumpfish caviar, golden whitefish caviar, or salmon red caviar, all sold in little jars in supermarkets. Otherwise, invest in some American farm-raised caviar or the even pricier imported sevruga, osetra, or beluga caviar.

1. **Boil round, red potatoes, the smallest you can find, until they're cooked through and tender.**

2. **Peel the potatoes, slice in half crosswise, and cut some potato off the base of each half, so the potato is steady when placed on a plate.**

3. **Using a melon baller, cut into the flat surface of each potato half and scoop out a little bowl in the middle.**

4. **Fill the hollow of each potato with lowfat sour cream and sprinkle the sour cream with caviar.**

For this elegant hors d'oeuvre, caviar is displayed on pale chartreuse Belgium endive.

1. **Wash a head of Belgium endive and cut it at the base to separate leaves.**

2. **Using a teaspoon, place a small dollop of lowfat sour cream at the wider end of each leaf and then sprinkle caviar on the sour cream.**

3. **Garnish the caviar and sour cream with a tiny sprig of dill.**

4. **On a round serving platter, arrange these like spokes, with the narrow end of the leaf pointing out.**

Getting some help: Ready-made appetizers

I often serve canned stuffed grape leaves and no one is the wiser. My guests sometimes even ask for the recipe. You can find heart-healthy, ready-made appetizers in supermarkets or natural foods stores. Offer some of the following on their own or add them to a few of your own appetizers:

- Roasted sweet red peppers
- Marinated artichoke hearts
- Smoked salmon
- Sliced veggies from the salad bar, to serve as crudités with a dip
- Stuffed tortellini (serve it on skewers)
- Freeze-dried vegetable crunchies, such as corn, peas, red bell peppers, carrots, and tomatoes, produced with no added fat and sold in natural food stores
- Canned stuffed grape leaves

Tasty Recipes to Impress Your Guests

The recipes in this section are attractive to the eye, and you and your guests will likely count them among your favorites for regular snacking. The Citrus-Scented Marinated Olives, in particular, are known to be highly addictive!

Some of the following recipes are hearty and healthy enough to be served as a main course as well as party munchies. You can even turn the Mushroom Pâté into a pasta sauce, as I explain in the recipe introduction. Use this section as inspiration — take a look at your favorite heart-healthy meals to see whether you can serve any of them as hors d'oeuvres at your next gathering.

☙ *Cinnamon and Spice Almonds*

Almonds have more of the monounsaturated fats, the cornerstone of the heart-healthy Mediterranean diet, than any other nut. Scent them with spices, add some raisins, and you've created a healthy treat. The small amount of butter in this recipe imparts its inimitable flavor without adding much saturated fat. When nuts are toasted in this way, they don't absorb much of the cooking oils because they already contain a large amount of fat. Serve this snack with cocktails or after-dinner coffee.

Preparation time: *5 minutes*

Cooking time: *10 minutes*

Yield: *3 cups (24 servings)*

1 tablespoon butter	*1 tablespoon ginger*
1 tablespoon unrefined safflower oil	*1½ teaspoons nutmeg*
3 cups raw almonds	*1½ cups raisins*
1 tablespoon cinnamon	*Salt*

1 In a skillet over medium heat, melt the butter and combine with the oil.

2 Add the almonds and toss to coat with the oil. Sprinkle the almonds with the cinnamon, ginger, and nutmeg and toss to combine ingredients. Toast, stirring occasionally, for 5 minutes.

3 Add the raisins and continue to cook the almond mixture until the nuts begin to brown, an additional 2 to 3 minutes. Season to taste with salt. Make sure to cool the nuts completely before storing.

Per serving: *Calories 151 (From Fat 91); Fat 10g (Saturated 0g); Cholesterol 1mg; Sodium 26mg; Carbohydrate 12g (Dietary Fiber 3g); Protein 4g.*

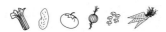

☝ Citrus-Scented Marinated Olives

Put one of these olives in your mouth, close your eyes, and you can taste summer in Provence! Let the Mediterranean flavors transport you. This recipe uses brine-cured olives, but if you want to cut back on salt, ordinary canned olives work fine as well. Use pitted ones so that more of the marinade can find its way into the olives. You can also marinate these olives in olive oil, but I use water here to cut back on calories and create a lighter taste.

Preparation time: *15 minutes, plus 3 days for the olives to marinate*

Marinade time: *3 days*

Yield: *3 cups olives (24 servings)*

1½ cups kalamata olives or other brine-cured olives	1 tablespoon grated orange peel
1½ cups cracked brine-cured green olives	1 tablespoon grated lemon peel
4 large cloves garlic, smashed	2 bay leaves
¼ cup orange juice	2 anchovies, minced, or 2 tablespoons anchovy paste
¼ cup fresh lemon juice	½ teaspoon dried thyme

1 Combine the olives, garlic, orange juice, lemon juice, orange peel, lemon peel, bay leaves, anchovies, and thyme in a glass jar with a tight-fitting lid.

2 Add enough water to the citrus marinade to cover the olives.

3 Seal the jar with the lid and shake the jar several times to distribute and combine the ingredients.

4 Refrigerate the olives for 3 days, shaking the jar once each day to keep the marinade well mixed.

Go-With: *Serve the olives with goat cheese and a baguette of French bread.*

Per serving: *Calories 44 (From Fat 36); Fat 4g (Saturated 0g); Cholesterol 0mg; Sodium 431mg; Carbohydrate 3g (Dietary Fiber 0g); Protein 0g.*

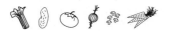

Skewered Scallop Seviche with Avocado

Seviche, popular in Latin America, is raw fish that has been marinated in citrus juice, usually lime. The acid in the fruit "cooks" the fish. Any white-fleshed fish or scallops can be prepared this way. Shellfish has a reputation for being high in cholesterol, but a serving of 4 skewers of these scallops contains only 16 mg of cholesterol.

Special tools: *36 bamboo skewers, 6 inches long*

Preparation time: *20 minutes, plus 4 hours marinating time*

Yield: *9 servings (about 4 skewers each)*

1½ cups fresh lime juice, or enough to cover the scallops

4 sprigs cilantro, stems removed and minced

1 tablespoon minced red onion

1 clove garlic, crushed and minced

½ pound tiny bay scallops, about 70, perfectly fresh

1 box (8 ounces) cherry tomatoes, washed

2 avocados

Salt and pepper

1 In a shallow 8-inch square baking dish, combine the juice, cilantro, onion, and garlic.

2 Rinse the scallops. If necessary, remove the tough, stark white hinge that attaches the scallop to the shell. Place the scallops in the lime juice marinade. Cover and refrigerate a minimum of 4 hours, or overnight. The scallops are "cooked" when they're opaque.

3 Cut each tomato in half crosswise. Peel and remove the seed of the avocados and cut them into ¾-inch cubes. The cubes need to be substantial enough so that they don't fall off the skewer. Drain the seviche and season to taste with salt and pepper.

4 Assemble the skewers by threading the components in this order: 1 scallop, 1 cube avocado, 1 scallop, and 1 cherry tomato half. Run the skewer through the center of the face of the tomato where it was cut and then out the top through the skin, so the tomato becomes a cap on the other foods.

5 On a round platter, arrange the skewers of seviche like spokes of a wheel, with the tomato caps at the center. Or use a horizontal tray and place the skewers in a row with the food colors forming stripes.

Per serving: *Calories 31 (From Fat 14); Fat 2g (Saturated 0g); Cholesterol 4mg; Sodium 54mg; Carbohydrate 2g (Dietary Fiber 1g); Protein 3g.*

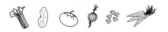

☉ Crudités with Mango Salsa and Creamy Avocado Dip

The inspiration for this recipe is a delicious combo dip I buy ready-made, a container with a layer of fresh guacamole topped with a layer of mango salsa. The combination of smooth and spicy is just right. The Creamy Avocado Dip included here is full of healthy monounsaturated fats and is high in folic acid, while the Mango Salsa gives you an effortless way to increase your fruit intake. For the crudités, try using only green and white vegetables, like I suggest here, for a designy, high-style look.

Preparation time: _20 minutes_

Yield: _20 servings_

1 head Boston lettuce, with the outside leaves still intact (see the tip at the end of the recipe)

1 large turnip

2 dozen slim spears of asparagus, trimmed and blanched

1 head endive, leaves separated and washed

1 cucumber, peeled, seeds removed, and sliced into spears

_1_ Taking the base of a head of Boston lettuce in one hand, gently open the leaves of the lettuce with the other hand, wiggling your fingers down between the leaves. (If the lettuce is sandy, submerge the opened head in a sink filled with water and briefly swish to loosen dirt. Drain upside down in an empty dish rack before proceeding.)

_2_ Meanwhile, peel the turnip and cut in ¼-inch rounds. Picture the turnip slice as the earth and cut a small V-shaped wedge at the North Pole and South Pole. Also make two V-shaped wedges at each end of the "equator."

_3_ Bring about an inch of water to boil in a skillet and add the asparagus. Cook until the asparagus is bright green and al dente, about 2 minutes. Remove with tongs, and submerge the asparagus spears in a bowl of cold water until they reach room temperature.

_4_ Tuck the turnip slices, asparagus, endive leaves, and cucumber between the lettuce leaves. Serve with the Mango Salsa and Creamy Avocado Dip.

Vary It! _If you decide your crudité composition is begging for more color, add carrot sticks._

Tip: _If the Boston lettuce on display has had the outside leaves removed, ask the produce manager where you shop to bring you a full and untrimmed head from the cartons of produce stored in the back._

Per serving: _Calories 8 (From Fat 1); Fat 0g (Saturated 0g); Cholesterol 0mg; Sodium 8mg; Carbohydrate 2g (Dietary Fiber 1g); Protein 1g._

Mango Salsa

This recipes lives and dies on whether the mango is sweet with a smooth texture, so chose your mango with care. When ripe, a mango yields to gentle pressure like a ripe avocado, and the stem end has a gentle aroma. Choose plump mangos, avoiding those with bruised or shriveled skin. This nonfat mix of healing fruits and vegetables also goes great with chicken and fish.

Preparation time: 15 minutes

Yield: About 3 cups (60 servings)

1 ripe mango, diced into ¼-inch pieces

1 cup sweet red pepper, cut into ¼-inch pieces

2 tablespoons minced red onion

1 fresh jalapeño chile, or to taste, seeded and minced

1 tablespoon minced cilantro

2 tablespoons lime juice (juice of 1 lime)

Salt

1 Put the mango, sweet red pepper, onion, chile, cilantro, and lime juice in a mixing bowl. Toss gently to combine the ingredients.

2 Season to taste with salt and serve immediately.

Per serving: Calories 16 (From Fat 9); Fat 1g (Saturated 0g); Cholesterol 0mg; Sodium 20mg; Carbohydrate 2g (Dietary Fiber 1g); Protein 0g.

Creamy Avocado Dip

Sour cream dips have just the right tartness to complement the sweetness of fresh, raw vegetables. Cut the saturated fat of the cream by making the dip with lowfat or nonfat sour cream, and as in this recipe, substituting some of the sour cream with avocado to add healthier fats.

Special tool: Food processor

Preparation time: 15 minutes

Yield: About 1½ cups (30 servings)

1 cup nonfat sour cream

¼ teaspoon ground cumin

1 avocado, peeled and cut into chunks

1 small clove garlic, minced

1 tablespoon chopped, fresh cilantro leaves (3 sprigs), plus extra for garnish

Salt and pepper

1 Put the sour cream in a food processor fitted with a metal blade.

2 Add the cumin to the sour cream in the processor, and then add the avocado, garlic, and cilantro. Process until smooth, scraping down the side of the processor bowl if necessary to incorporate all the ingredients.

3 Season to taste with salt and pepper. Transfer the dip to a small serving bowl and garnish with chopped cilantro. Serve immediately. (The dip can also be prepared earlier the same day you plan to serve it. Press plastic wrap onto the surface of the dip so that no air comes in contact with the avocado in the dip to keep it from turning brown. Refrigerate until ready to serve and add the cilantro garnish right before serving.)

Per serving: Calories 19 (From Fat 9); Fat 1g (Saturated 0g); Cholesterol 1mg; Sodium 31mg; Carbohydrate 2g (Dietary Fiber 0g); Protein 0g.

☞ Mushroom Pâté

With its hearty texture, rich brown hues, and a dash of sherry, this vegetarian mushroom pâté is much more than a passable substitute for the regular pork and liver versions. Instead, cashews are added as a source of oils. This pâté is such a winner that I experimented thinning it with a little white wine and making it into a pestolike pasta sauce, served with penne. It worked!

Special tool: *Food processor*

Preparation time: *30 minutes, plus 4 hours chilling time*

Cooking time: *20 minutes*

Yield: *12 to 15 servings of 2 tablespoons each*

5 tablespoons unrefined safflower oil

2 large shallots, chopped (½ cup)

2 cloves garlic, crushed and chopped

1¼ pounds fresh shiitake mushrooms, stemmed and coarsely chopped

1 cup roasted salted cashews

1 tablespoon finely chopped fresh basil

1 tablespoon finely chopped fresh parsley, plus sprigs for garnish

2 tablespoons sherry

Salt and pepper

1 In a large, heavy skillet over medium heat, heat 4 tablespoons of the oil and add the shallots, garlic, and mushrooms. Cook until the mixture begins to brown and all the liquid evaporates, stirring frequently, 15 to 20 minutes, depending on the moisture content of the mushrooms. Remove the skillet from the heat.

2 In a food processor fitted with a metal blade, chop the cashews until they have a fine texture. Add the remaining 1 tablespoon oil and continue to process to make a coarse paste.

3 Add the mushroom mixture, basil, parsley, and sherry. Pulse the processor on and off until the pâté has a coarse texture. Season to taste with the salt and pepper.

4 Transfer the mushroom pâté to a small ceramic loaf pan, or a bowl lined with plastic wrap so you can easily pop out the pâté. Cover and chill 4 hours. Serve in the loaf pan, or turn the pâté out of the bowl and garnish with sprigs of parsley. Enjoy on crostini.

Per serving: *Calories 85 (From Fat 66); Fat 7g (Saturated 1g); Cholesterol 0mg; Sodium 50mg; Carbohydrate 4g (Dietary Fiber 1g); Protein 2g.*

Part V
The Part of Tens

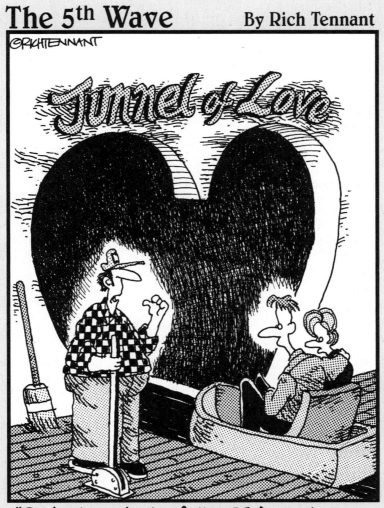

The 5th Wave   By Rich Tennant

"Be just a minute, folks. We've got some LDL clogging up the passages. Once we get them unclogged, you'll be on your way."

In this part . . .

*W*ell, here you are. You've reached the place that helps make a *For Dummies* book a *For Dummies* book. Personally, I'm nuts about lists. I have lists of things to do today, tomorrow, and next week; I have grocery lists, telephone lists, and, well, you get the picture. But if you don't get the picture, just flip through the following pages, and you soon will. I've put together four chapters that contain really useful lists for controlling cholesterol. If my editor hadn't said, "Stop!" there would have been more. What can I say? I tried.

Chapter 15

Ten Clicks to Reliable Cholesterol Information

*R*ules are made to be broken, so this Part of Tens is actually a Part of Seventeens (which is to say, 11 entries with 17 different links to cholesterol info). The plain fact is that the Internet has too many ultra-good, cholesterol-centered Web sites for me to whittle them all down to a measly list of ten. Enjoy the bonus sites listed here, as well as the other cholesterol info sites scattered throughout the chapters in this book.

Keep two things in mind when surfing the medical Web:

1. Be cautious. Absolutely anyone can dream up a Web page, so you're not always guaranteed accurate information. When choosing among sources, exercise good judgment. Look for a reputable name and reasonable advice, not pie-in-the-sky (even if it's a low-fat and cholesterol-free pie) recommendations. The sites listed in this chapter meet those guidelines. So click to your heart's content. Or rather, to its health.

2. Things change on the Web, more quickly and more often than you may expect. If you can't find a site listed here or if when you do find it, the contents don't match the listing, just go with the flow. After all, the new stuff may be even better than the last round.

The American Heart Association

www.cholesterollowdown.org

You can also reach the American Heart Association's Cholesterol Low Down by calling up the basic AHA site (www.amheart.org), clicking on the site map, and scrolling to Cholesterol Low Down under Healthy Life Style. Or, as with other big sites that have smaller sections on cholesterol, you can get where you're going by clicking on the address above.

The Cholesterol Low Down is the American Heart Association's national cholesterol education program whose primary aims are to urge us all to see the doctor, determine our cholesterol numbers, and set out on a five-step plan for long-term heart health. Accordingly, this page has five buttons to click: Getting Started, Adjust Your Diet, Get Active, Check Your Progress, and Keep it Up (and Down).

Each button leads to a well-designed page with concise directions. For example, click Adjust Your Diet and you get a page pointing you toward subsections such as Eating to Lower Your Cholesterol, How to Shop, Fat Facts, and (goody!) Recipe of the Month. All in all, this information is pretty much the kind of solid info you've come to expect from people who spend their professional lives worrying about your heart.

Brand Name Cholesterol-Lowering Drugs

www.caduet.com

www.crestor.com

www.lipitor.com

www.pravachol.com

www.vytorin.com

www.zocor.com

You've got questions. These sites have answers about the medical drugs most frequently prescribed for lowering cholesterol. The general format includes information similar to that found on other sites. The hot stuff on these is the occasional offer of a free course of the med via a coupon you take to your doctor who writes a prescription that you hand to the pharmacist. What? You thought they were going to send it through the mail?

Of course, you can also access online information about these drugs by typing their generic names into the search box of any search engine. Table 15-1 lists brand-name drugs and their generic equivalents.

Table 15-1	Brand Name/Generic Anti-Cholesterol Drugs
Brand Name	*Generic Name*
Caduet	Amlodipine and atorvastatin
Crestor	Rosuvastatin
Lipitor	Atorvastatin
Pravachol	Pravastatin
Vytorin	Ezetimibe and simvastatin
Zetia	Ezetimibe
Zocor	Simvastatin

Center for Drug Evaluation and Research

www.fda.gov/cder/drug/default.htm

As its Web address indicates, the Center for Drug Evaluation and Research (CDER) is a division of the Food and Drug Administration (FDA). The CDER Web site offers valuable information and evaluations of drug products, including those used to lower cholesterol levels.

For another path to cholesterol-specific medications, you can go to the main FDA homepage at www.fda.gov and type **cholesterol-lowering drugs** in the search box. You get millions of documents and pages of articles on everything even faintly linked to these medicines. The site is pure heaven for hypochondriacs. No, no, I didn't mean you!

Centers for Disease Control and Prevention (CDC)

www.cdc.gov/cholesterol

You can go to the homepage for the CDC (www.cdc.gov) and try to maneuver your way through to the page devoted to cholesterol, a workout in itself. Or you can simply go right to the cholesterol page with the address above. Me? I chose the second path. But then, I get my workout on a balance board every day, so who needs all that extra clicking? Either way, the CDC cholesterol page gives you what this agency is famous for — facts, statistics, and prevention strategies. And, of course, the latest news and press releases. Neat.

The Mayo Clinic

www.mayohealth.org

When it comes to consumer-health communications, the Mayo Clinic is true blue, just as cozy and user-friendly as all get out. I typed **cholesterol** into the search box and up popped more than 200 essays on cholesterol. Most relevant? The first 50, from High Blood Cholesterol to Heart Attack.

For people fuzzy about cholesterol facts, the Mayo Clinic's absolute claim to fame, on exhibit here, is its intelligent, balanced, and easily accessible presentation of serious technical stuff. Not to mention its sly (maybe unintentional) sense of medical humor. For example, did I mention that in its list of cholesterol-related essays the Mayo Clinic lists "Heart attack" right after "Erectile Dysfunction: A sign of heart disease?" Hmmmmm.

MedicineNet.com

www.medicinenet.com

MedicineNet.com — don't you just love the spiffy capital *N* right there in the middle? — is a doctor-owned, doctor-maintained Web site with a newsy point of view. Medical info junkies may browse through all the topics or choose the cholesterol-specific info, which dishes up a tasty smorgasbord of cholesterol bits and bytes.

When I typed **cholesterol** into the search bar, I got back a list of more than 1,000 cholesterol-related articles on

- ✔ Diseases and conditions
- ✔ Health and living
- ✔ Ask the experts
- ✔ Medications
- ✔ Procedures and tests
- ✔ Health news

I also received general tips for living well while controlling my cholesterol. Frankly, I figure if you read them all, you can wave good-bye to your doctor and hang up your own shingle to treat your own cholesterol conditions. Just kidding.

MedlinePlus.com

`www.nlm.nih.gov/medlineplus/cholesterol.html`

MedlinePlus is a service of the National Library of Medicine and the National Institutes of Health. Right there on the homepage is an alphabet that gives you access to absolutely tons of information about practically any medical subject that crosses your mind. You can access cholesterol information directly with the address above, or you can go to the homepage at — what else? — `http://medlineplus.gov`, click C, and then pick your way through to Cholesterol.

Either way, you get to look at Basics, Research, Overviews, Latest News, Diagnosis/Symptoms, Treatment, Prevention/Screening, Alternative Therapy, Nutrition, Disease Management, and Specific Management. But, as Thomas P. "Tip" O'Neill, one-time Speaker of the U.S. House of Representatives used to say, "All politics is local." The same goes for cholesterol: If yours is worrisome, you want help right in your hometown. So my favorite click on this site is the one labeled Go Local. Click here, choose one of the 19 states listed either from a drop-down list or an interactive map, and you can wander through resources as far as the eye can see — or the typing finger takes you. The only complaint: How come they don't list all 50 states? For now, the simple answer is, what you see is what you get. But check back later: And, no, I have no answer right now.

National Cholesterol Education Program

www.nhlbi.nih.gov/about/ncep/index.htm

www.nhlbi.nih.gov/guidelines/cholesterol/index.htm

The National Heart, Lung, and Blood Institute (NHLBI) launched the National Cholesterol Education Program (NCEP) in November 1985 with a goal of reducing illness and death from coronary heart disease (CHD) in the United States by reducing the percent of Americans with high blood cholesterol.

Through educational efforts directed at health professionals and the public, the NCEP aims to raise awareness and understanding about high blood cholesterol as a risk factor for CHD and the benefits of lowering cholesterol levels as a means of preventing CHD.

The first Web site listed above takes you directly to NCEP. The second provides access directly to the latest cholesterol guidelines:

- The executive summary of the 2001 *Third Report of the Expert Panel on Detection, Evaluation, and Treatment of High Blood Cholesterol in Adults,* also known as Adult Treatment Panel III (or ATP III for short)
- The full ATP III
- The ATP III Update 2004: *Implications of Recent Clinical Trials for the ATP III Guidelines*

These reports are widely considered the official word on cholesterol evaluation and treatment for most high-powered health groups, such as the American Heart Association — and for your doctor, too. (For a dissenting view to the ATP III Update, check out Chapter 12.)

Other goodies on this second site include information about cholesterol-lowering drugs and conditions that may increase the risk of elevated cholesterol levels. The "fun part" is an interactive calculator that enables you to predict your ten-year risk of heart attack based on your cholesterol level and other personal risk factors.

National Heart, Lung, and Blood Institute

www.nhlbi.nih.gov

You got a taste of NHLBI from the first list of Web sites in this chapter that sent you to ATP III. Now, open up the door to a ton of statistics and snippets of health information about (what else?) your heart, your lungs, and your blood.

Before you leave this site, take note of something special: a link to studies seeking patients. Before a new medicine or treatment method is approved by the Food and Drug Administration, there must be proof that it's "safe and efficacious." (Translation: It won't kill you, and it does work.)

Much of the required proof comes from government-sponsored trials. To find out more about trials currently in progress, run your mouse over to the left side of the page to the headline Clinical Trials, then go down one line, and click NHLBI Studies Conducted at NIH in Bethesda, MD, to pull up various ongoing studies. Check this out to see if you want to join a trial to assess the potential of a new treatment program.

Stedman's Online Medical Dictionary

www.stedmans.com/section.cfm/45

Listen, making your way through medical terms, including the various forms of cholesterol, can be a daunting task. Stedman's is the *ne plus ultra* (Latin for, "nothing better than this") medical look-up book. On this version, you can type in a whole word, search by the first two letters of the word, or search backwards, meaning you can type in a keyword or definition and get the exact word you're looking for. So do it!

WebMD

www.webmd.com

This site is just terrific. Go to the homepage, type **cholesterol** into the search box, click Enter, and there's no end to the things you can discover.

The medical experts who run this site keep adding information on cholesterol guidelines, cholesterol-lowering drugs, and cholesterol-control diets. You name it, and it's here. Best of all, the material is accessible, reliable, and . . . well, you fill in whatever good word comes to mind.

Chapter 16

Ten Nutrition Web Sites

A s with every other list of Web sites I've compiled for my *For Dummies* books (*Nutrition For Dummies* and *Weight Loss Kit For Dummies,* Wiley Publishing, Inc.), if my editors had made this section the Part of 100s, I could have easily met the goal.

When you're looking for reliable nutrition guidelines and information, the ten Web sites listed in this chapter are the cream of the crop, or better yet, the highest-grade skim milk. Each of the sites is an old friend I've come to lean on. Each has something special to offer. If I've missed your particular favorite, or you find a site that you think is especially useful, don't hesitate to let me know, perhaps for inclusion in the next edition of this book. Just e-mail the info to www.dummies.com/register.

In the meantime, eat well and, as the song says, be happy.

Watch out for curves on the information superhighway. For reasons known only to their webmasters, even successful Web sites are susceptible to change without notice. What was there last week can disappear into some parallel Internet universe, never to be found again. If the appearance of a site listed in this book changes, just snoop around the site a bit for the info you need. If the site disappears altogether, try looking up key words, such as **USDA** or **cholesterol**, via a universal search engine like www.google.com.

The American Cancer Society

www.cancer.org

Yes, the American Cancer Society (ACS) Web site is dedicated primarily to information about cancer: definitions, treatments, research, and support services. Yes, most of the nutrition news you find here is available elsewhere. But this site's defined focus provides easy access to other cancer-related topics.

Even, yes, again, cholesterol. Try it: Type **cholesterol** into the search bar on the ACS homepage, and bingo! You've opened a grab bag of ACS information about cholesterol's effect on your body and your risk of various kinds of cancer.

Until now, the ACS was barely a blip on the screen of nutrition sources. Today, with a growing number of well-designed studies to demonstrate that some foods and diet regimens — not to mention some drugs, such as those used to lower cholesterol — may affect your risk of certain types of cancer, the ACS Web site offers solid reporting on this area of nutritional research.

American Council on Science and Health, and the Center for Science in the Public Interest

www.acsh.org

www.cspinet.org

This two-for-one special gives you nonprofit, consumer-friendly organizations whose Web sites provide news releases, position papers, and highly reliable information about nutrition issues and your health.

Your bonus is that the American Council on Science and Health (ACSH) and the Center for Science in the Public Interest (CSPI) are usually on opposite sides of any nutritional issue. For example, the CSPI spearheaded the drive against the fat substitute Olestra, while the ACSH contended that the substitute was useful in some foods for some people. This kind of disagreement ensures that typing in the same search word or phrase, such as **low cholesterol,** on both sites provides you with the pros *and* cons associated with that topic.

Neither site is overly fancy. But both provide straight talk on specific issues, such as which fast foods have the most artery-clogging trans fatty acids (boo) and the least saturated fats (yea) or why tobacco is bad for you (maybe the only subject on which these guys agree).

The sites also feature online membership enrollment and order forms for publications, like the list-filled *Nutrition Action Healthletter* from the CSPI or the well-sourced and footnoted reports from the ACSH. The ACSH site takes on a cool and calm personality, while the CSPI resembles a hot-button advocate. In practice, both are solid and respectable as all get out.

The American Dietetic Association

www.eatright.org

The American Dietetic Association (ADA), which shares initials with the American Diabetes Association, is the world's largest membership association of nutrition professionals. Its Web site is jam-packed with food and diet tips, guidelines, research, policies, and stats.

The ADA homepage displays seven bright green boxes, each labeled with a subject. Food & Nutrition Information has diet tips. Shop Online is a guide to ADA publications. Media is fun if you're addicted to press releases. Careers & Students, Conferences & Events, Advocacy & the Profession, and Professional Development are clearly for association members.

The most useful choice for folks trying to figure out exactly how to create a cholesterol-busting meal plan may be the button up and to the right that says Find a Nutrition Professional. Click that link, and you get a page asking you to accept the Association's conditions. Say yes, and you move on to a page where more clicks get you info explaining how to find a dietitian in your area.

If you can bend your brain around the much-too-adorable Net address (Eatright? Give me a break!), this site is a true treasure. And golly gee, who wouldn't love having a personal dietitian to lead the way through the maze of conflicting fat and cholesterol directives?

The American Heart Association

www.americanheart.org

The American Heart Association (AHA) site is a must-see on any cholesterol tour of the Web. True, most of the info here is geared to reducing the obesity-related risks of heart disease. However, the AHA also dishes up solid advice for anyone looking for basic nutritional information and the lowdown on cholesterol. But boy oh boy, do they make you work to get to it! The multiple clicks will give your clicking finger a charley horse — but your brain (and you heart, of course) will appreciate the exercise.

For example, the homepage has 18 subjects you can investigate, ranging from Heart Attack/Stroke Warning Signs at the top to Local Info at the bottom. Click on Healthy Lifestyle (in the middle of the column), and you get several more choices. Pick Diet & Nutrition, and you receive the following six options:

- ✔ Dietary Recommendations
- ✔ No-Fad Diet
- ✔ Nutrition Facts
- ✔ Smart Shopping
- ✔ Delicious Decisions
- ✔ Face the Fats

I'm not saying this isn't all good stuff. I'm just saying, I'm exhausted. The best bet is simply to noodle around the site.

The Food Allergy & Anaphylaxis Network

www.foodallergy.org

The Food Allergy & Anaphylaxis Network (FAAN) is a nonprofit, membership organization (individuals can join for $30 per year) whose participants include families, doctors, dietitians, nurses, support groups, and food manufacturers in the United States, Canada, and Europe. The group provides education about food allergies, as well as support and coping strategies for people who are allergic to specific foods. The site's best feature, an e-mail allergy-alert system, is free.

Open the FAAN homepage, and you can easily log on to updates, daily tips, newsletter excerpts, and all the usual service-oriented goodies. To start receiving allergy alerts, click on the Special Allergy Alerts link, fill out the electronic form, and zap it off. Performing this quick task connects you to an early-warning system of allergy-linked news and information about product recalls, such as a July 2007 recall of dark chocolate bars whose label didn't list milk, a potential allergen. This no-nonsense, highly accessible site can help you avoid such incidents.

The Food and Drug Administration

www.fda.gov

Entering the FDA Web site is like opening the door to the world's biggest toy store. The virtual shelves contain so much stuff that you hardly know what to grab first. Luckily, all the toys are free in this store. You can linger here happily for days (weeks, years, or maybe forever) following the maze of cross-references and sources.

As you can see by its name, the first concern of the Food and Drug Administration is what you eat. Yes, the homepage offers information about medicines for people and pets, poisons and their side effects, medical devices (think pacemaker), and FDA field operations (rules and regulations enforcement). They even have a place to report an adverse event ("I took that antibiotic and got hives!"). But for foodies, food is the main event.

To access the food part of the site:

1. **Go to the homepage.**

2. **Click Food in the column on the left side of the page.**

   Say, "Wow!" What you get is access to a page for the Center for Food Safety and Applied Nutrition. Say, "Wow!" again because this covers everything. And I mean everything.

3. **Now, browse to your heart's content.**

Food and Nutrition Information Center

www.nal.usda.gov/fnic

The Food and Nutrition Information Center (FNIC) houses one of several nutrition-related data collections in the U.S. Department of Agriculture's National Agricultural Library. Like the basic Food and Drug Administration (FDA) Web site (see the preceding section), the FNIC site is chock-full of facts. You can dive in and swim around for hours without coming up for air.

But getting to exactly the info nugget you need can take a couple of clicks. Be patient, it's worth it. After you get to the homepage, find the link to the resources list. Click on it to bring up a long list of possibilities.

Browse as you please, but click the nutrition and cardiovascular diseases link when you're ready to fight cholesterol. Up pops a list of, well, *resources:* books, cookbooks, magazines, and newsletters, all dedicated to teaching you how to plan a diet that lowers your cholesterol and reduces your risk of heart disease. Click on the items that look interesting. Now wasn't that worth the clicks?

The U.S. Department of Agriculture Nutrient Database

www.nal.usda.gov/fnic/cgi-bin/nut_search.pl

The U.S. Department of Agriculture Nutrient Database is the ultimate nutrition chart. Cholesterol, calories, vitamins — you name it, and this site measures it.

The simple fact is that you just can't plan a low-cholesterol, controlled-fat diet (or any other diet for that matter) without this chart, which serves up nutrition data on more than 5,000 foods and breaks the information down according to different sizes, portions, and different methods of preparation (boiled, broiled, fried, dried, and so on).

Each entry on the list is a snapshot of a specific food serving ("raw apple with skin," for example) that shows how much the serving weighs and how much of these it contains:

- Calcium
- Carbohydrates
- Cholesterol
- Dietary fiber
- Fat
- Folate
- Food energy (calories)
- Iron
- Magnesium
- Niacin
- Phosphorus
- Potassium

✔ Protein

✔ Riboflavin (vitamin B2)

✔ Saturated, monounsaturated, and polyunsaturated fat

✔ Sodium

✔ Thiamin (vitamin B1)

✔ Vitamin A

✔ Vitamin B6

✔ Vitamin B12

✔ Vitamin C

✔ Water (as a percentage of the serving's weight)

Here's how to find the food you're looking for:

1. **Type its name into the empty search box and then press Enter.**

   For example, **apple.**

2. **Ignore the fancy stuff. Scroll down and click something basic.**

   Up comes a list of possibilities such as "Baby food, juice, apple and grape" or "Baby food, apples and turkey, strained." In this case, clicking "Apples, raw, with skin" brings up a new screen listing various forms of raw apples such as "100 grams edible portion" or "1 cup, quartered or chopped" or "1 large (3¼" diameter) (approx 2 per pound)."

3. **Click the box in front of the serving you prefer and click the Submit button.**

   There you are — calories and nutrients for one large apple, including cholesterol, dietary fiber, and the different kinds of fats.

The Weight Control Information Network

`www.niddk.nih.gov/health/nutrit/win.htm`

Weight control is an important path to controlling cholesterol, so the Weight Control Information Network (WIN) site belongs on your must-see list. The homepage for this site, which is maintained by the National Institutes of Health (NIH) and the National Institute of Diabetes and Digestive and Kidney Diseases (NIDDK), gives you access to a database with articles, books, and audiovisual material related to weight loss, plus a wealth of statistics on weight and weight maintenance, and NIH research studies.

In fact, the list of information is so complete you could lose weight just lifting it.

Chapter 17

Ten Cholesterol Myths

. . . .

In This Chapter
▶ Quantifying cholesterol's risks for women and kids
▶ Fooling around with fiber facts
▶ Getting it right on red meat
▶ Fighting cholesterol with Woody Allen and the Duchess of Windsor

. . . .

*I*n the words of the queen in Lewis Carroll's classic tale, *Alice's Adventures in Wonderland,* "I've believed as many as six impossible things before breakfast." Who hasn't?

For example, everyone *knows* that (a) chocolate is bad for your heart, (b) margarine is better than butter, and (c) women don't need to worry about cholesterol. Except (a) it isn't, (b) it isn't, and (c) I'm getting ahead of myself. In short, this chapter uncovers the truth hiding behind several common misperceptions about cholesterol.

Most of the Cholesterol in Your Body Comes from Food

Yes, you get some cholesterol from food, but the surprising fact is that most of the waxy material floating through your bloodstream is made right in your very own body. Your liver processes the proteins, fats, and carbs you eat to churn out about 1 gram (1,000 milligrams) of cholesterol every day.

Your body uses a lot of this homemade cholesterol to perform various functions such as enabling your brain cells to shoot messages back and forth. (Check out Chapter 2 for the other uses.) But when you bring in additional cholesterol from food, trouble may loom.

To keep your cholesterol level within healthy bounds, the *Dietary Guidelines for Americans,* from our good friends at the U.S. Department of Agriculture (USDA) and the U.S. Department of Health and Human Services (HHS), recommend that you consume no more than 300 milligrams of cholesterol a day from food.

But here's a surprise: Overall, the total amount of fat and saturated fat in your diet now seems to be more important than the amount of cholesterol in the foods you eat in determining your cholesterol level. Which leads me nicely into the very next myth.

All Fatty Foods Raise Your Cholesterol

Wrong. Why? Because — here comes some good info — all dietary fats are not alike. The difference lies in *saturation,* the number of hydrogen atoms attached to the carbon atoms on dietary-fat molecules. I won't waste your time by reprinting the entire fat/saturation spiel I present in Chapter 5.

Suffice it to say that saturated fatty acids, commonly known as "sat fats," increase the amount of fat in your blood, including the amount of *low-density lipoproteins* (LDLs), the "bad" particles that ferry cholesterol into your arteries.

On the other hand, monounsaturated fatty acids and polyunsaturated fatty acids, like those found in high-fat plant foods such as nuts and avocados (see Chapter 6), may actually reduce the amount of fats in your blood, including LDLs.

But before you go getting too excited, keep these facts in mind:

✔ All fats are relatively high in calories. (They contain twice as many calories per gram as proteins and carbs.)

✔ A higher-calorie diet promotes weight gain.

✔ Weight gain raises cholesterol.

The moral of this little tale? Not all dietary fats are "bad," but a little goes a long way.

Women Never Have to Worry about Their Cholesterol

Ah, if only it were true. Women do tend to have lower cholesterol levels than men do from adolescence right through middle age. One protective weapon in a woman's cholesterol-fighting arsenal seems to be the female body's continuous, natural stream of estrogen.

Researchers have made this deduction from the fact that a woman's cholesterol level rises with the onset of menopause and the slowdown in her natural production of estrogen.

Older women are actually more likely than older men to have high cholesterol, but women do have one other lifelong advantage in the heart game. Their blood vessels are more elastic — that is, they are more likely than a man's blood vessels to stay wide open — which may help protect against high blood pressure and a heart-stopping blood clot.

Children Have No Cholesterol Problems

Ah, if only this were true, too. Infants require fatty acids, including saturated fatty acids, to promote and sustain proper growth and development, including the growth and development of nerve and brain cells (see Chapter 2, please).

In the 1980s, when overzealous parents sought to protect their babies by feeding them formulas made of skim milk, a disastrous epidemic of babies who failed to grow and develop as normally expected occurred.

Today, the American Heart Association (AHA) and the American Academy of Pediatrics (AAP) recommend a food plan with sufficient amounts of all fats for children up to the age of 2. After that, the kiddy cholesterol squad gets tough with the tykes.

According to the AHA, by age 12, as many as seven out of every ten American children have fatty deposits in their arteries. To counter this trend, the AHA recommends testing cholesterol levels in any child older than 2 who has a family history of coronary artery disease in parents or grandparents younger than 55.

Eating More Dietary Fiber Lowers Blood Cholesterol

The answer to this myth is another, "Not necessarily." As you can see in Chapter 5, there are two kinds of dietary fiber, insoluble and soluble.

Insoluble dietary fiber is the rough stuff — cellulose, lignin, and hemicellulose — in leaves, grasses, twigs, seeds, and bran (the hard outer covering of grains).

Human beings literally don't have the stomach for insoluble fiber. To pull nutrients out of insoluble fibers, animals need a very long gut and sometimes more than one stomach — a physical setup common to animals such as cows but not to us.

Soluble dietary fiber — gums and pectins — is found in the flesh of grains, fruits, and veggies. Examples include pectin in apples and beta glucan, the gum that makes oatmeal sticky. (Beans are also a good source of beta glucan.)

Soluble dietary fiber sops up cholesterol. Insoluble dietary fiber doesn't. Increasing your consumption of insoluble dietary fiber, which moves food through your intestinal tract faster, will reduce your risk of constipation, but it won't lower your cholesterol.

Increasing your consumption of soluble dietary fiber will turn those cholesterol numbers downward, but only by about 10 percent (or less). Listen, nothing's perfect.

Cholesterol Is the Only Thing That Leads to Plaque in Your Arteries

Actually, no. An amino acid called *homocysteine* may be equally at fault. Your body makes homocysteine as a byproduct of digesting proteins.

Homocysteine circulates into your arteries, and it can rough up the interior surface of the vessels, producing miniscule chinks and ledges for cholesterol to cling to.

After cholesterol latches on the arterial wall, it attracts more cholesterol particles and other cellular debris, building teeny-weeny little piles of junk that become plaque. Alert: Heart attack looms.

As you can see in Chapter 2, a diet rich in the B vitamin folate appears to reduce homocysteine levels, thus reducing the risk of a heart attack. One group of foods truly packed with folic acid is green, leafy veggies. (Turn back to Chapter 2 — yes, again — for a list of foods high in folic acid.)

Red Meat Has More Cholesterol Than Chicken or Turkey

No. Although red meat, even lean beef, has more total fat per ounce and up to five times as much saturated fat as chicken or turkey, dark chicken or turkey (the succulent leg and thigh) may deliver more cholesterol per ounce.

Go figure. Better yet, you can check out the figures in Table 17-1.

Table 17-1	Red Meat versus Chicken and Turkey		
Food (3 oz)	*Total Fat*	*Saturated Fat*	*Cholesterol*
Turkey (Roast)			
White meat	4 g	0.9 g	58.5 mg
Dark meat	6 g	2.0 g	72 mg
Chicken (Roast)			
White meat	3.6 g	1.1 g	43.8 mg
Dark meat	8.4 g	2.3 g	78 mg
Beef (Roast)			
Lean beef	12 g	5 g	69 mg

Source: *U.S. Department of Agriculture.*

A Heart Attack Is the Only Health Risk Associated with High Cholesterol

Alas, no. Plaque buildup is not specific to the coronary arteries. A person with high cholesterol may also develop plaque deposits in the arteries that feed blood to the brain.

Cerebral thrombosis, the most common form of stroke, occurs when a blood clot (thrombus) forms in a cerebral blood vessel, blocking the vessel and depriving brain cells of blood and oxygen. According to the American Heart Association, cerebral thrombosis is most common in arteries already damaged or narrowed by plaque.

This is not a trivial matter. According to the American Heart Association/American Stroke Association *Heart Disease and Stroke Statistics, 2007 Update,* in 2004, stroke was to blame for 1 of every 16 deaths in the United States.

The Centers for Disease Control and Prevention's National Center for Health Statistics ranks stroke as the third leading cause of death for Americans, right up there behind heart disease and cancer. Here are the facts concerning stroke in the United States:

✔ On average, every three to four minutes someone in America dies of a stroke.

✔ In 2004, 150,147 Americans suffered a fatal stroke.

✔ More women than men die after having a stroke; in 2004, the numbers were 91,487 women versus 58,660 men.

✔ Of the people who suffer a stroke, 4.5 percent are younger than 60.

Finally, here is a cholesterol fact to ruin your romantic evening. Most of us worry about cholesterol's effects on coronary arteries, but the truth is cholesterol doesn't differentiate between a coronary blood vessel and one in any other part of the body, like the penis.

Yes, you read that right. High cholesterol may cause plaque buildup that blocks the blood vessels carrying blood to the penis. A reduction in blood flow to the penis caused by a blocked vessel in the leg or penis itself would "certainly" affect a man's ability to sustain erection, says one urologist at the male sexual dysfunction clinic at Johns Hopkins Medical Centers in Baltimore, Maryland.

Chew on that one the next time you plan dinner for your beloved — if your beloved is male, of course.

Changing Your Diet Is the Only Way to Control Your Cholesterol

No again. In fact, this book includes one whole chapter (Chapter 8) on how regular exercise lowers cholesterol, a second one (Chapter 7) on the virtues of weight control, a third (Chapter 9) on why you should stop smoking right now, and last but not least, a fourth (Chapter 10) describing the cholesterol-control benefits of consuming alcohol in moderation.

You Can Never Be Too Rich or Too Thin, and Your Cholesterol Can Never Be Too Low

I'm a writer, a class of workers rarely overburdened with too much cash, so I'm not going to argue with the first part of that heading. But I am a nutrition writer, so I know that excessive thinness can be a sign of poor health or the result of an eating disorder such as anorexia nervosa or bulimia.

As for cholesterol, believe it or not, too low can be as problematic as too high. For example, if your cholesterol suddenly takes a nosedive into the basement below 100 mg/dL, your doctor may not be smiling when he brings you the news. *Hypocholesterolemia* — very low cholesterol — can signal danger ahead. What kind of danger? Malnutrition, an overactive thyroid, cirrhosis of the liver, and certain forms of cancer (colon cancer and liver cancer are good guesses).

Having consistently low cholesterol is not always a guarantee of long life. In the late 1990s, in a survey of 3,500 Japanese American male residents of Hawaii, researchers found a higher death rate among the men with the lowest cholesterol levels (about 149 mg/dL) than among men whose cholesterol levels circled around the supposedly borderline 232 mg/dL mark.

Since then, both American and British medical journals have published reports that state a total cholesterol level below 160 mg/dL appears to be tied to a higher risk of death from the diseases and conditions I mention above, especially in men who drink, smoke, and have high blood pressure. That is, if they don't take matters into their own hands first:

✔ A relatively early study (1966) reported in the prestigious *British Medical Journal* carried results of a French survey of data for 6,393 men showing that those with low cholesterol had an incidence of suicide three times higher than the incidence among men with middling or high cholesterol.

✔ Moving right ahead, in 1999, the *British Journal of Psychiatry* published a report from Finland's Public Health Institute in which men with very low cholesterol were more likely than men with high cholesterol to be hospitalized for depression.

Thin quiz

Wait. Before you go, who's thought to have first said that quote about never being too rich or too thin?

a. Paris Hilton and Nicole Richie

b. The Duchess of Windsor

c. Fergie, the Duchess of York

d. King Lear

Answer: (b) The Duchess of Windsor, also known as Wallis Warfield Simpson, the "original" Camilla Parker Bowles. To marry Wallis, a divorced woman, King Edward VIII gave up the British throne on December 11, 1936, to King George the VI, the father of Queen Elizabeth II, the mother of Prince Charles, and mother-in-law first to Princess Diana and then to Ms. Parker Bowles. Whether Wallis actually uttered the rich/thin words, the second part is still bad advice, health-wise.

Some researchers suggest these increased rates of depression and suicide may occur because low-fat or low-cholesterol diets reduce the levels of a brain chemical called serotonin that promotes a feeling of well-being.

In the end, one is left to ponder the strangeness of life and the weirdly prescient message in Woody Allen's character who, in the 1973 movie, *Sleeper,* wakes up in the year 2173 to discover that hamburgers, French fries, and milkshakes are health food. In 2007? Not so much.

Chapter 18

Ten (Okay, Eleven) "Eureka!" Cholesterol Moments

- -

In This Chapter

▶ Announcing the bad news about saturated fats

▶ Naming cholesterol as a heart risk

▶ Tuning up with Mr. Fit

▶ Pinning the rap on LDLs

▶ Introducing cholesterol-buster meds

- -

This chapter is a handy guide to a half-century's worth of advances in the science of protecting your heart by keeping your arteries clean and your body in tip-top shape.

As you read through the list, think about all those people who spent their time sitting at lab benches or adding up statistics to enhance your possibility of living a full, rich life. Clearly, a heartfelt, "Thanks a lot," is in order.

Finding the "Wow!" factor

The word *eureka* loosely translates from the Greek as, "Oh, boy, look what I discovered," a statement most commonly attributed to the ancient Greek mathematician Archimedes.

Sitting in his bath one day, Old Archie suddenly realized that he could calculate the volume of an irregularly shaped solid object, such as himself, by immersing the object into water and measuring how much liquid it displaced.

Some versions of the Archimedes tale say that right after shouting *"Heureka!"* (Greek for "Eureka!"), Archimedes leaped out of the tub and ran starkers through the streets of his native Syracuse. Whether his fellow citizens shouted *"Heureka!"* upon seeing him is lost to history.

1957: The Prudent Diet

The Prudent Diet was the brainchild of the Diet and Coronary Heart Disease Study Project of the Bureau of Nutrition at the New York City Department of Health.

Well before the establishment decided that the risk of heart attack may be lowered by reducing the intake of foods high in saturated fats while emphasizing unsaturated fats, the New Yorkers (whom I'm proud to say included my uncle, Seymour H. Rinzler, MD) said, "Let's try it."

Boy, were they ever right. By the end of the fourth year of the study, the incidence of heart attack among the middle-aged, often-overweight male participants was far below the numbers that researchers had predicted.

As a result, the Prudent Diet became the role model for the American Heart Association's Step I and Step II eating plans (check 'em out in Chapter 4), and a new approach to eating your way to a healthy heart was born.

1958: Introducing Cholesterol Busters

Cholestyramine (brand name: Questran, Questran Light) was the first cholesterol-lowering drug approved by the U.S. Food and Drug Administration (FDA).

This prescription drug sops up natural digestive juices and bile acids found in your intestines and eliminates them from your body. Because you need bile compounds to digest food, your body responds by converting cholesterol into bile, thus lowering the amount of cholesterol in your blood vessels. (Read the whole story in Chapter 12.)

Cholestyramine is almost 50 years old, and although some of its market has been taken over by the statin drugs (see "1986: Unveiling Statins" later in this chapter), it's still selling. Two years ago, cholestyramine's manufacturer appealed to the FDA for permission to sell it as an over-the-counter product rather than a prescription drug. The FDA nixed the idea.

1971: Naming Cholesterol an Official Risk Factor for Heart Attack

Framingham, Massachusetts, is a small industrial town about 20 miles west of Boston. I mean no disrespect to its hardworking inhabitants when I say that you would probably never have heard of Framingham if a team of Boston

University Medical School researchers hadn't set up shop there shortly after World War II. But they did. And they recruited most of the town's nearly 30,000 citizens as volunteers in a study of who gets heart disease and why.

Within 20 years, an analysis of hundreds, maybe even thousands, of tests performed on the Framingham residents produced statistics showing a relationship between high serum (blood) cholesterol and the risk of heart attack. Here are the numbers:

Cholesterol Level	Percentage of People with Heart Attack
<200 mg/dL	10
200–239 mg/dL	12
>240 mg/dL	18

Do those figures look familiar? You bet they do. Just check out the current breakdown for high, medium, and low cholesterol levels in Chapter 3.

More to the point, these numbers led the Framingham researchers and the National Heart Institute to create the first task force on arteriosclerosis, another big step on the road to the general public becoming interested in controlling cholesterol. Yeah, team!

1971: MRFIT Gets Going

The Multiple Risk Factor Intervention Trial (MRFIT) was an eight-year (1974–1982) study in which 250 scientists at 28 medical centers across the United States interviewed 361,662 middle-aged men to get 12,866 volunteers.

The volunteers were thought to be at high risk for heart attack based on risk factors such as age, smoking habits, a high-cholesterol diet, high blood pressure, and obesity.

The guys were divided into two groups: One group was taught to modify their behavior; the other was left to their own devices. At the end of the trial, the big news was that nonsmokers with lower cholesterol and lower blood pressure were less likely to have a heart attack. Today we take that for granted.

1984: Indicting Hypercholesterolemia

In 1984, a 14-member panel of distinguished scientists gathered at the National Heart, Lung, and Blood Institute for a Consensus Development Conference to analyze the existing studies on cholesterol and heart disease and invite testimony relating to evidence linking the risk factor to the disease.

What they heard was so convincing that they certified *hypercholesterolemia* — a nine-syllable way to say *high cholesterol* — as a medical condition worthy of treatment. And just like that, practically overnight, millions of people who once considered themselves healthy had something to worry about. Ain't science great?

1985: Recognizing the Risk from LDLs

For years, cholesterol researchers plodded along thinking plain old high cholesterol was the basic risk factor for heart disease. They also wondered why some people with sky-high cholesterol readings never had heart attacks.

Joseph L. Goldstein and Michael S. Brown of the University of Texas Health Center in Dallas changed all that on October 14, 1985, when they won the Nobel Prize for identifying LDLs as the true risk factor in the cholesterol game. Bravo, Goldstein and Brown!

1985–1987: Establishing the National Cholesterol Education Program

The National Cholesterol Education Program (NCEP) was created in 1985, released to an advisory panel in 1986, and announced to the American public in 1987. Based on the Framingham stats (see "1971: Naming Cholesterol an Official Risk Factor for Heart Attack" earlier in this chapter), the NCEP formally designated levels of cholesterol as "high" (>240 mg/dL), "borderline high" (200–239 mg/dL), and "desirable" (<200 mg/dL).

This classification formally declared more than 25 percent of all Americans as being at risk of heart attack from high cholesterol. Wow! Who knew?

1986: Unveiling Statins

Statin is shorthand for a class of drugs that lowers cholesterol at the source by interrupting your liver's natural production of this fatty substance. The first two statins — pravastatin (Pravachol) and simvastatin (Zocor) — appeared in 1986. The third, lovastatin (Mevacor), came online the following year.

For the full story on statins, check out Chapter 12. For the *big problem* with statins, run your finger down to "2001: Baycol Bombs."

1988, 1993, 2001: ATP I, ATP II, ATP III

The National Cholesterol Education Program's *Expert Panel on Detection, Evaluation, and Treatment of High Blood Cholesterol in Adults* report is one whale of a mouthful, so the whole thing is commonly called ATP (adult treatment panel), which certainly slides more easily off the tongue.

ATP I, published in 1988, focused on prevention and offered tips for warding off heart disease in healthy people with high cholesterol. The report also identified LDLs as a primary target, advising people whose LDLs are higher than "normal" to work with their doctors to reduce their risk for heart disease by lowering LDLs.

ATP II came out in 1993. Once again, the report stressed the importance of getting LDLs down into a healthy range, but ATP II added something new. Moving from prevention for healthy people to the management of existing heart disease, the report urged people who'd already had a heart attack to lower their LDLs, preferably to 100 mg/dL (or less).

ATP III, the current version, appeared in 2001. The advice to lower LDLs is still included, but once again, the National Cholesterol Education Program has come up with something new. The report identifies a new condition called *metabolic syndrome* (multiple risk factors, such as high blood pressure, obesity, smoking, and high cholesterol) as an important warning of heart disease ahead.

ATP III also offers a version of a medical crystal ball — a risk-factor-based formula that enables you to determine whether you should be on cholesterol-busting drugs (see Chapter 12) and guesstimate your odds of having a heart attack in the next ten years. If you're brave enough to face the future, you can do the math in Chapter 3.

2001: Baycol Bombs

Baycol, the brand name for the drug cerivastatin, was introduced by Bayer A.G. in 1997 and, as you can see from the date on this entry, taken off the market a scant four years later.

One side effect of statin drugs, a class of cholesterol-lowering drugs, is rhabdomyolysis — the destruction of muscle cells. If enough muscle cells are destroyed, the debris may pile up in your kidneys, triggering kidney failure. Among Baycol users, the incidence of cell damage was ten times greater than it was for people using other statins, and the effect was far more likely to be fatal.

By August 7, 2001, when Bayer took Baycol off the market, at least 31 deaths were linked to the medication in the United States, and the FDA had reports of nine more abroad. As of 2007, the number of deaths attributed to Baycol worldwide has climbed past the 100 mark.

For more details on Baycol and the risks associated with other statins, turn to Chapter 12. The lesson to take away from this short set of paragraphs is simple: Never take any drug without reading the fine print.

2001–2004: Anti-Cholesterol Combo Pills

When it comes to therapeutic drugs, time marches on and so do the innovations. In 2001, Kos Pharmaceuticals introduced Advicor, the first anti-cholesterol combination pill. Advicor contains extended-release niacin (believed to raise HDLs, the "good" cholesterol) and the statin drug lovastatin (Lipitor). Three years later, Merck/Schering-Plough released Vytorin, a combo that includes ezetimibe (a drug that reduces the body's absorption of fats, including cholesterol) plus the statin drug simvastatin (Zocor). And Pfizer introduced Caduet, which contains the anti-hypertension drug amlodipine (Norvasc) plus the statin lovastatin (Lipitor).

The good news about these two-fers is that a person who needs two drugs can get them both in a single pill. The bad news is that the pill provides the risk of two drugs along with the benefits.

Whether the benefits outweigh the risks for a specific patient is a question only that person (and his doctor) can decide. For investors, the answer is crystal clear. In 2006, Advicor scored $116 million in sales; by summer 2007, Vytorin was a $2 billion/year blockbuster; and Caduet sales are predicted to hit $1.1 billion by 2008. Eureka!

Appendix

Calories and Other Nutrients in Food

．．．

*F*or Dummies books are special because they are (a) accessible and (b) complete. Really complete. Really, really complete. This appendix is about as good as it gets.

You get a printed chart showing the important nutrients in several hundred every day foods — useful information when you're fighting the battle against cholesterol.

You also get instructions on how to access and use the totally wonderful U.S. Department of Agriculture Nutrient Database, the (shhhh!) secret source of every nutrition expert's info on foods. This database contains over 6,000 food entries.

The Nutrition Chart

The really long chart shows a standard set of nutrients for several hundred common foods. The abbreviations used in this chart (and in all nutrient descriptions) are

- ✔ g = gram
- ✔ mg = milligram
- ✔ mcg = micrograms
- ✔ IU = International Units

The listing for the large apple (skin on), with numbers rounded off, looks like this:

Description and Serving

Apple, 1 large, raw	3½" diameter
Grams	212
Water [g]	178
Calories [kcal]	125
Fat (total) [g]	0.8
Fat (saturated) [g]	0.1
Fat (monounsaturated) [g]	0
Fat (polyunsaturated) [g]	0.2
Cholesterol [mg]	0
Protein [g]	0.4
Carbohydrates [g]	32
Fiber [g]	5.7
Calcium [mg]	14.8
Phosphorus [mg]	14.8
Iron [mg]	0.4
Sodium [mg]	0
Potassium [mg]	243.8
Magnesium [mg]	10.6
Zinc [mg]	0.1
Copper [mg]	0.1
Vitamin A [IU]	112.4
Thiamin [mg]	0.04
Riboflavin [mg]	0.03

Description and Serving	
Niacin [mg]	0.2
Vitamin B6 [mg]	0.1
Folate [mcg]	5.9
Vitamin B12 [mcg]	0
Vitamin C [mg]	12.1

The order of the nutrients shown in this chart does not match the order on the complete USDA Nutrient Database, but it's sensible in grouping the fats together.

The USDA Nutrient Database

The USDA nutrient database is the nutritional equivalent of the Nile River, the source from which our nutrient information flows. Accessing the database begins with an address: www.nal.usda.gov/fnic/cgi-bin/nut_search. pl. Click here and you're in nutrition heaven — surrounded by bits and bytes of data for over 6,000 foods and servings, each listed by its exact name and size. When you connect to the entry you want, the chart that pops up on the screen will look a little like the listings I include here but with *a lot* more information.

NDB#	Description & Serving	Grams	Water	Calories	Fat	Fat: Saturated	Fat: Monounsaturated	Fat: Polyunsaturated	Cholesterol	Protein	Carbohydrates	Fiber	Calcium
		g	kcal	g	g	g	g	mg	g	g	g	mg

Beans (legumes) and bean products

NDB#	Description & Serving	Grams	Water	Calories	Fat	Fat: Saturated	Fat: Monounsaturated	Fat: Polyunsaturated	Cholesterol	Protein	Carbohydrates	Fiber	Calcium
16015	Black beans, cooked, boiled, wo/salt 1 cup	172	113.07	227.04	0.93	0.24	0.08	0.4	0	15.24	40.78	14.96	46.44
16053	Broadbeans (fava beans), cooked, boiled, wo/salt 1 cup	170	121.62	187	0.68	0.11	0.13	0.28	0	12.92	33.41	9.18	61.2
16058	Chickpeas (garbanzo beans, bengal gm), seeds, canned 1 cup	240	167.26	285.6	2.74	0.28	0.62	1.22	0	11.88	54.29	10.56	76.8
16025	Great northern beans, cooked, boiled, wo/salt 1 cup	177	122.13	208.86	0.8	0.25	0.04	0.33	0	14.74	37.33	12.39	120.36
16028	Kidney beans, all types, cooked, boiled, wo/salt 1 cup	177	118.48	224.79	0.89	0.13	0.07	0.49	0	15.35	40.37	11.33	49.56
16070	Lentils, cooked, boiled, wo/salt 1 cup	198	137.89	229.68	0.75	0.1	0.13	0.35	0	17.86	39.88	15.64	37.62
16072	Lima beans, lrg, cooked, boiled, wo/salt 1 cup	188	131.21	216.2	0.71	0.17	0.06	0.32	0	14.66	39.27	13.16	31.96
16038	Navy beans, cooked, boiled, wo/salt 1 cup	182	114.99	258.44	1.04	0.27	0.09	0.45	0	15.83	47.88	11.65	127.4
16086	Peas, split, cooked, boiled, wo/salt 1 cup	196	136.2	231.28	0.76	0.11	0.16	0.32	0	16.35	41.38	16.27	27.44
16090	Peanuts, all types, dry-roasted, w/salt 1 oz	28.35	0.44	165.85	14.08	1.95	6.99	4.45	0	6.71	6.1	2.27	15.31
16097	Peanut butter, chunk style, w/salt 2 tablespoons	32	0.36	188.48	15.98	3.07	7.54	4.53	0	7.7	6.91	2.11	13.12
16098	Peanut butter, smooth style, w/salt 2 tablespoons	32	0.39	189.76	16.33	3.31	7.77	4.41	0	8.07	6.17	1.89	12.16
16109	Soybeans, cooked, boiled, wo/salt 1 cup	172	107.59	297.56	15.43	2.23	3.41	8.71	0	28.62	17.06	10.32	175.44
16120	Soy milk, fluid 1 cup	245	228.51	80.85	4.68	0.52	0.8	2.04	0	6.74	4.43	3.19	9.8
16123	Soy sauce made from soy & wheat (shoyu) 1 tablespoon	16	11.37	8.48	0.01	0	0	0.01	0	0.83	1.36	0.13	2.72
16124	Soy sauce made from soy (tamari) 1 tablespoon	18	11.88	10.8	0.02	0	0	0.01	0	1.89	1	0.14	3.6
16114	Tempeh 1 cup	166	91.22	330.34	12.75	1.84	2.81	7.19	0	31.46	28.27	0	154.38
16127	Tofu, raw, regular 1 cup (½" cubes)	248	209.68	188.48	11.85	1.71	2.62	6.69	0	20.04	4.66	2.98	260.4
16046	White beans, small, cooked, boiled, wo/salt 1 cup	179	113.2	254.18	1.15	0.3	0.1	0.49	0	16.06	46.2	18.62	130.67

NDB#	Phosphorus	Iron	Sodium	Potassium	Magnesium	Zinc	Copper	Vitamin A	Thiamin	Riboflavin	Niacin	Vitamin B6	Folate	Vitamin B12	Vitamin C
	mg	mg	mg	mg	mg	mg	mg	IU	mg	mg	mg	mg	mcg	mcg	mg

Beans (legumes) and bean products

NDB#	Phosphorus	Iron	Sodium	Potassium	Magnesium	Zinc	Copper	Vitamin A	Thiamin	Riboflavin	Niacin	Vitamin B6	Folate	Vitamin B12	Vitamin C
16015	240.8	3.61	1.72	610.6	120.4	1.93	0.36	10.32	0.42	0.1	0.87	0.12	255.94	0	0
16053	212.5	2.55	8.5	455.6	73.1	1.72	0.44	25.5	0.16	0.15	1.21	0.12	176.97	0	0.51
16058	216	3.24	717.6	412.8	69.6	2.54	0.42	57.6	0.07	0.08	0.33	1.14	160.32	0	9.12
16025	292.05	3.77	3.54	692.07	88.5	1.56	0.44	1.77	0.28	0.1	1.21	0.21	180.89	0	2.3
16028	251.34	5.2	3.54	713.31	79.65	1.89	0.43	0	0.28	0.1	1.02	0.21	229.39	0	2.12
16070	356.4	6.59	3.96	730.62	71.28	2.51	0.5	15.84	0.33	0.14	2.1	0.35	357.98	0	2.97
16072	208.68	4.49	3.76	955.04	80.84	1.79	0.44	0	0.3	0.1	0.79	0.3	156.23	0	0
16038	285.74	4.51	1.82	669.76	107.38	1.93	0.54	3.64	0.37	0.11	0.97	0.3	254.62	0	1.64
16086	194.04	2.53	3.92	709.52	70.56	1.96	0.35	13.72	0.37	0.11	1.74	0.09	127.2	0	0.78
16090	101.49	0.64	230.49	186.54	49.9	0.94	0.19	0	0.12	0.03	3.83	0.07	41.19	0	0
16097	101.44	0.61	155.52	239.04	50.88	0.89	0.16	0	0.04	0.04	4.38	0.14	29.44	0	0
16098	118.08	0.59	149.44	214.08	50.88	0.93	0.04	0	0.03	0.03	4.29	0.15	23.68	0	0
16109	421.4	8.84	1.72	885.8	147.92	1.98	0.7	15.48	0.27	0.49	0.69	0.4	92.54	0	2.92
16120	120.05	1.42	29.4	345.45	46.55	0.56	0.29	78.4	0.39	0.17	0.36	0.1	3.68	0	0
16123	17.6	0.32	914.4	28.8	5.44	0.06	0.02	0	0.01	0.02	0.54	0.03	2.48	0	0
16124	23.4	0.43	1005.48	38.16	7.2	0.08	0.02	0	0.01	0.03	0.71	0.04	3.28	0	0
16114	341.96	3.75	9.96	609.22	116.2	3	1.11	1138.76	0.22	0.18	7.69	0.5	86.32	1.66	0
16127	240.56	13.29	17.36	300.08	255.44	1.98	0.48	210.8	0.2	0.13	0.48	0.12	37.2	0	0.25
16046	302.51	5.08	3.58	828.77	121.72	1.95	0.27	0	0.42	0.11	0.49	0.23	245.05	0	0

NDB#	Description & Serving	Grams	Water	Calories	Fat	Fat. Saturated	Fat. Monounsaturated	Fat. Polyunsaturated	Cholesterol	Protein	Carbohydrates	Fiber	Calcium
		g	kcal	g	g	g	g	mg	g	g	g	mg	

Beverages

Alcohol beverages

14037	Alcoholic bev, distilled, all (gin, rum, vodka, whiskey) 80 proof												
	1 fl oz	27.8	18.51	64.22	0	0	0	0	0	0	0	0	0
14550	Alcoholic bev (gin, rum, vodka, whiskey) 86 proof												
	1 fl oz	27.8	17.76	69.5	0	0	0	0	0	0	0.03	0	0
14533	Alcoholic bev, distilled, all 100 proof												
	1 fl oz	27.8	15.99	82.01	0	0	0	0	0	0	0	0	0
14003	Beer, reg												
	1 can (12 fl oz)	356	328.59	145.96	0	0	0	0	0	1.07	13.17	0.71	17.8
14006	Beer, light												
	1 can (12 fl oz)	354	337.01	99.12	0	0	0	0	0	0.71	4.6	0	17.7
14096	Wine, red												
	1 wine glass (3.5 fl oz)	103	91.16	74.16	0	0	0	0	0	0.21	1.75	0	8.24
14104	Wine, rosé												
	1 wine glass (3.5 fl oz)	103	91.57	73.13	0	0	0	0	0	0.21	1.44	0	8.24
14106	Wine, white												
	1 wine glass (3.5 fl oz)	103	92.29	70.04	0	0	0	0	0	0.1	0.82	0	9.27

Carbonated beverages

14121	Club soda												
	1 can (16 fl oz)	474	473.53	0	0	0	0	0	0	0	0	0	23.7
14400	Cola												
	1 can (16 fl oz)	492	439.85	201.72	0	0	0	0	0	0	51.17	0	14.76
14416	Cola, lo cal, w/asprt												
	1 can (16 fl oz)	474	473.05	4.74	0	0	0	0	0	0.47	0.47	0	18.96
14166	Cola, lo cal, or pepper-types, w/saccharin												
	1 can (16 fl oz)	474	473.05	0	0	0	0	0	0	0	0.47	0	18.96
14136	Ginger ale												
	1 can (16 fl oz)	488	445.06	165.92	0	0	0	0	0	0	42.46	0	14.64
14155	Tonic water												
	1 bottle (11 fl oz)	336	306.1	114.24	0	0	0	0	0	0	29.57	0	3.36

Coffee and tea

14209	Coffee, brewed, prep w/tap water												
	1 cup (8 fl oz)	237	235.34	4.74	0	0	0	0	0	0.24	0.95	0	4.74
14215	Coffee, instant, reg, prep w/water												
	6 fl oz	179	177.21	3.58	0	0	0	0	0	0.18	0.72	0	5.37
14219	Coffee, instant, decaffeinated, pdr, prep w/water												
	1 cup (6 fl oz)	179	177.21	3.58	0	0	0	0	0	0.18	0.72	0	5.37

NDB#	Phosphorus	Iron	Sodium	Potassium	Magnesium	Zinc	Copper	Vitamin A	Thiamin	Riboflavin	Niacin	Vitamin B6	Folate	Vitamin B12	Vitamin C
	mg	mg	mg	mg	mg	mg	mg	IU	mg	mg	mg	mg	mcg	mcg	mg
Beverages															
14037	1.11	0.01	0.28	0.56	0	0.01	0.01	0	0	0	0	0	0	0	0
14550	1.11	0.01	0.28	0.56	0	0.01	0.01	0	0	0	0	0	0	0	0
14533	1.11	0.01	0.28	0.56	0	0.01	0.01	0	0	0	0	0	0	0	0
14003	42.72	0.11	17.8	89	21.36	0.07	0.03	0	0.02	0.09	1.61	0.18	21.36	0.07	0
14006	42.48	0.14	10.62	63.72	17.7	0.11	0.08	0	0.03	0.11	1.39	0.12	14.51	0.04	0
14096	14.42	0.44	5.15	115.36	13.39	0.09	0.02	0	0.01	0.03	0.08	0.04	2.06	0.01	0
14104	15.45	0.39	5.15	101.97	10.3	0.06	0.05	0	0	0.02	0.08	0.02	1.13	0.01	0
14106	14.42	0.33	5.15	82.4	10.3	0.07	0.02	0	0	0.01	0.07	0.01	0.21	0	0
14121	0	0.05	99.54	9.48	4.74	0.47	0.03	0	0	0	0	0	0	0	0
14400	59.04	0.15	19.68	4.92	4.92	0.05	0.05	0	0	0	0	0	0	0	0
14416	42.66	0.14	28.44	0	4.74	0.38	0.05	0	0.02	0.11	0	0	0	0	0
14166	52.14	0.19	75.84	9.48	4.74	0.24	0.12	0	0	0	0	0	0	0	0
14136	0	0.88	34.16	4.88	4.88	0.24	0.09	0	0	0	0	0	0	0	0
14155	0	0.03	13.44	0	0	0.34	0.02	0	0	0	0	0	0	0	0
14209	2.37	0.12	4.74	127.98	11.85	0.05	0.02	0	0	0	0.53	0	0.24	0	0
14215	5.37	0.09	5.37	64.44	7.16	0.05	0.01	0	0	0	0.51	0	0	0	0
14219	5.37	0.07	5.37	62.65	7.16	0.05	0.01	0	0	0.03	0.5	0	0	0	0

NDB#	Description & Serving	Grams	Water	Calories	Fat	Fat: Saturated	Fat: Monounsaturated	Fat: Polyunsaturated	Cholesterol	Protein	Carbohydrates	Fiber	Calcium
		g	kcal	g	g	g	g	mg	g	g	g	mg
14237	Coffee sub, crl grain bev, prep w/water 1 cup (8 fl oz)	240	236.88	12	0	0.02	0.01	0.05	0	0.24	2.4	0	7.2
14355	Tea, brewed, prep w/tap water 1 cup (8 fl oz)	237	236.29	2.37	0	0	0	0.01	0	0	0.71	0	0
14381	Tea, herb, other than chamomile, brewed 1 cup (8 fl oz)	178	177.47	1.78	0	0	0	0.01	0	0	0.36	0	3.56
14545	Tea, herb, chamomile, brewed 1 cup (8 fl oz)	237	236.29	2.37	0	0	0	0.01	0	0	0.47	0	4.74

Dairy products

Butter

NDB#	Description & Serving	Grams	Water	Calories	Fat	Fat: Saturated	Fat: Monounsaturated	Fat: Polyunsaturated	Cholesterol	Protein	Carbohydrates	Fiber	Calcium
01145	Butter, without salt 1 tablespoon	14.2	2.55	101.81	11.52	7.17	3.33	0.43	31.08	0.12	0.01	0	3.34

Cheese

NDB#	Description & Serving	Grams	Water	Calories	Fat	Fat: Saturated	Fat: Monounsaturated	Fat: Polyunsaturated	Cholesterol	Protein	Carbohydrates	Fiber	Calcium
01004	Blue 1 oz	28.35	12.02	100.09	8.15	5.29	2.21	0.23	21.32	6.07	0.66	0	149.57
01007	Camembert 1 wedge	38	19.68	113.83	9.21	5.8	2.67	0.28	27.36	7.52	0.18	0	147.29
01009	Cheddar 1 cup, diced	132	48.51	531.4	43.74	27.84	12.4	1.24	138.47	32.87	1.69	0	952.12
01011	Colby 1 cup, diced	132	50.42	519.62	42.39	26.69	12.25	1.26	125.27	31.36	3.39	0	903.67
01012	Cottage cheese, creamed, lrg curd 1 cup (not packed)	210	165.82	217.03	9.47	5.99	2.7	0.29	31.29	26.23	5.63	0	126
01014	Cottage cheese, uncrmd, dry, lrg or sml curd 1 cup (not packed)	145	115.67	122.66	0.61	0.4	0.16	0.02	9.72	25.04	2.68	0	45.97
01015	Cottage cheese, 2% fat 1 cup (not packed)	226	179.24	202.68	4.36	2.76	1.24	0.13	18.98	31.05	8.2	0	154.81
01016	Cottage cheese, 1% fat 1 cup (not packed)	226	186.4	163.62	2.31	1.46	0.66	0.07	9.94	28	6.15	0	137.63
01017	Cream cheese 1 tablespoon	14.5	7.79	50.61	5.06	3.19	1.43	0.18	15.91	1.09	0.39	0	11.59
01186	Cream cheese, fat free 100 grams	100	75.53	96	1.36	0.9	0.33	0.06	8	14.41	5.8	0	185
01018	Edam 1 oz	28.35	11.78	101.1	7.88	4.98	2.3	0.19	25.29	7.08	0.41	0	207.24
01019	Feta 1 oz	28.35	15.65	74.72	6.03	4.24	1.31	0.17	25.23	4.03	1.16	0	139.62
01157	Goat cheese, semisoft type 1 oz	28.35	12.9	103.19	8.46	5.85	1.93	0.2	22.4	6.12	0.72	0	84.48

NDB#	Phosphorus	Iron	Sodium	Potassium	Magnesium	Zinc	Copper	Vitamin A	Thiamin	Riboflavin	Niacin	Vitamin B6	Folate	Vitamin B12	Vitamin C
	mg	mg	mg	mg	mg	mg	mg	IU	mg	mg	mg	mg	mcg	mcg	mg
14237	16.8	0.14	9.6	57.6	9.6	0.07	0.02	0	0.02	0	0.52	0.03	0.72	0	0
14355	2.37	0.05	7.11	87.69	7.11	0.05	0.02	0	0	0.03	0	0	12.32	0	0
14381	0	0.14	1.78	16.02	1.78	0.07	0.03	0	0.02	0.01	0	0	1.07	0	0
14545	0	0.19	2.37	21.33	2.37	0.09	0.04	47.4	0.02	0.01	0	0	1.42	0	0

Dairy products

NDB#	Phosphorus	Iron	Sodium	Potassium	Magnesium	Zinc	Copper	Vitamin A	Thiamin	Riboflavin	Niacin	Vitamin B6	Folate	Vitamin B12	Vitamin C
01145	3.24	0.02	1.56	3.69	0.28	0.01	0	434.24	0	0	0.01	0	0.4	0.02	0
01004	109.83	0.09	395.57	72.66	6.5	0.75	0.01	204.4	0.01	0.11	0.29	0.05	10.32	0.35	0
01007	131.7	0.13	319.85	70.9	7.59	0.9	0.01	350.74	0.01	0.19	0.24	0.09	23.63	0.49	0
01009	675.97	0.9	819.06	129.89	36.67	4.11	0.04	1397.88	0.04	0.5	0.11	0.1	24.02	1.09	0
01011	602.58	1	797.54	166.98	34.08	4.05	0.06	1364.88	0.02	0.5	0.12	0.1	24.02	1.09	0
01012	276.78	0.29	850.08	177.03	11.05	0.78	0.06	342.3	0.04	0.34	0.26	0.14	25.62	1.31	0
01014	150.8	0.33	18.56	46.98	5.71	0.68	0.04	43.5	0.04	0.21	0.22	0.12	21.46	1.2	0
01015	340.13	0.36	917.56	217.41	13.56	0.95	0.06	158.2	0.05	0.42	0.33	0.17	29.61	1.61	0
01016	302.39	0.32	917.56	193.23	12.07	0.86	0.06	83.62	0.05	0.37	0.29	0.15	28.02	1.43	0
01017	15.14	0.17	42.85	17.31	0.93	0.08	0	206.92	0	0.03	0.01	0.01	1.91	0.06	0
01186	434	0.18	545	163	14	0.88	0.05	930	0.05	0.17	0.16	0.05	37	0.55	0
01018	151.84	0.12	273.58	53.21	8.44	1.06	0.01	259.69	0.01	0.11	0.02	0.02	4.59	0.44	0
01019	95.6	0.18	316.41	17.52	5.45	0.82	0.01	126.72	0.04	0.24	0.28	0.12	9.07	0.48	0
01157	106.31	0.46	146	44.79	8.22	0.19	0.16	378.19	0.02	0.19	0.33	0.02	0.57	0.06	0

NDB#	Description & Serving	Grams	Water	Calories	Fat	Fat: Saturated	Fat: Monounsaturated	Fat: Polyunsaturated	Cholesterol	Protein	Carbohydrates	Fiber	Calcium
		g	kcal	gm	g	g	g	mg	g	g	g	mg	
01022	Gouda 1 oz	28.35	11.75	101.01	7.78	4.99	2.2	0.19	32.32	7.07	0.63	0	198.39
01023	Gruyere 1 cup, diced	132	43.81	545.09	42.69	24.97	13.26	2.29	145.2	39.35	0.48	0	1334.52
01024	Limburger 1 oz	28.35	13.73	92.71	7.73	4.75	2.44	0.14	25.52	5.68	0.14	0	140.81
01025	Monterey 1 cup, diced	132	54.13	492.79	39.97	25.17	11.55	1.19	117.48	32.31	0.9	0	985.25
01026	Mozzarella, whole milk 1 oz	28.35	15.35	79.77	6.12	3.73	1.86	0.22	22.23	5.51	0.63	0	146.57
01026	Mozzarella, part skim milk 1 oz	28.35	15.25	72.08	4.51	2.87	1.28	0.13	16.39	6.88	0.79	0	183.06
01030	Muenster 1 cup, diced	132	55.14	486.22	39.65	25.23	11.5	0.87	126.19	30.9	1.48	0	946.84
01031	Neufchatel 1 oz	28.35	17.64	73.67	6.64	4.19	1.92	0.18	21.57	2.82	0.83	0	21.35
01032	Parmesan, grated 1 tablespoon	5	0.88	22.79	1.5	0.95	0.44	0.03	3.94	2.08	0.19	0	68.79
01034	Port de salut 1 cup, diced	132	59.99	464.14	37.22	22.03	12.33	0.96	162.36	31.39	0.75	0	857.74
01035	Provolone 1 oz	28.35	11.61	99.65	7.55	4.84	2.1	0.22	19.53	7.25	0.61	0	214.3
01036	Ricotta, whole milk ½ cup	124	88.91	215.68	16.1	10.29	4.5	0.48	62.74	13.96	3.77	0	256.68
01037	Ricotta, part skim milk 1 cup	246	183.05	339.62	19.46	12.12	5.69	0.64	75.77	28.02	12.64	0	669.12
01038	Romano 1 oz	28.35	8.76	109.61	7.64	4.85	2.22	0.17	29.48	9.02	1.03	0	301.59
01039	Roquefort 1 oz	28.35	11.16	104.62	8.69	5.46	2.4	0.37	25.52	6.11	0.57	0	187.62
01040	Swiss 1 cup, diced	132	49.12	496.01	36.23	23.47	9.6	1.28	121.04	37.53	4.46	0	1268.39
Eggs													
01123	Egg, whole, raw, fresh 1 extra large	58	43.69	86.42	5.81	1.8	2.21	0.79	246.5	7.24	0.71	0	28.42
01124	Egg, white, raw, fresh 1 large egg white	33.4	29.33	16.7	0	0	0	0	0	3.51	0.34	0	2
01125	Egg, yolk, raw, fresh 1 large egg yolk	16.6	8.1	59.43	5.12	1.59	1.95	0.7	212.65	2.78	0.3	0	22.74

NDB#	Phosphorus	Iron	Sodium	Potassium	Magnesium	Zinc	Copper	Vitamin A	Thiamin	Riboflavin	Niacin	Vitamin B6	Folate	Vitamin B12	Vitamin C
	mg	mg	mg	mg	mg	mg	mg	IU	mg	mg	mg	mg	mcg	mcg	mg
01022	154.88	0.07	232.27	34.16	8.22	1.11	0.01	182.57	0.01	0.09	0.02	0.02	5.93	0.44	0
01023	799	0.22	443.52	106.92	47.4	5.15	0.04	1609.08	0.08	0.37	0.14	0.11	13.73	2.11	0
01024	111.42	0.04	226.8	36.29	5.95	0.6	0.01	363.16	0.02	0.14	0.04	0.02	16.3	0.29	0
01025	586.08	0.95	707.92	106.52	35.65	3.96	0.04	1254	0.02	0.51	0.12	0.1	24.02	1.09	0
01026	105.09	0.05	105.77	19.02	5.27	0.63	0.01	224.53	0	0.07	0.02	0.02	1.98	0.19	0
01026	131.26	0.06	132.11	23.73	6.58	0.78	0.01	165.56	0.01	0.09	0.03	0.02	2.49	0.23	0
01030	617.36	0.54	828.56	177.41	36.1	3.71	0.04	1478.4	0.02	0.42	0.14	0.07	15.97	1.94	0
01031	38.64	0.08	113.23	32.35	2.15	0.15	0	321.49	0	0.06	0.04	0.01	3.2	0.07	0
01032	40.36	0.05	93.08	5.36	2.54	0.16	0	35.05	0	0.02	0.02	0.01	0.4	0.07	0
01034	475.2	0.57	704.88	179.26	32.1	3.43	0.03	1759.56	0.02	0.32	0.08	0.07	24.02	1.98	0
01035	140.64	0.15	248.2	39.21	7.82	0.92	0.01	231.05	0.01	0.09	0.04	0.02	2.95	0.41	0
01036	196.04	0.47	104.28	129.7	14.01	1.44	0.03	607.6	0.02	0.24	0.13	0.05	15.13	0.42	0
01037	449.2	1.08	306.76	307.5	36.33	3.3	0.08	1062.72	0.05	0.46	0.19	0.05	32.23	0.72	0
01038	215.46	0.22	340.2	24.47	11.6	0.73	0.01	161.88	0.01	0.1	0.02	0.02	1.93	0.32	0
01039	111.16	0.16	512.85	25.71	8.37	0.59	0.01	296.82	0.01	0.17	0.21	0.04	13.89	0.18	0
01040	798.07	0.22	343.2	146.12	47.4	5.15	0.04	1115.4	0.03	0.48	0.12	0.11	8.45	2.21	0
01123	103.24	0.84	73.08	70.18	5.8	0.64	0.01	368.3	0.04	0.29	0.04	0.08	27.26	0.58	0
01124	4.34	0.01	54.78	47.76	3.67	0	0	0	0	0.15	0.03	0	1	0.07	0
01125	81.01	0.59	7.14	15.6	1.49	0.52	0	322.87	0.03	0.11	0	0.07	24.24	0.52	0

NDB#	Description & Serving	Grams g	Water kcal	Calories g	Fat g	Fat: Saturated g	Fat: Monounsaturated g	Fat: Polyunsaturated mg	Cholesterol g	Protein g	Carbohydrates g	Fiber mg	Calcium
Milk and cream													
Milk													
01077	Milk, whole, 3.3% fat 1 cup	244	214.7	149.92	8.15	5.07	2.35	0.3	33.18	8.03	11.37	0	291.34
01079	Milk, lowfat, 2% fat, w/ vit A 1 cup	244	217.67	121.2	4.68	2.92	1.35	0.17	18.3	8.13	11.71	0	296.7
01082	Milk, lowfat, 1% fat, w/ vit A 1 cup	244	219.8	102.15	2.59	1.61	0.75	0.1	9.76	8.03	11.66	0	300.12
01085	Milk, skim, w/ vit A 1 cup	245	222.46	85.53	0.44	0.29	0.12	0.02	4.41	8.35	11.88	0	302.33
01088	Milk, bttrmlk, cultured, from skim milk 1 cup	245	220.82	98.99	2.16	1.34	0.62	0.08	8.58	8.11	11.74	0	285.18
01154	Milk, dry, skim, non-fat sol, reg, w/ vit A 1 cup	120	3.79	434.8	0.92	0.6	0.24	0.04	23.52	43.39	62.38	0	1508.28
01090	Milk, dry, whole 1 cup	128	3.16	634.69	34.19	21.43	10.14	0.85	124.29	33.69	49.18	0	1167.87
01095	Milk, canned, cond, swtnd 1 cup	306	83.11	981.58	26.62	16.79	7.43	1.03	103.73	24.2	166.46	0	867.51
01153	Milk, canned, evap, whole, w/ vit A 1 fl oz	31.5	23.32	42.33	2.38	1.45	0.74	0.08	9.26	2.15	3.16	0	82.15
01097	Milk, canned, evap, skim 1 cup	256	203.26	199.48	0.51	0.31	0.16	0.02	9.22	19.33	29.06	0	741.12
01106	Milk, goat 1 cup	244	212.35	167.9	10.1	6.51	2.71	0.36	27.82	8.69	10.86	0	325.74
Cream													
01049	Cream, half and half 1 tablespoon	15	12.09	19.55	1.73	1.07	0.5	0.06	5.54	0.44	0.65	0	15.74
01052	Cream, light whipping 1 cup, fluid (yields 2 cups whipped)	239	151.77	698.88	73.87	46.22	21.73	2.11	265.29	5.19	7.07	0	165.87
01053	Cream, heavy whipping 1 cup, fluid (yields 2 cups whipped)	238	137.35	820.58	88.06	54.82	25.43	3.27	326.3	4.88	6.64	0	153.75
01053	Cream, heavy whipping 1 tablespoon	15	10.28	36.56	3.75	2.33	1.08	0.14	13.13	0.37	0.52	0	13.53
01056	Cream, sour, cultured 1 cup	230	163.19	492.79	48.21	30.01	13.92	1.79	102.12	7.27	9.82	0	267.72
01056	Cream, sour, cultured 1 tablespoon	12	8.51	25.71	2.52	1.57	0.73	0.09	5.33	0.38	0.51	0	13.97
01074	Cream, sour, imitation, cultured 1 cup	230	163.65	479.46	44.9	40.92	1.35	0.13	0	5.52	15.25	0	5.75

NDB#	Phosphorus	Iron	Sodium	Potassium	Magnesium	Zinc	Copper	Vitamin A	Thiamin	Riboflavin	Niacin	Vitamin B6	Folate	Vitamin B12	Vitamin C
	mg	mg	mg	mg	mg	mg	mg	IU	mg	mg	mg	mg	mcg	mcg	mg

Milk and cream

NDB#	Phosphorus	Iron	Sodium	Potassium	Magnesium	Zinc	Copper	Vitamin A	Thiamin	Riboflavin	Niacin	Vitamin B6	Folate	Vitamin B12	Vitamin C
01077	227.9	0.12	119.56	369.66	32.79	0.93	0.02	307.44	0.09	0.4	0.2	0.1	12.2	0.87	2.29
01079	232.04	0.12	121.76	376.74	33.35	0.95	0.02	500.2	0.1	0.4	0.21	0.1	12.44	0.89	2.32
01082	234.73	0.12	123.22	380.88	33.72	0.95	0.02	500.2	0.1	0.41	0.21	0.1	12.44	0.9	2.37
01085	247.21	0.1	126.18	405.72	27.83	0.98	0.03	499.8	0.09	0.34	0.22	0.1	12.74	0.93	2.4
01088	218.54	0.12	257.01	370.69	26.83	1.03	0.03	80.85	0.08	0.38	0.14	0.08	12.25	0.54	2.4
01154	1161.84	0.38	642.36	2152.92	132	4.9	0.05	2637.6	0.5	1.86	1.14	0.43	60	4.84	8.11
01090	992.64	0.6	475.26	1702.27	108.17	4.28	0.1	1180.16	0.36	1.54	0.83	0.39	47.36	4.16	11.06
01095	775.1	0.58	388.62	1136.48	78.49	2.88	0.05	1003.68	0.28	1.27	0.64	0.16	34.27	1.36	7.96
01153	63.79	0.06	33.33	95.48	7.62	0.24	0.01	125.06	0.01	0.1	0.06	0.02	2.49	0.05	0.59
01097	498.94	0.74	294.4	848.64	69.12	2.3	0.04	1003.52	0.12	0.79	0.45	0.14	22.02	0.61	3.17
01106	270.11	0.12	121.51	498.74	34.09	0.73	0.11	451.4	0.12	0.34	0.68	0.11	1.46	0.16	3.15
01049	14.28	0.01	6.11	19.44	1.53	0.08	0	65.1	0.01	0.02	0.01	0.01	0.38	0.05	0.13
01052	146.03	0.07	81.98	231.35	17.28	0.6	0.02	2693.53	0.06	0.3	0.1	0.07	8.84	0.47	1.46
01053	148.51	0.07	89.49	179.45	16.73	0.55	0.01	3498.6	0.05	0.26	0.09	0.06	8.81	0.43	1.38
01053	10.59	0.01	5.55	17.18	1.26	0.04	0	141.3	0	0.02	0.01	0	0.35	0.03	0.11
01056	195.27	0.14	122.59	331.2	25.83	0.62	0.04	1817	0.08	0.34	0.15	0.04	24.84	0.69	1.98
01056	10.19	0.01	6.4	17.28	1.35	0.03	0	94.8	0	0.02	0.01	0	1.3	0.04	0.1
01074	102.35	0.9	234.6	369.15	14.67	2.71	0.13	0	0	0	0	0	0	0	0

NDB#	Description & Serving	Grams	Water	Calories	Fat	Fat: Saturated	Fat: Monounsaturated	Fat: Polyunsaturated	Cholesterol	Protein	Carbohydrates	Fiber	Calcium
		g	kcal	g	g	g	g	mg	g	g	g	mg	
Ice cream, ice milk													
19270	Ice cream, chocolate ½ cup (4 fl oz)	66	36.76	142.56	7.26	4.49	2.12	0.27	22.44	2.51	18.61	0.79	71.94
19271	Ice cream, strawberry ½ cup (4 fl oz)	66	39.6	126.72	5.54	3.43	0	0	19.14	2.11	18.22	0.2	79.2
19095	Ice cream, vanilla ½ cup (4 fl oz)	66	40.26	132.66	7.26	4.48	2.09	0.27	29.04	2.31	15.58	0	84.48
19088	Ice milk, vanilla ½ cup (4 fl oz)	66	45.01	91.74	2.84	1.74	0.81	0.11	9.24	2.51	14.98	0	91.74
Yogurt													
01116	Yogurt, plain, whole milk 1 cup (8 fl oz)	245	215.36	150.48	7.96	5.14	2.19	0.23	31.12	8.5	11.42	0	295.72
01117	Yogurt, plain, lowfat 1 cup (8 fl oz)	245	208.42	155.05	3.8	2.45	1.04	0.11	14.95	12.86	17.25	0	447.37
01118	Yogurt, plain, skim milk 1 cup (8 fl oz)	245	208.81	136.64	0.44	0.28	0.12	0.01	4.41	14.04	18.82	0	487.8
Fats and oils													
Fats													
04542	Chicken fat 1 tablespoon	12.8	0.03	115.25	12.77	3.81	5.72	2.68	10.88	0	0	0	0
04002	Lard 1 tablespoon	12.8	0	115.46	12.8	5.02	5.77	1.43	12.16	0	0	0	0.01
04071	Margarine, reg, hard, corn (hydr) 1 teaspoon	4.7	0.74	33.78	3.78	0.62	2.15	0.85	0	0.04	0.04	0	1.41
04092	Margarine, soft, corn (hydr & reg) 1 teaspoon	4.7	0.76	33.67	3.78	0.66	1.49	1.47	0	0.04	0.02	0	1.25
04585	Margarine blend, 60% corn oil & 40% butter 1 tablespoon	14.2	2.24	101.96	11.46	4.04	4.65	2.26	12.5	0.12	0.09	0	3.98
Oils													
04529	Almond oil 1 tablespoon	13.6	0	120.22	13.6	1.12	9.51	2.37	0	0	0	0	0
04582	Canola oil 1 tablespoon	14	0	123.76	14	0.99	8.25	4.14	0	0	0	0	0
04518	Corn, salad or cooking oil 1 tablespoon	13.6	0	120.22	13.6	1.73	3.29	7.98	0	0	0	0	0
04053	Olive, salad or cooking oil 1 tablespoon	13.5	0	119.34	13.5	1.82	9.95	1.13	0	0	0	0	0.02
04042	Peanut, salad or cooking oil 1 tablespoon	13.5	0	119.34	13.5	2.28	6.24	4.32	0	0	0	0	0.01

NDB#	Phosphorus	Iron	Sodium	Potassium	Magnesium	Zinc	Copper	Vitamin A	Thiamin	Riboflavin	Niacin	Vitamin B6	Folate	Vitamin B12	Vitamin C
	mg	mg	mg	mg	mg	mg	mg	IU	mg	mg	mg	mg	mcg	mcg	mg
19270	70.62	0.61	50.16	164.34	19.14	0.38	0.09	274.56	0.03	0.13	0.15	0.04	10.56	0.19	0.46
19271	66	0.14	39.6	124.08	9.24	0.22	0.02	211.2	0.03	0.17	0.11	0.03	7.92	0.2	5.08
19095	69.3	0.06	52.8	131.34	9.24	0.46	0.02	269.94	0.03	0.16	0.08	0.03	3.3	0.26	0.4
19088	71.94	0.07	56.1	139.26	9.9	0.29	0.01	108.9	0.04	0.17	0.06	0.04	3.96	0.44	0.53
01116	232.51	0.12	113.68	378.77	28.37	1.45	0.02	301.35	0.07	0.35	0.18	0.08	18.13	0.91	1.3
01117	351.58	0.2	171.99	572.81	42.75	2.18	0.03	161.7	0.11	0.52	0.28	0.12	27.44	1.38	1.96
01118	383.43	0.22	187.43	624.51	46.8	2.38	0.04	17.15	0.12	0.57	0.3	0.13	29.89	1.5	2.13

Fats and oils

NDB#	Phosphorus	Iron	Sodium	Potassium	Magnesium	Zinc	Copper	Vitamin A	Thiamin	Riboflavin	Niacin	Vitamin B6	Folate	Vitamin B12	Vitamin C
04542	0	0	0	0	0	0	0	0	0	0	0	0	0	0	0
04002	0	0	0	0	0	0.01	0	0	0	0	0	0	0	0	0
04071	1.08	0	44.34	1.99	0.12	0	0	167.84	0	0	0	0	0.06	0	0.01
04092	0.95	0	50.7	1.77	0.11	0	0	167.84	0	0	0	0	0.05	0	0.01
04585	3.27	0.01	127.37	5.11	0.28	0	0	507.08	0	0	0	0	0.28	0.01	0.01
04529	0	0	0	0	0	0	0	0	0	0	0	0	0	0	0
04582	0	0	0	0	0	0	0	0	0	0	0	0	0	0	0
04518 0	0	0	0	0	0	0	0	0	0	0	0	0	0	0	
04053	0.16	0.05	0.01	0	0	0.01	0	0	0	0	0	0	0	0	0
04042	0	0	0.01	0	0.01	0	0	0	0	0	0	0	0	0	0

NDB#	Description & Serving	Grams	Water	Calories	Fat	Fat: Saturated	Fat: Monounsaturated	Fat: Polyunsaturated	Cholesterol	Protein	Carbohydrates	Fiber	Calcium
		g	kcal	g	g	g	g	mg	g	g	g	mg
04058	Sesame, salad or cooking oil 1 tablespoon	13.6	0	120.22	13.6	1.93	5.4	5.67	0	0	0	0	0
04044	Soybean, salad or cooking oil (hydrognated) 1 tablespoon	13.6	0	120.22	13.6	1.96	3.17	7.87	0	0	0	0	0.01
04038	Wheat germ oil 1 tablespoon	13.6	0	120.22	13.6	2.56	2.05	8.39	0	0	0	0	0

Fruits and fruit juices

NDB#	Description & Serving	Grams	Water	Calories	Fat	Fat: Saturated	Fat: Monounsaturated	Fat: Polyunsaturated	Cholesterol	Protein	Carbohydrates	Fiber	Calcium
09003	Apples, raw, with skin 3½" diameter	212	178	125	0.8	0.1	0	0.2	0	0.4	32	5.7	14.8
09011	Apples, dried, sulfured, uncooked 1 cup	86	27.31	208.98	0.28	0.04	0.01	0.08	0	0.8	56.67	7.48	12.04
09400	Apple juice, canned or bottled, unsweetened, w/ vit C 1 cup	248	218.07	116.56	0.27	0.05	0.01	0.08	0	0.15	28.97	0.25	17.36
09021	Apricots, raw 1 cup, halves	155	133.84	74.4	0.6	0.04	0.26	0.12	0	2.17	17.24	3.72	21.7
09024	Apricots, canned, juice pk, w/skin, sol & liquids 1 cup, halves	244	211.35	117.12	0.1	0.01	0.04	0.02	0	1.54	30.11	3.9	29.28
09032	Apricots, dried, sulfured, uncooked 1 half	3.5	1.09	8.33	0.02	0	0.01	0	0	0.13	2.16	0.32	1.58
09403	Apricot nectar, canned, w/ vit C 1 cup	251	213.02	140.56	0.23	0.02	0.1	0.04	0	0.93	36.12	1.51	17.57
09038	Avocados, raw, California 1 fruit, without skin and seeds	173	125.53	306.21	29.98	4.48	19.4	3.53	0	3.65	11.95	8.48	19.03
09039	Avocados, raw, Florida 1 fruit, without skin and seeds	304	242.38	340.48	26.96	5.34	14.8	4.5	0	4.83	27.09	16.11	33.44
09040	Bananas, raw 1 cup, sliced	150	111.39	138	0.72	0.28	0.06	0.13	0	1.55	35.15	3.6	9
09042	Blackberries, raw 1 cup	144	123.32	74.88	0.56	0.02	0.05	0.32	0	1.04	18.37	7.63	46.08
09050	Blueberries, raw 1 pint, as purchased	402	340.13	225.12	1.53	0.13	0.22	0.67	0	2.69	56.8	10.85	24.12
09063	Cherries, sour, red, raw 1 cup with pits	103	0	0	0	0	0	0	0	0	0	0	0
09070	Cherries, sweet, raw 1 cup, with pits	117	94.49	84.24	1.12	0.25	0.31	0.34	0	1.4	19.36	2.69	17.55
09083	Currants, European black, raw 1 cup	112	91.8	70.56	0.46	0.04	0.06	0.2	0	1.57	17.23	0	61.6
09085	Currants, zante, dried 1 cup	144	27.66	407.52	0.39	0.04	0.07	0.26	0	5.88	106.68	9.79	123.84
09087	Dates, domestic, nat & dry 1 cup, pitted, chopped	178	40.05	489.5	0.8	0.34	0.27	0.06	0	3.51	130.85	13.35	56.96

NDB#	Phosphorus	Iron	Sodium	Potassium	Magnesium	Zinc	Copper	Vitamin A	Thiamin	Riboflavin	Niacin	Vitamin B6	Folate	Vitamin B12	Vitamin C
	mg	mg	mg	mg	mg	mg	mg	IU	mg	mg	mg	mg	mcg	mcg	mg
04058	0	0	0	0	0	0	0	0	0	0	0	0	0	0	0
04044	0.03	0	0	0	0	0	0	0	0	0	0	0	0	0	0
04038	0	0	0	0	0	0	0	0	0	0	0	0	0	0	0

Fruits and fruit juices

NDB#	Phosphorus	Iron	Sodium	Potassium	Magnesium	Zinc	Copper	Vitamin A	Thiamin	Riboflavin	Niacin	Vitamin B6	Folate	Vitamin B12	Vitamin C
09003	14.8	0.4	0	243.8	10.6	0.1	0.1	112.4	0.04	0.03	0.2	0.1	5.9	0	12.1
09011	32.68	1.2	74.82	387	13.76	0.17	0.16	0	0	0.14	0.8	0.11	0	0	3.35
09400	17.36	0.92	7.44	295.12	7.44	0.07	0.05	2.48	0.05	0.04	0	0.07	0.25	0	103.17
09021	29.45	0.84	1.55	458.8	12.4	0.4	0.14	4048.6	0.05	0.06	0.93	0.08	13.33	0	15.5
09024	48.8	0.73	9.76	402.6	24.4	0.27	0.13	4126.04	0.04	0.05	0.84	0.13	4.15	0	11.96
09032	4.1	0.16	0.35	48.23	1.65	0.03	0.02	253.4	0	0.01	0.1	0.01	0.36	0	0.08
09403	22.59	0.95	7.53	286.14	12.55	0.23	0.18	3303.16	0.02	0.04	0.65	0.06	3.26	0	136.54
09038	72.66	2.04	20.76	1096.82	70.93	0.73	0.46	1058.76	0.19	0.21	3.32	0.48	113.32	0	13.67
09038	118.56	1.61	15.2	1483.52	103.36	1.28	0.76	1860.48	0.33	0.37	5.84	0.85	162.03	0	24.02
09040	30	0.47	1.5	594	43.5	0.24	0.16	121.5	0.07	0.15	0.81	0.87	28.65	0	13.65
09042	30.24	0.82	0	282.24	28.8	0.39	0.2	237.6	0.04	0.06	0.58	0.08	48.96	0	30.24
09050	40.2	0.68	24.12	357.78	20.1	0.44	0.25	402	0.19	0.2	1.44	0.14	25.73	0	52.26
09063	0	0	0	0	0	0	0	0	0	0	0	0	0	0	0
09070	22.23	0.46	0	262.08	12.87	0.07	0.11	250.38	0.06	0.07	0.47	0.04	4.91	0	8.19
09083	66.08	1.72	2.24	360.64	26.88	0.3	0.1	257.6	0.06	0.06	0.34	0.07	0	0	202.72
09085	180	4.69	11.52	1284.48	59.04	0.95	0.67	105.12	0.23	0.2	2.33	0.43	14.69	0	6.77
09087	71.2	2.05	5.34	1160.56	62.3	0.52	0.51	89	0.16	0.18	3.92	0.34	22.43	0	0

NDB#	Description & Serving	Grams	Water	Calories	Fat	Fat, Saturated	Fat, Monounsaturated	Fat, Polyunsaturated	Cholesterol	Protein	Carbohydrates	Fiber	Calcium
		g	kcal	g	g	g	g	mg	g	g	g	mg	
09088	Elderberries, raw 1 cup	145	115.71	105.85	0.73	0.03	0.12	0.36	0	0.96	26.68	10.15	55.1
09094	Figs, dried, uncooked 1 fig	19	5.4	48.45	0.22	0.04	0.05	0.11	0	0.58	12.42	1.77	27.36
09109	Gooseberries, canned, light syrup pk, sol & liquids 1 cup	252	201.85	183.96	0.5	0.03	0.05	0.28	0	1.64	47.25	6.05	40.32
09111	Grapefruit, raw, pink & red & white, all areas 1 cup sections with juice	230	209.05	73.6	0.23	0.03	0.03	0.06	0	1.45	18.58	2.53	27.6
09123	Grapefruit juice, canned, unsweetened 1 cup	247	222.55	93.86	0.25	0.03	0.03	0.06	0	1.28	22.13	0.25	17.29
09131	Grapes, American type (slipskin), raw 1 cup	92	74.8	57.96	0.32	0.1	0.01	0.09	0	0.58	15.78	0.92	12.88
09132	Grapes, European type (adherent skin), raw 1 cup, seedless	160	128.9	113.6	0.93	0.3	0.04	0.27	0	1.06	28.43	1.6	17.6
09135	Grape juice, canned or bottled, unsweetened, wo/vit C 1 cup	253	212.82	154.33	0.2	0.06	0.01	0.06	0	1.42	37.85	0.25	22.77
09139	Guavas, common, raw 1 cup, strawberry	244	210.08	124.44	1.46	0.42	0.13	0.62	0	2	28.99	13.18	48.8
09148	Kiwi fruit, (Chinese gooseberries), fresh, raw 1 large fruit, without skin	91	75.58	55.51	0.4	0.03	0.04	0.22	0	0.9	13.54	3.09	23.66
09149	Kumquats, raw 1 fruit, without refuse	19	15.52	11.97	0.02	0	0	0	0	0.17	3.12	1.25	8.36
09152	Lemon juice, raw 1 fl oz	30.5	27.67	7.63	0	0	0	0	0	0.12	2.63	0.12	2.14
09160	Lime juice, raw 1 fl oz	30.8	27.78	8.32	0.03	0	0	0.01	0	0.14	2.78	0.12	2.77
09176	Mangos, raw 1 fruit, without refuse	207	169.14	134.55	0.56	0.14	0.21	0.11	0	1.06	35.19	3.73	20.7
09181	Melons, cantaloupe, raw 1 cup, balls	177	158.91	61.95	0.5	0.13	0.01	0.19	0	1.56	14.8	1.42	19.47
09184	Melons, honeydew, raw 1 cup, diced (approx 20 pieces per cup)	170	152.42	59.5	0.17	0.04	0	0.07	0	0.78	15.61	1.02	10.2
09191	Nectarines, raw 1 fruit (2½" dia)	136	117.34	66.64	0.63	0.07	0.24	0.31	0	1.28	16.02	2.18	6.8
09193	Olives, ripe, canned (small-extra lrg) 1 large	4.4	3.52	5.06	0.47	0.06	0.35	0.04	0	0.04	0.28	0.14	3.87
09194	Olives, ripe, canned (jumbo-super colossal) 1 jumbo	8.3	7	6.72	0.57	0.08	0.42	0.05	0	0.08	0.47	0.21	7.8
09201	Oranges, raw, California, Valencias 1 fruit (2⅝" dia, sphere)	121	104.47	59.29	0.36	0.04	0.07	0.07	0	1.26	14.39	3.03	48.4
09202	Oranges, raw, California, navels 1 fruit (2⅞" dia)	140	121.53	64.4	0.13	0.02	0.02	0.03	0	1.44	16.28	3.36	56
09203	Oranges, raw, Florida 1 fruit (2⅝" dia, sphere)	141	122.87	64.86	0.3	0.04	0.05	0.06	0	0.99	16.27	3.38	60.63

NDB#	Phosphorus	Iron	Sodium	Potassium	Magnesium	Zinc	Copper	Vitamin A	Thiamin	Riboflavin	Niacin	Vitamin B6	Folate	Vitamin B12	Vitamin C
	mg	mg	mg	mg	mg	mg	mg	IU	mg	mg	mg	mg	mcg	mcg	mg
09088	56.55	2.32	8.7	406	7.25	0.16	0.09	870	0.1	0.09	0.73	0.33	8.7	0	52.2
09094	12.92	0.42	2.09	135.28	11.21	0.1	0.06	25.27	0.01	0.02	0.13	0.04	1.43	0	0.15
09109	17.64	0.83	5.04	194.04	15.12	0.28	0.55	347.76	0.05	0.13	0.39	0.03	8.06	0	25.2
09111	18.4	0.21	0	319.7	18.4	0.16	0.11	285.2	0.08	0.05	0.58	0.1	23.46	0	79.12
09123	27.17	0.49	2.47	377.91	24.7	0.22	0.09	17.29	0.1	0.05	0.57	0.05	25.69	0	72.12
09131	9.2	0.27	1.84	175.72	4.6	0.04	0.04	92	0.08	0.05	0.28	0.1	3.59	0	3.68
09132	20.8	0.42	3.2	296	9.6	0.08	0.14	116.8	0.15	0.09	0.48	0.18	6.24	0	17.28
09135	27.83	0.61	7.59	333.96	25.3	0.13	0.07	20.24	0.07	0.09	0.66	0.16	6.58	0	0.25
09139	61	0.76	7.32	692.96	24.4	0.56	0.25	1932.48	0.12	0.12	2.93	0.35	34.16	0	447.74
09148	36.4	0.37	4.55	302.12	27.3	0.15	0.14	159.25	0.02	0.05	0.46	0.08	34.58	0	89.18
09149	3.61	0.07	1.14	37.05	2.47	0.02	0.02	57.38	0.02	0.02	0.1	0.01	3.04	0	7.11
09152	1.83	0.01	0.31	37.82	1.83	0.02	0.01	6.1	0.01	0	0.03	0.02	3.93	0	14.03
09160	2.16	0.01	0.31	33.57	1.85	0.02	0.01	3.08	0.01	0	0.03	0.01	2.53	0	9.02
09176	22.77	0.27	4.14	322.92	18.63	0.08	0.23	8060.58	0.12	0.12	1.21	0.28	28.98	0	57.34
09181	30.09	0.37	15.93	546.93	19.47	0.28	0.07	5706.48	0.06	0.04	1.02	0.2	30.09	0	74.69
09184	17	0.12	17	460.7	11.9	0.12	0.07	68	0.13	0.03	1.02	0.1	10.2	0	42.16
09191	21.76	0.2	0	288.32	10.88	0.12	0.1	1000.96	0.02	0.06	1.35	0.03	5.03	0	7.34
09193	0.13	0.15	38.37	0.35	0.18	0.01	0.01	17.73	0	0	0	0	0	0	0.04
09194	0.25	0.28	74.53	0.75	0.33	0.02	0.02	28.72	0	0	0	0	0	0	0.12
09201	20.57	0.11	0	216.59	12.1	0.07	0.04	278.3	0.11	0.05	0.33	0.08	46.71	0	58.69
09202	26.6	0.17	1.4	249.2	14	0.08	0.08	256.2	0.12	0.06	0.41	0.1	47.18	0	80.22
09203	16.92	0.13	0	238.29	14.1	0.11	0.05	282	0.14	0.06	0.56	0.07	24.39	0	63.45

NDB#	Description & Serving	Grams	Water	Calories	Fat	Fat, Saturated	Fat, Monounsaturated	Fat, Polyunsaturated	Cholesterol	Protein	Carbohydrates	Fiber	Calcium
		g	g	kcal	g	g	g	g	mg	g	g	g	mg
09206	Orange juice, raw 1 cup	248	218.98	111.6	0.5	0.06	0.09	0.1	0	1.74	25.79	0.5	27.28
09218	Tangerines (mandarin oranges), raw 1 large (2½" dia)	98	85.85	43.12	0.19	0.02	0.03	0.04	0	0.62	10.97	2.25	13.72
09219	Tangerines (mandarin oranges), canned, juice pk 1 cup	249	222.88	92.13	0.07	0.01	0.01	0.01	0	1.54	23.83	1.74	27.39
09226	Papayas, raw 1 cup, cubes	140	124.36	54.6	0.2	0.06	0.05	0.04	0	0.85	13.73	2.52	33.6
09229	Papaya nectar, canned 1 cup	250	212.55	142.5	0.38	0.12	0.1	0.09	0	0.43	36.28	1.5	25
09231	Passion fruit (granadilla), purple, raw 1 fruit, without refuse	18	13.13	17.46	0.13	0.01	0.02	0.07	0	0.4	4.21	1.87	2.16
09236	Peaches, raw 1 large (2¾" dia) (approx 2½ per lb)	157	137.63	67.51	0.14	0.02	0.05	0.07	0	1.1	17.43	3.14	7.85
09246	Peaches, dried, sulfured, uncooked 1 half	13	4.13	31.07	0.1	0.01	0.04	0.05	0	0.47	7.97	1.07	3.64
09251	Peach nectar, canned, wo/ vit C 1 cup	249	213.24	134.46	0.05	0	0.02	0.03	0	0.67	34.66	1.49	12.45
09252	Pears, raw 1 medium (approx 2½ per lb)	166	139.12	97.94	0.66	0.04	0.14	0.16	0	0.65	25.08	3.98	18.26
09259	Pears, dried, sulfured, uncooked 1 half with liquid	76	20.28	199.12	0.48	0.03	0.1	0.11	0	1.42	52.97	5.7	25.84
09265	Persimmons, native, raw 1 fruit, without refuse	25	16.1	31.75	0.1	0	0	0	0	0.2	8.38	0	6.75
09266	Pineapple, raw 1 cup, diced	155	134.08	75.95	0.67	0.05	0.07	0.23	0	0.6	19.2	1.86	10.85
09273	Pineapple juice, canned, unsweetened, wo/ vit C 1 cup	250	213.83	140	0.2	0.01	0.02	0.07	0	0.8	34.45	0.5	42.5
09278	Plantains, cooked 1 cup, slices	154	103.64	178.64	0.28	0.11	0.02	0.05	0	1.22	47.97	3.54	3.08
09279	Plums, raw 1 fruit (2⅛" dia)	66	56.23	36.3	0.41	0.03	0.27	0.09	0	0.52	8.59	0.99	2.64
09286	Pomegranates, raw 1 pomegranate (3⅜" dia)	154	124.69	104.72	0.46	0.06	0.07	0.1	0	1.46	26.44	0.92	4.62
09287	Prickly pears, raw 1 fruit	103	90.18	42.23	0.53	0.07	0.08	0.22	0	0.75	9.86	3.71	57.68
09291	Prunes, dried, uncooked 1 prune	8.4	2.72	20.08	0.04	0	0.03	0.01	0	0.22	5.27	0.6	4.28
09294	Prune juice, canned 1 cup	256	207.97	181.76	0.08	0.01	0.05	0.02	0	1.56	44.67	2.56	30.72
09296	Quinces, raw 1 fruit, without refuse	92	77.1	52.44	0.09	0.01	0.03	0.05	0	0.37	14.08	1.75	10.12
09298	Raisins, seedless 1 cup, packed	165	25.44	495	0.76	0.25	0.03	0.22	0	5.31	130.56	6.6	80.85

NDB#	Phosphorus	Iron	Sodium	Potassium	Magnesium	Zinc	Copper	Vitamin A	Thiamin	Riboflavin	Niacin	Vitamin B6	Folate	Vitamin B12	Vitamin C
	mg	mg	mg	mg	mg	mg	mg	IU	mg	mg	mg	mg	mcg	mcg	mg
09206	42.16	0.5	2.48	496	27.28	0.12	0.11	496	0.22	0.07	0.99	0.1	75.14	0	124
09218	9.8	0.1	0.98	153.86	11.76	0.24	0.03	901.6	0.1	0.02	0.16	0.07	19.99	0	30.18
09219	24.9	0.67	12.45	331.17	27.39	1.27	0.08	2121.48	0.2	0.07	1.11	0.1	11.45	0	85.16
09226	7	0.14	4.2	359.8	14	0.1	0.02	397.6	0.04	0.04	0.47	0.03	53.2	0	86.52
09229	0	0.85	12.5	77.5	7.5	0.38	0.03	277.5	0.02	0.01	0.38	0.02	5.25	0	7.5
09231	12.24	0.29	5.04	62.64	5.22	0.02	0.02	126	0	0.02	0.27	0.02	2.52	0	5.4
09236	18.84	0.17	0	309.29	10.99	0.22	0.11	839.95	0.03	0.06	1.55	0.03	5.34	0	10.36
09246	15.47	0.53	0.91	129.48	5.46	0.07	0.05	281.19	0	0.03	0.57	0.01	0.04	0	0.62
09251	14.94	0.47	17.43	99.6	9.96	0.2	0.17	642.42	0.01	0.03	0.72	0.02	3.49	0	13.2
09252	18.26	0.42	0	207.5	9.96	0.2	0.18	33.2	0.03	0.07	0.17	0.03	12.12	0	6.64
09259	44.84	1.6	4.56	405.08	25.08	0.3	0.28	2.28	0.01	0.11	1.04	0.05	0	0	5.32
09265	6.5	0.63	0.25	77.5	0	0	0	0	0	0	0	0	0	0	16.5
09266	10.85	0.57	1.55	175.15	21.7	0.12	0.17	35.65	0.14	0.06	0.65	0.13	16.43	0	23.87
09273	20	0.65	2.5	335	32.5	0.28	0.23	12.5	0.14	0.06	0.64	0.24	57.75	0	26.75
09278	43.12	0.89	7.7	716.1	49.28	0.2	0.1	1399.86	0.07	0.08	1.16	0.37	40.04	0	16.79
09279	6.6	0.07	0	113.52	4.62	0.07	0.03	213.18	0.03	0.06	0.33	0.05	1.45	0	6.27
09286	12.32	0.46	4.62	398.86	4.62	0.18	0.11	0	0.05	0.05	0.46	0.16	9.24	0	9.39
09287	24.72	0.31	5.15	226.6	87.55	0.12	0.08	52.53	0.01	0.06	0.47	0.06	6.18	0	14.42
09291	6.64	0.21	0.34	62.58	3.78	0.04	0.04	166.91	0.01	0.01	0.16	0.02	0.31	0	0.28
09294	64	3.02	10.24	706.56	35.84	0.54	0.17	7.68	0.04	0.18	2.01	0.56	1.02	0	10.5
09296	15.64	0.64	3.68	181.24	7.36	0.04	0.12	36.8	0.02	0.03	0.18	0.04	2.76	0	13.8
09298	160.05	3.43	19.8	1239.15	54.45	0.45	0.51	13.2	0.26	0.15	1.35	0.41	5.45	0	5.45

NDB#	Description & Serving	Grams	Water	Calories	Fat	Fat: Saturated	Fat: Monounsaturated	Fat: Polyunsaturated	Cholesterol	Protein	Carbohydrates	Fiber	Calcium
		g	kcal	g	g	g	g	mg	g	g	g	mg	
09302	Raspberries, raw 1 cup	123	106.48	60.27	0.68	0.02	0.07	0.38	0	1.12	14.23	8.36	27.06
09309	Rhubarb, frozen, uncooked 1 cup, diced	137	128.11	28.77	0.15	0.04	0.03	0.07	0	0.75	6.99	2.47	265.78
09316	Strawberries, raw 1 cup, halves	152	139.19	45.6	0.56	0.03	0.08	0.28	0	0.93	10.67	3.5	21.28
09326	Watermelon, raw 1 cup, balls	154	140.93	49.28	0.66	0.07	0.16	0.22	0	0.95	11.06	0.77	12.32

Grain products

Breads

NDB#	Description & Serving	Grams	Water	Calories	Fat	Fat: Saturated	Fat: Monounsaturated	Fat: Polyunsaturated	Cholesterol	Protein	Carbohydrates	Fiber	Calcium
18001	Bagels, plain, enriched, w/calcium propionate (incl onion, poppy, sesame) 1 bagel (3" dia)	57	18.58	156.75	0.91	0.13	0.07	0.4	0	5.99	30.44	1.31	42.18
18007	Bagels, oat bran 1 bagel (3" dia)	57	18.75	145.35	0.68	0.11	0.14	0.28	0	6.1	30.38	2.05	6.84
18079	Bread crumbs, dry, grated, plain 1 cup	108	6.7	426.6	5.83	1.36	2.26	1.68	0	13.5	78.3	2.59	245.16
18080	Breadsticks, plain 1 small stick (approx 4¼" long)	5	0.31	20.6	0.48	0.07	0.19	0.18	0	0.6	3.42	0.15	1.1
18347	Dinner rolls, wheat 1 roll (1 oz)	28.35	10.49	77.4	1.79	0.43	0.92	0.3	0	2.44	13.04	1.07	49.9
18258	English muffins, plain, enriched, w/ca prop (incl sourdough) 1 muffin	57	24	133.95	1.03	0.15	0.17	0.51	0	4.39	26.22	1.54	99.18
18266	English muffins, whole-wheat 1 muffin	66	30.16	133.98	1.39	0.22	0.34	0.55	0	5.81	26.66	4.42	174.9
18349	French rolls 1 roll	38	13.22	105.26	1.63	0.37	0.75	0.32	0	3.27	19.08	1.22	34.58
18029	French or Vienna bread (incl sourdough) 1 large slice (5" × 2½" × 1")	35	12.01	95.9	1.05	0.22	0.43	0.24	0	3.08	18.17	1.05	26.25
18350	Hamburger or hot dog, plain rolls 1 roll	43	14.62	122.98	2.19	0.51	1.07	0.39	0	3.66	21.63	1.16	59.77
18353	Hard (incl kaiser) rolls 1 roll (3½" dia)	57	17.67	167.01	2.45	0.35	0.65	0.98	0	5.64	30.04	1.31	54.15
18033	Italian bread 1 large slice (4½" × 3¼" × ¾")	30	10.71	81.3	1.05	0.26	0.24	0.42	0	2.64	15	0.81	23.4
18035	Mixed-grain (incl whole-grain, 7-grain) bread 1 large slice	32	12.06	80	1.22	0.26	0.49	0.3	0	3.2	14.85	2.05	29.12
18041	Pita, white, enriched bread 1 large pita (6½" dia)	60	19.26	165	0.72	0.1	0.06	0.32	0	5.46	33.42	1.32	51.6
18042	Pita, whole-wheat bread 1 large pita (6½" dia)	64	19.58	170.24	1.66	0.26	0.22	0.68	0	6.27	35.2	4.74	9.6

NDB#	Phosphorus	Iron	Sodium	Potassium	Magnesium	Zinc	Copper	Vitamin A	Thiamin	Riboflavin	Niacin	Vitamin B6	Folate	Vitamin B12	Vitamin C
	mg	mg	mg	mg	mg	mg	mg	IU	mg	mg	mg	mg	mcg	mcg	mg
09302	14.76	0.7	0	186.96	22.14	0.57	0.09	159.9	0.04	0.11	1.11	0.07	31.98	0	30.75
09309	16.44	0.4	2.74	147.96	24.66	0.14	0.03	146.59	0.04	0.04	0.28	0.03	11.23	0	6.58
09316	28.88	0.58	1.52	252.32	15.2	0.2	0.07	41.04	0.03	0.1	0.35	0.09	26.9	0	86.18
09326	13.86	0.26	3.08	178.64	16.94	0.11	0.05	563.64	0.12	0.03	0.31	0.22	3.39	0	14.78

Grain products

NDB#	Phosphorus	Iron	Sodium	Potassium	Magnesium	Zinc	Copper	Vitamin A	Thiamin	Riboflavin	Niacin	Vitamin B6	Folate	Vitamin B12	Vitamin C
18001	54.72	2.03	304.38	57.57	16.53	0.5	0.09	0	0.31	0.18	2.6	0.03	12.54	0	0
18007	94.05	1.76	288.99	116.28	32.49	1.19	0.07	2.28	0.19	0.19	1.69	0.12	26.22	0	0.11
18079	158.76	6.61	930.96	238.68	49.68	1.32	0.18	1.08	0.83	0.47	7.4	0.11	27	0.02	0
18347	6.05	0.21	32.85	6.2	1.6	0.04	0.01	0	0.03	0.03	0.26	0	1.5	0	0
18347	33.45	1.01	96.39	37.71	11.91	0.29	0.04	0	0.12	0.08	1.15	0.02	4.25	0	0
18258	75.81	1.43	264.48	74.67	11.97	0.4	0.07	0	0.25	0.16	2.21	0.02	21.09	0.02	0.06
18266	186.12	1.62	420.42	138.6	46.86	1.06	0.14	0	0.2	0.09	2.25	0.11	32.34	0	0
18349	31.92	1.03	231.42	43.32	7.6	0.29	0.07	1.52	0.2	0.11	1.65	0.02	12.54	0	0
18029	36.75	0.89	213.15	39.55	9.45	0.3	0.07	0	0.18	0.12	1.66	0.02	10.85	0	0
18350	37.84	1.36	240.8	60.63	8.6	0.27	0.05	0	0.21	0.13	1.69	0.02	11.61	0.01	0
18353	57	1.87	310.08	61.56	15.39	0.54	0.09	0	0.27	0.19	2.42	0.03	8.55	0	0
18033	30.9	0.88	175.2	33	8.1	0.26	0.06	0	0.14	0.09	1.31	0.01	9	0	0
18035	56.32	1.11	155.84	65.28	16.96	0.41	0.08	0	0.13	0.11	1.4	0.11	15.36	0.02	0.1
18041	58.2	1.57	321.6	72	15.6	0.5	0.1	0	0.36	0.2	2.78	0.02	14.4	0	0
18042	115.2	1.85	340.48	108.8	44.16	0.97	0.18	0	0.22	0.05	1.82	0.15	22.4	0	0

NDB#	Description & Serving	Grams	Water	Calories	Fat	Fat: Saturated	Fat: Monounsaturated	Fat: Polyunsaturated	Cholesterol	Protein	Carbohydrates	Fiber	Calcium
		g	kcal	kcal	g	g	g	g	mg	g	g	g	mg
18044	**Pumpernickel bread** 1 regular slice	26	9.85	65	0.81	0.11	0.24	0.32	0	2.26	12.35	1.69	17.68
18047	**Raisin, enriched bread** 1 large slice	32	10.75	87.68	1.41	0.35	0.73	0.22	0	2.53	16.74	1.38	21.12
18060	**Rye bread** 1 slice	32	11.94	82.88	1.06	0.2	0.42	0.26	0	2.72	15.46	1.86	23.36
18064	**Wheat (incl wheat berry) bread** 1 slice	25	9.28	65	1.03	0.22	0.43	0.23	0	2.28	11.8	1.08	26.25
18069	**White bread, commly prep (incl soft bread crumbs)** 1 cup, crumbs	45	16.52	120.15	1.62	0.36	0.73	0.33	0.45	3.69	22.28	1.04	48.6
18360	**Taco shells, baked** 1 large (6½" dia)	21	1.26	98.28	4.75	0.7	1.99	1.81	0	1.51	13.1	1.58	33.6
18363	**Tortillas, rtb or -fry, corn** 1 medium tortilla (approx 6" dia)	26	11.47	57.72	0.65	0.09	0.17	0.29	0	1.48	12.12	1.35	45.5
18364	**Tortillas, rtb or -fry, flour** 1 medium tortilla (approx 6" dia)	32	8.58	104	2.27	0.35	0.92	0.89	0	2.78	17.79	1.06	40
Crackers													
18214	**Cheese, regular** 1 cup, bite size	62	1.92	311.86	15.69	5.81	5.58	3	8.06	6.26	36.08	1.49	93.62
18215	**Cheese, sandwich-type w/pnut butter filling** 1 sandwich	7	0.27	33.74	1.62	0.36	0.85	0.31	0.35	0.88	3.99	0.2	5.53
18216	**Crispbread, rye** 1 crispbread or cracker	10	0.61	36.6	0.13	0.01	0.02	0.06	0	0.79	8.22	1.65	3.1
18217	**Matzoh, plain** 1 matzoh	28.35	1.22	111.98	0.4	0.06	0.04	0.17	0	2.84	23.73	0.85	3.69
18220	**Melba toast, plain** 1 cup, pieces	30	1.53	117	0.96	0.13	0.23	0.38	0	3.63	22.98	1.89	27.9
18226	**Rye, wafers, plain** 1 cracker (4½" × 2½" × ⅛")	11	0.55	36.74	0.1	0.01	0.02	0.04	0	1.06	8.84	2.52	4.4
18228	**Saltines (incl oyster, soda, soup)** 1 cup, oyster crackers	45	1.85	195.3	5.31	0.95	2.91	0.83	0	4.14	32.18	1.35	53.55
18232	**Wheat, regular** 1 Euphrates	4	0.12	18.92	0.82	0.15	0.47	0.12	0	0.34	2.6	0.18	1.96
Flours and meals													
20011	**Buckwheat flour, whole-groat** 1 cup	120	13.38	402	3.72	0.81	1.14	1.14	0	15.14	84.71	12	49.2
20322	**Cornmeal, degermed, enriched, white** 1 cup	138	15.99	505.08	2.28	0.31	0.57	0.98	0	11.7	107.2	10.21	6.9
20022	**Cornmeal, degermed, enriched, yellow** 1 cup	138	15.99	505.08	2.28	0.31	0.57	0.98	0	11.7	107.2	10.21	6.9

NDB#	Phosphorus	Iron	Sodium	Potassium	Magnesium	Zinc	Copper	Vitamin A	Thiamin	Riboflavin	Niacin	Vitamin B6	Folate	Vitamin B12	Vitamin C
	mg	mg	mg	mg	mg	mg	mg	IU	mg	mg	mg	mg	mcg	mcg	mg
18044	46.28	0.75	174.46	54.08	14.04	0.38	0.07	0	0.09	0.08	0.8	0.03	8.84	0	0
18047	34.88	0.93	124.8	72.64	8.32	0.23	0.06	0.64	0.11	0.13	1.11	0.02	10.88	0	0.16
18060	40	0.91	211.2	53.12	12.8	0.36	0.06	1.28	0.14	0.11	1.22	0.02	16.32	0	0.06
18064	37.5	0.83	132.5	50.25	11.5	0.26	0.05	0	0.1	0.07	1.03	0.02	10.25	0	0
18069	42.3	1.36	242.1	53.55	10.8	0.28	0.06	0	0.21	0.15	1.79	0.03	15.3	0.01	0
18360	52.08	0.53	77.07	37.59	22.05	0.29	0.03	73.5	0.05	0.01	0.28	0.08	1.26	0	0
18363	81.64	0.36	41.86	40.04	16.9	0.24	0.04	62.92	0.03	0.02	0.39	0.06	3.9	0	0
18364	39.68	1.06	152.96	41.92	8.32	0.23	0.09	0	0.17	0.09	1.14	0.02	3.84	0	0
18214	135.16	2.96	616.9	89.9	22.32	0.7	0.13	100.44	0.35	0.27	2.9	0.34	15.5	0.29	0
18215	22.68	0.2	69.44	17.15	4.06	0.08	0.02	22.33	0.03	0.02	0.46	0.1	1.75	0	0
18216	26.9	0.24	26.4	31.9	7.8	0.24	0.03	0	0.02	0.01	0.1	0.02	2.2	0	0
	25.23	0.9	0.57	31.75	7.09	0.19	0.02	0	0.11	0.08	1.1	0.03	3.97	0	0
18220	58.8	1.11	248.7	60.6	17.7	0.6	0.09	0	0.12	0.08	1.23	0.03	7.8	0	0
18226	36.74	0.65	87.34	54.45	13.31	0.31	0.05	2.53	0.05	0.03	0.17	0.03	4.95	0	0.01
18232	47.25	2.43	585.9	57.6	12.15	0.35	0.09	0	0.25	0.21	2.36	0.02	13.95	0	0
18232	8.8	0.18	31.8	7.32	2.48	0.06	0.01	0	0.02	0.01	0.2	0.01	0.72	0	0
20011	404.4	4.87	13.2	692.4	301.2	3.74	0.62	0	0.5	0.23	7.38	0.7	64.8	0	0
20322	115.92	5.7	4.14	223.56	55.2	0.99	0.11	0	0.99	0.56	6.95	0.35	66.24	0	0
20022	115.92	5.7	4.14	223.56	55.2	0.99	0.11	569.94	0.99	0.56	6.95	0.35	66.24	0	0

NDB#	Description & Serving	Grams	Water	Calories	Fat	Fat: Saturated	Fat: Monounsaturated	Fat: Polyunsaturated	Cholesterol	Protein	Carbohydrates	Fiber	Calcium
		g	g	kcal	g	g	g	g	mg	g	g	g	mg
20320	Cornmeal, whole-grain, white 1 cup	122	12.52	441.64	4.38	0.62	1.16	2	0	9.91	93.81	8.91	7.32
20020	Cornmeal, whole-grain, yellow 1 cup	122	12.52	441.64	4.38	0.62	1.16	2	0	9.91	93.81	8.91	7.32
18236	Cracker meal 1 cup	115	8.74	440.45	1.96	0.31	0.17	0.83	0	10.7	93.04	2.94	26.45
20090	Rice flour, brown 1 cup	158	18.91	573.54	4.39	0.88	1.59	1.57	0	11.42	120.84	7.27	17.38
20061	Rice flour, white 1 cup	158	18.79	578.28	2.24	0.61	0.7	0.6	0	9.4	126.61	3.79	15.8
20063	Rye flour, dark 1 cup	128	14.17	414.72	3.44	0.4	0.42	1.54	0	17.96	87.99	28.93	71.68
20064	Rye flour, medium 1 cup	102	10.05	361.08	1.81	0.2	0.21	0.78	0	9.58	79.04	14.89	24.48
20065	Rye flour, light 1 cup	102	8.96	374.34	1.39	0.15	0.16	0.58	0	8.56	81.83	14.89	21.42
20076	Wheat flour, durum 1 cup	192	21	650.88	4.74	0.87	0.66	1.88	0	26.27	136.57	0	65.28
20080	Wheat flour, whole-grain 1 cup	120	12.32	406.8	2.24	0.39	0.28	0.93	0	16.44	87.08	14.64	40.8
20081	Wheat flour, white, all-purpose, enriched, bleached 1 cup	125	14.9	455	1.23	0.19	0.11	0.52	0	12.91	95.39	3.38	18.75
20581	Wheat flour, white, all-purpose, enriched, unbleached 1 cup	125	14.9	455	1.23	0.19	0.11	0.52	0	12.91	95.39	3.38	18.75
Grains and cereals													
20006	Barley, pearled, cooked 1 cup	157	108.02	193.11	0.69	0.15	0.09	0.34	0	3.55	44.31	5.97	17.27
20010	Buckwheat groats, roasted, cooked 1 cup	168	127.06	154.56	1.04	0.23	0.32	0.32	0	5.68	33.5	4.54	11.76
20013	Bulgur, cooked 1 cup	182	141.52	151.06	0.44	0.08	0.06	0.18	0	5.61	33.82	8.19	18.2
08161	Corn grits, white, regquick, enriched, cooked w/water, w/salt 1 cup	242	206.43	145.2	0.48	0.07	0.12	0.19	0	3.39	31.46	0.48	0
08164	Corn grits, yellow, regquick, enriched, cooked w/water, wo/salt (corn) 1 cup	242	206.43	145.2	0.48	0.07	0.12	0.19	0	3.39	31.46	0.48	0
20029	Couscous, cooked 1 cup, cooked	157	113.93	175.84	0.84	0.15	0.12	0.34	0	5.95	36.46	2.2	12.56
08174	Farina, unenr, cooked w/water, wo/salt, (wheat) 1 cup	233	204.81	116.5	0.23	0.02	0.02	0.07	0	3.26	24.7	3.26	4.66
20030	Hominy, canned, white 1 cup	165	136.17	118.8	1.45	0.2	0.38	0.66	0	2.44	23.53	4.13	16.5
20330	Hominy, canned, yellow 1 cup	160	132.05	115.2	1.41	0.2	0.37	0.64	0	2.37	22.82	4	16

NDB#	Phosphorus	Iron	Sodium	Potassium	Magnesium	Zinc	Copper	Vitamin A	Thiamin	Riboflavin	Niacin	Vitamin B6	Folate	Vitamin B12	Vitamin C
	mg	*mg*	*mg*	*mg*	*mg*	*mg*	*mg*	*IU*	*mg*	*mg*	*mg*	*mg*	*mcg*	*mcg*	*mg*
20320	294.02	4.21	42.7	350.14	154.94	2.22	0.24	0	0.47	0.25	4.43	0.37	30.99	0	0
20020	294.02	4.21	42.7	350.14	154.94	2.22	0.24	572.18	0.47	0.25	4.43	0.37	30.99	0	0
18236	119.6	5.34	32.2	132.25	27.6	0.79	0.26	0	0.8	0.54	6.56	0.04	25.3	0	0
20090	532.46	3.13	12.64	456.62	176.96	3.87	0.36	0	0.7	0.13	10.02	1.16	25.28	0	0
20061	154.84	0.55	0	120.08	55.3	1.26	0.21	0	0.22	0.03	4.09	0.69	6.32	0	0
20063	808.96	8.26	1.28	934.4	317.44	7.19	0.96	0	0.4	0.32	5.47	0.57	76.8	0	0
20064	211.14	2.16	3.06	346.8	76.5	2.03	0.29	0	0.29	0.12	1.76	0.27	19.38	0	0
20065	197.88	1.84	2.04	237.66	71.4	1.79	0.26	0	0.34	0.09	0.82	0.24	22.44	0	0
20076	975.36	6.76	3.84	827.52	276.48	7.99	1.06	0	0.8	0.23	12.94	0.8	83.14	0	0
20080	415.2	4.66	6	486	165.6	3.52	0.46	0	0.54	0.26	7.64	0.41	52.8	0	0
20081	135	5.8	2.5	133.75	27.5	0.88	0.18	0	0.98	0.62	7.38	0.06	32.5	0	0
20581	135	5.8	2.5	133.75	27.5	0.88	0.18	0	0.98	0.62	7.38	0.06	32.5	0	0
20006	84.78	2.09	4.71	146.01	34.54	1.29	0.16	10.99	0.13	0.1	3.24	0.18	25.12	0	0
20010	117.6	1.34	6.72	147.84	85.68	1.02	0.25	0	0.07	0.07	1.58	0.13	23.52	0	0
20013	72.8	1.75	9.1	123.76	58.24	1.04	0.14	0	0.1	0.05	1.82	0.15	32.76	0	0
08161	29.04	1.55	539.66	53.24	9.68	0.17	0.03	0	0.24	0.15	1.96	0.06	2.42	0	0
08164	29.04	1.55	0	53.24	9.68	0.17	0.03	145.2	0.24	0.15	1.96	0.06	2.42	0	0
20029	34.54	0.6	7.85	91.06	12.56	1.37	0.22	0	0.33	0.14	5.19	0.27	79.2	0	0
08174	27.96	0.05	0	30.29	4.66	0.16	0.03	0	0.02	0.02	0.23	0.02	4.66	0	0
20030	57.75	1.02	346.5	14.85	26.4	1.73	0.05	0	0	0.01	0.05	0.01	1.65	0	0
20330	56	0.99	336	14.4	25.6	1.68	0.05	176	0	0.01	0.05	0.01	1.6	0	0

NDB#	Description & Serving	Grams	Water	Calories	Fat	Fat: Saturated	Fat: Monounsaturated	Fat: Polyunsaturated	Cholesterol	Protein	Carbohydrates	Fiber	Calcium
		g	kcal	g	g	g	g	mg	g	g	g	mg	
20032	Millet, cooked 1 cup	240	171.38	285.6	2.4	0.41	0.44	1.22	0	8.42	56.81	3.12	7.2
20034	Oat bran, cooked 1 cup	219	183.96	87.6	1.88	0.36	0.64	0.74	0	7.03	25.05	5.69	21.9
08121	Oats, reg & quick & instant, wo/fort, cooked w/water, wo/salt (oats) 1 cup	234	199.6	145.08	2.34	0.42	0.75	0.87	0	6.08	25.27	3.98	18.72
08123	Oats, instant, fort, plain, prep w/water (oats) 1 cup, cooked	234	200.07	138.06	2.34	0.42	0.75	0.87	0	5.85	23.87	3.98	215.28
20037	Rice, brown, long-grain, cooked 1 cup	195	142.53	216.45	1.76	0.35	0.64	0.63	0	5.03	44.77	3.51	19.5
20041	Rice, brown, medium-grain, cooked 1 cup	195	142.27	218.4	1.62	0.32	0.59	0.58	0	4.52	45.84	3.51	19.5
20345	Rice, white, long-grain, reg, cooked, enriched, w/salt 1 cup	158	108.14	205.4	0.44	0.12	0.14	0.12	0	4.25	44.51	0.63	15.8
20055	Rice, white, glutinous, cooked 1 cup, cooked	174	133.34	168.78	0.33	0.07	0.12	0.12	0	3.51	36.7	1.74	3.48
20066	Semolina, enriched 1 cup	167	21.16	601.2	1.75	0.25	0.21	0.72	0	21.18	121.63	6.51	28.39
20067	Sorghum 1 cup	192	17.66	650.88	6.34	0.88	1.91	2.63	0	21.7	143.29	0	53.76
08084	Wheat germ, toasted, plain 1 cup	113	6.33	431.66	12.09	2.07	1.7	7.48	0	32.88	56.05	14.58	50.85
08084	Wheat germ, toasted, plain 1 oz	28.35	1.59	108.3	3.03	0.52	0.43	1.88	0	8.25	14.06	3.66	12.76
08145	Whole wheat hot nat crl, cooked w/water, wo/salt, (wheat) 1 cup	242	202.31	150.04	0.97	0.15	0.14	0.49	0	4.84	33.15	3.87	16.94
20089	Wild rice, cooked 1 cup	164	121.25	165.64	0.56	0.08	0.08	0.35	0	6.54	35	2.95	4.92
Pasta													
20100	Macaroni, cooked, enriched 1 cup elbow shaped	140	92.39	197.4	0.94	0.13	0.11	0.38	0	6.68	39.68	1.82	9.8
20108	Macaroni, whole-wheat, cooked 1 cup elbow shaped	140	94.01	173.6	0.76	0.14	0.11	0.3	0	7.46	37.16	3.92	21
20110	Noodles, egg, cooked, enriched 1 cup	160	109.92	212.8	2.35	0.5	0.69	0.65	52.8	7.6	39.74	1.76	19.2
20112	Noodles, egg, spinach, cooked, enriched 1 cup	160	109.63	211.2	2.51	0.58	0.79	0.56	52.8	8.06	38.8	3.68	30.4
20113	Noodles, Chinese, chow mein 1 cup	45	0.33	237.15	13.84	1.97	3.46	7.8	0	3.77	25.89	1.76	9
20115	Noodles, Japanese, soba, cooked 1 cup	114	83.23	112.86	0.11	0.02	0.03	0.04	0	5.77	24.44	0	4.56

NDB#	Phosphorus	Iron	Sodium	Potassium	Magnesium	Zinc	Copper	Vitamin A	Thiamin	Riboflavin	Niacin	Vitamin B6	Folate	Vitamin B12	Vitamin C
	mg	mg	mg	mg	mg	mg	mg	IU	mg	mg	mg	mg	mcg	mcg	mg
20032	240	1.51	4.8	148.8	105.6	2.18	0.39	0	0.25	0.2	3.19	0.26	45.6	0	0
20034	260.61	1.93	2.19	201.48	87.6	1.16	0.14	0	0.35	0.07	0.32	0.05	13.14	0	0
08121	177.84	1.59	2.34	131.04	56.16	1.15	0.13	37.44	0.26	0.05	0.3	0.05	9.36	0	0
08123	175.5	8.33	376.74	131.04	56.16	1.15	0.13	1996.02	0.7	0.37	7.23	0.98	198.9	0	0
20037	161.85	0.82	9.75	83.85	83.85	1.23	0.2	0	0.19	0.05	2.98	0.28	7.8	0	0
20041	150.15	1.03	1.95	154.05	85.8	1.21	0.16	0	0.2	0.02	2.59	0.29	7.8	0	0
20345	67.94	1.9	603.56	55.3	18.96	0.77	0.11	0	0.26	0.02	2.33	0.15	4.74	0	0
20055	13.92	0.24	8.7	17.4	8.7	0.71	0.09	0	0.03	0.02	0.5	0.05	1.74	0	0
20066	227.12	7.28	1.67	310.62	78.49	1.75	0.32	0	1.35	0.95	10	0.17	120.24	0	0
20067	551.04	8.45	11.52	672	0	0	0	0	0.46	0.27	5.62	0	0	0	0
08084	1294.98	10.27	4.52	1070.11	361.6	18.84	0.7	0	1.89	0.93	6.32	1.11	397.76	0	6.78
08084	324.89	2.58	1.13	268.47	90.72	4.73	0.18	0	0.47	0.23	1.58	0.28	99.79	0	1.7
08145	166.98	1.5	0	171.82	53.24	1.16	0.2	0	0.17	0.12	2.15	0.18	26.62	0	0
20089	134.48	0.98	4.92	165.64	52.48	2.2	0.2	0	0.09	0.14	2.11	0.22	42.64	0	0

Pasta

NDB#	Phosphorus	Iron	Sodium	Potassium	Magnesium	Zinc	Copper	Vitamin A	Thiamin	Riboflavin	Niacin	Vitamin B6	Folate	Vitamin B12	Vitamin C
20100	75.6	1.96	1.4	43.4	25.2	0.74	0.14	0	0.29	0.14	2.34	0.05	9.8	0	0
20108	124.6	1.48	4.2	61.6	42	1.13	0.23	0	0.15	0.06	0.99	0.11	7	0	0
20110	110.4	2.54	11.2	44.8	30.4	0.99	0.14	32	0.3	0.13	2.38	0.06	11.2	0.14	0
20112	91.2	1.74	19.2	59.2	38.4	1.01	0.13	164.8	0.39	0.2	2.36	0.18	33.6	0.22	0
20113	72.45	2.13	197.55	54	23.4	0.63	0.08	38.25	0.26	0.19	2.68	0.05	9.9	0	0
20115	28.5	0.55	68.4	39.9	10.26	0.14	0.01	0	0.11	0.03	0.58	0.05	7.98	0	0

NDB#	Description & Serving	Grams	Water	Calories	Fat	Fat. Saturated	Fat. Monounsaturated	Fat. Polyunsaturated	Cholesterol	Protein	Carbohydrates	Fiber	Calcium
		g	kcal	g	g	g	g	mg	g	g	g	mg	
20121	Spaghetti, cooked, enriched, wo/ salt 1 cup	140	92.39	197.4	0.94	0.13	0.11	0.38	0	6.68	39.68	2.38	9.8
20127	Spaghetti, spinach, cooked 1 cup	140	95.4	182	0.88	0.13	0.1	0.36	0	6.41	36.61	0	42
20125	Spaghetti, whole-wheat, cooked 1 cup	140	94.01	173.6	0.76	0.14	0.11	0.3	0	7.46	37.16	6.3	21

Herbs, spices, and condiments

NDB#	Description & Serving	Grams	Water	Calories	Fat	Fat. Saturated	Fat. Monounsaturated	Fat. Polyunsaturated	Cholesterol	Protein	Carbohydrates	Fiber	Calcium
02001	Allspice, ground 1 teaspoon	1.9	0.16	4.99	0.17	0.05	0.01	0.04	0	0.12	1.37	0.41	12.55
02002	Anise seed 1 teaspoon	2.1	0.2	7.08	0.33	0.01	0.21	0.07	0	0.37	1.05	0.31	13.56
02003	Basil, ground 1 teaspoon	1.4	0.09	3.52	0.06	0	0.01	0.03	0	0.2	0.85	0.57	29.59
02004	Bay leaf, crumbled 1 teaspoon	0.6	0.03	1.88	0.05	0.01	0.01	0.01	0	0.05	0.45	0.16	5.01
02005	Caraway seed 1 teaspoon	2.1	0.21	6.99	0.31	0.01	0.15	0.07	0	0.42	1.05	0.8	14.47
02006	Cardamon, ground 1 teaspoon	2	0.17	6.23	0.13	0.01	0.02	0.01	0	0.22	1.37	0.56	7.66
11935	Catsup 1 tablespoon	15	9.99	15.6	0.05	0.01	0.01	0.02	0	0.23	4.09	0.2	2.85
02007	Celery seed 1 teaspoon	2	0.12	7.84	0.51	0.04	0.32	0.07	0	0.36	0.83	0.24	35.33
02008	Chervil, dried 1 teaspoon	0.6	0.04	1.42	0.02	0	0.01	0.01	0	0.14	0.29	0.07	8.08
02009	Chili powder 1 teaspoon	2.6	0.2	8.16	0.44	0.08	0.09	0.19	0	0.32	1.42	0.89	7.23
11615	Chives, freeze-dried 1 tablespoon	0.2	0	0.62	0.01	0	0	0	0	0.04	0.13	0.05	1.63
11156	Chives, raw 1 teaspoon, chopped	1	0.91	0.3	0.01	0	0	0	0	0.03	0.04	0.03	0.92
02010	Cinnamon, ground 1 teaspoon	2.3	0.22	6.01	0.07	0.01	0.01	0.01	0	0.09	1.84	1.25	28.25
02011	Cloves, ground 1 teaspoon	2.1	0.14	6.78	0.42	0.11	0.03	0.15	0	0.13	1.29	0.72	13.56
02012	Coriander leaf, dried 1 teaspoon	0.6	0.04	1.67	0.03	0	0.01	0	0	0.13	0.31	0.06	7.48
02013	Coriander seed 1 teaspoon	1.8	0.16	5.36	0.32	0.02	0.24	0.03	0	0.22	0.99	0.75	12.76
02014	Cumin seed 1 teaspoon	2.1	0.17	7.87	0.47	0.03	0.29	0.07	0	0.37	0.93	0.22	19.54
02015	Curry powder 1 teaspoon	2	0.19	6.5	0.28	0.04	0.11	0.05	0	0.25	1.16	0.66	9.56

NDB#	Phosphorus	Iron	Sodium	Potassium	Magnesium	Zinc	Copper	Vitamin A	Thiamin	Riboflavin	Niacin	Vitamin B6	Folate	Vitamin B12	Vitamin C
	mg	mg	mg	mg	mg	mg	mg	IU	mg	mg	mg	mg	mcg	mcg	mg
20121	75.6	1.96	1.4	43.4	25.2	0.74	0.14	0	0.29	0.14	2.34	0.05	9.8	0	0
20127	151.2	1.46	19.6	81.2	86.8	1.51	0.29	212.8	0.14	0.14	2.14	0.13	16.8	0	0
20125	124.6	1.48	4.2	61.6	42	1.13	0.23	0	0.15	0.06	0.99	0.11	7	0	0

Herbs, spices, and condiments

NDB#	Phosphorus	Iron	Sodium	Potassium	Magnesium	Zinc	Copper	Vitamin A	Thiamin	Riboflavin	Niacin	Vitamin B6	Folate	Vitamin B12	Vitamin C
02001	2.15	0.13	1.46	19.84	2.56	0.02	0.01	10.26	0	0	0.05	0.01	0.68	0	0.74
02002	9.24	0.78	0.33	30.26	3.57	0.11	0.02	6.53	0.01	0.01	0.06	0.01	0.21	0	0.44
02003	6.86	0.59	0.48	48.06	5.91	0.08	0.02	131.25	0	0	0.1	0.02	3.84	0	0.86
02004	0.68	0.26	0.14	3.18	0.72	0.02	0	37.11	0	0	0.01	0.01	1.08	0	0.28
02005	11.93	0.34	0.36	28.37	5.42	0.12	0.02	7.62	0.01	0.01	0.08	0.01	0.21	0	0.44
02006	3.55	0.28	0.37	22.38	4.57	0.15	0.01	0	0	0	0.02	0	0	0	0.42
11935	5.85	0.11	177.9	72.15	3.3	0.03	0.03	152.4	0.01	0.01	0.21	0.03	2.25	0	2.27
02007	10.93	0.9	3.2	28	8.8	0.14	0.03	1.04	0.01	0.01	0.06	0.01	0.2	0	0.34
02008	2.7	0.19	0.5	28.44	0.78	0.05	0	35.1	0	0	0.03	0.01	1.64	0	0.3
02009	7.88	0.37	26.26	49.82	4.42	0.07	0.01	908.1	0.01	0.02	0.21	0.05	2.6	0	1.67
11615	1.04	0.04	0.14	5.92	1.28	0.01	0	136.6	0	0	0.01	0	0.22	0	1.32
11156	0.58	0.02	0.03	2.96	0.42	0.01	0	43.53	0	0	0.01	0	1.05	0	0.58
02010	1.41	0.88	0.61	11.5	1.28	0.05	0.01	5.98	0	0	0.03	0.01	0.67	0	0.65
02011	2.21	0.18	5.1	23.14	5.54	0.02	0.01	11.13	0	0.01	0.03	0.03	1.95	0	1.7
02012	2.89	0.25	1.27	26.8	4.16	0.03	0.01	35.1	0.01	0.01	0.06	0.01	1.64	0	3.4
02013	7.36	0.29	0.64	22.81	5.94	0.08	0.02	0	0	0.01	0.04	0	0	0	0.38
02014	10.47	1.39	3.52	37.54	7.68	0.1	0.02	26.67	0.01	0.01	0.1	0.01	0.21	0	0.16
02015	6.98	0.59	1.04	30.86	5.08	0.08	0.02	19.72	0.01	0.01	0.07	0.01	3.08	0	0.23

NDB#	Description & Serving	Grams	Water	Calories	Fat	Fat: Saturated	Fat: Monounsaturated	Fat: Polyunsaturated	Cholesterol	Protein	Carbohydrates	Fiber	Calcium
		g	kcal	g	g	g	g	mg	g	g	g	mg	
02016	Dill seed 1 teaspoon	2.1	0.16	6.4	0.31	0.02	0.2	0.02	0	0.34	1.16	0.44	31.83
02017	Dill weed, dried 1 teaspoon	1	0.07	2.53	0.04	0	0	0	0	0.2	0.56	0.14	17.84
02045	Dill weed, fresh 5 sprigs	1	0.86	0.43	0.01	0	0.01	0	0	0.03	0.07	0.02	2.08
11957	Fennel, bulb, raw 1 cup, sliced	87	78.48	26.97	0.17	0	0	0	0	1.08	6.34	2.7	42.63
02018	Fennel seed 1 teaspoon	2	0.18	6.9	0.3	0.01	0.2	0.03	0	0.32	1.05	0.8	23.93
02019	Fenugreek seed 1 teaspoon	3.7	0.33	11.95	0.24	0.05	0	0	0	0.85	2.16	0.91	6.5
11215	Garlic, raw 1 teaspoon	2.8	1.64	4.17	0.01	0	0	0.01	0	0.18	0.93	0.06	5.07
02021	Ginger, ground 1 teaspoon	1.8	0.17	6.25	0.11	0.03	0.02	0.02	0	0.16	1.27	0.23	2.09
02022	Mace, ground 1 teaspoon	1.7	0.14	8.08	0.55	0.16	0.19	0.07	0	0.11	0.86	0.34	4.29
02023	Marjoram, dried 1 teaspoon	0.6	0.05	1.63	0.04	0	0.01	0.03	0	0.08	0.36	0.24	11.94
02024	Mustard seed, yellow 1 teaspoon	3.3	0.23	15.49	0.95	0.05	0.65	0.18	0	0.82	1.15	0.49	17.2
02025	Nutmeg, ground 1 teaspoon	2.2	0.14	11.54	0.8	0.57	0.07	0.01	0	0.13	1.08	0.46	4.06
02026	Onion powder 1 teaspoon	2.1	0.11	7.28	0.02	0	0	0.01	0	0.21	1.69	0.12	7.62
02027	Oregano, ground 1 teaspoon	1.5	0.11	4.59	0.15	0.04	0.01	0.08	0	0.17	0.97	0.64	23.64
02028	Paprika 1 teaspoon	2.1	0.2	6.07	0.27	0.04	0.03	0.17	0	0.31	1.17	0.44	3.72
02029	Parsley, dried 1 teaspoon	0.3	0.03	0.83	0.01	0	0.01	0	0	0.07	0.15	0.09	4.4
11297	Parsley, raw 1 tablespoon	3.8	3.33	1.37	0.03	0.01	0.01	0	0	0.11	0.24	0.13	5.24
02030	Pepper, black 1 teaspoon	2.1	0.22	5.36	0.07	0.02	0.02	0.02	0	0.23	1.36	0.56	9.17
02031	Pepper, red or cayenne 1 teaspoon	1.8	0.14	5.72	0.31	0.06	0.05	0.15	0	0.22	1.02	0.49	2.67
02032	Pepper, white 1 teaspoon	2.4	0.27	7.1	0.05	0.02	0.02	0.01	0	0.25	1.65	0.63	6.37
11937	Pickles, cucumber, dill 1 cup (about 23 slices)	155	142.09	27.9	0.29	0.07	0	0.12	0	0.96	6.4	1.86	13.95
11940	Pickle, cucumber, sweet 1 cup, sliced	170	110.94	198.9	0.44	0.11	0.01	0.18	0	0.63	54.08	1.87	6.8
11941	Pickle, cucumber, sour 1 large (4" long)	135	127.01	14.85	0.27	0.07	0	0.11	0	0.45	3.04	1.62	0

NDB#	Phosphorus	Iron	Sodium	Potassium	Magnesium	Zinc	Copper	Vitamin A	Thiamin	Riboflavin	Niacin	Vitamin B6	Folate	Vitamin B12	Vitamin C
	mg	mg	mg	mg	mg	mg	mg	IU	mg	mg	mg	mg	mcg	mcg	mg
02016	5.81	0.34	0.41	24.91	5.37	0.11	0.02	1.11	0.01	0.01	0.06	0.01	0.21	0	0.44
02017	5.43	0.49	2.08	33.08	4.51	0.03	0	58.5	0	0	0.03	0.01	0	0	0.5
02045	0.66	0.07	0.61	7.38	0.55	0.01	0	77.18	0	0	0.02	0	1.5	0	0.85
11957	43.5	0.63	45.24	360.18	14.79	0.17	0.06	116.58	0.01	0.03	0.56	0.04	23.49	0	10.44
02018	9.75	0.37	1.76	33.88	7.7	0.07	0.02	2.7	0.01	0.01	0.12	0	0	0	0.42
02019	10.96	1.24	2.49	28.48	7.05	0.09	0.04	2.22	0.01	0.01	0.06	0	2.11	0	0.11
11215	4.28	0.05	0.48	11.23	0.7	0.03	0.01	0	0.01	0	0.02	0.03	0.09	0	0.87
02021	2.66	0.21	0.58	24.17	3.31	0.08	0.01	2.65	0	0	0.09	0.02	0.7	0	0.13
02022	1.87	0.24	1.36	7.87	2.77	0.04	0.04	13.6	0.01	0.01	0.02	0.01	1.29	0	0.36
02023	1.84	0.5	0.46	9.13	2.08	0.02	0.01	48.41	0	0	0.02	0.01	1.64	0	0.31
02024	27.74	0.33	0.15	22.52	9.85	0.19	0.01	2.05	0.02	0.01	0.26	0.01	2.51	0	0.1
02025	4.68	0.07	0.36	7.69	4.03	0.05	0.02	2.24	0.01	0	0.03	0.01	1.67	0	0.07
02026	7.14	0.05	1.12	19.81	2.55	0.05	0	0	0.01	0	0.01	0.03	3.49	0	0.31
02027	3	0.66	0.22	25.03	4.05	0.07	0.01	103.55	0.01	0	0.09	0.02	4.11	0	0.75
02028	7.24	0.5	0.71	49.23	3.88	0.09	0.01	1272.68	0.01	0.04	0.32	0.04	2.23	0	1.49
02029	1.05	0.29	1.36	11.41	0.75	0.01	0	70.02	0	0	0.02	0	0.54	0	0.37
11297	2.2	0.24	2.13	21.05	1.9	0.04	0.01	197.6	0	0	0.05	0	5.78	0	5.05
02030	3.64	0.61	0.92	26.44	4.06	0.03	0.02	3.99	0	0.01	0.02	0.01	0.21	0	0.44
02031	5.28	0.14	0.54	36.25	2.74	0.04	0.01	748.98	0.01	0.02	0.16	0.04	1.91	0	1.38
02032	4.22	0.34	0.12	1.74	2.16	0.03	0.02	0	0	0	0.01	0.01	0.24	0	0.5
11937	32.55	0.82	1987.1	179.8	17.05	0.22	0.12	509.95	0.02	0.04	0.09	0.02	1.55	0	2.95
11940	20.4	1	1596.3	54.4	6.8	0.14	0.18	214.2	0.02	0.05	0.3	0.03	1.7	0	2.04
11941	18.9	0.54	1630.8	31.05	5.4	0.03	0.11	195.75	0	0.01	0	0.01	0.96	0	1.35

NDB#	Description & Serving	Grams	Water	Calories	Fat	Fat: Saturated	Fat: Monounsaturated	Fat: Polyunsaturated	Cholesterol	Protein	Carbohydrates	Fiber	Calcium
		g	kcal	g	g	g	g	mg	g	g	g	mg
11945	Pickle relish, sweet 1 tablespoon	15	9.31	19.5	0.07	0.01	0.03	0.02	0	0.06	5.26	0.17	0.45
11943	Pimento, canned 1 tablespoon	12	11.17	2.76	0.04	0.01	0	0.02	0	0.13	0.61	0.23	0.72
02033	Poppy seed 1 teaspoon	2.8	0.19	14.93	1.25	0.14	0.18	0.86	0	0.51	0.66	0.28	40.56
02034	Poultry seasoning 1 teaspoon	1.5	0.14	4.61	0.11	0.05	0.02	0.03	0	0.14	0.98	0.17	14.94
02035	Pumpkin pie spice 1 teaspoon	1.7	0.14	5.81	0.21	0.11	0.02	0.01	0	0.1	1.18	0.25	11.59
02036	Rosemary, dried 1 teaspoon	1.2	0.11	3.98	0.18	0.1	0	0	0	0.06	0.77	0.51	15.36
02063	Rosemary, fresh 1 teaspoon	0.7	0.47	0.92	0.04	0.02	0.01	0.01	0	0.02	0.14	0.1	2.22
02037	Saffron 1 teaspoon	0.7	0.08	2.17	0.04	0.01	0	0.01	0	0.08	0.46	0.03	0.78
02038	Sage, ground 1 teaspoon	0.7	0.06	2.2	0.09	0.05	0.01	0.01	0	0.07	0.43	0.28	11.56
02047	Salt, table 1 tablespoon	18	0.04	0	0	0	0	0	0	0	0	0	4.32
02039	Savory, ground 1 teaspoon	1.4	0.13	3.81	0.08	0.05	0	0	0	0.09	0.96	0.64	29.84
02066	Spearmint, dried 1 teaspoon	0.5	0.06	1.43	0.03	0.01	0	0.02	0	0.1	0.26	0.15	7.44
02041	Tarragon, ground 1 teaspoon	1.6	0.12	4.73	0.12	0.03	0.01	0.06	0	0.36	0.8	0.12	18.23
02049	Thyme, fresh 1 teaspoon	0.8	0.52	0.81	0.01	0	0	0	0	0.04	0.2	0.11	3.24
02042	Thyme, ground 1 teaspoon	1.4	0.11	3.87	0.1	0.04	0.01	0.02	0	0.13	0.9	0.52	26.45
02043	Turmeric, ground 1 teaspoon	2.2	0.25	7.79	0.22	0.07	0.04	0.05	0	0.17	1.43	0.46	4.02
02050	Vanilla extract 1 tablespoon	13	6.84	37.44	0.01	0	0	0	0	0.01	1.64	0	1.43
02048	Vinegar, cider 1 tablespoon	15	14.07	2.1	0	0	0	0	0	0	0.89	0	0.9

Meat

Beef

NDB#	Description & Serving	Grams	Water	Calories	Fat	Fat: Saturated	Fat: Monounsaturated	Fat: Polyunsaturated	Cholesterol	Protein	Carbohydrates	Fiber	Calcium
13369	Brisket, flat half, lean & fat, 0" fat, braised 3 oz	85	49.08	182.75	8	2.85	3.53	0.31	80.75	25.91	0	0	4.25
13034	Chuck, arm pot rst, lean & fat, ¼" fat, braised 3 oz	85	40.79	282.2	20.24	7.97	8.68	0.77	84.15	23.32	0	0	8.5
13073	Rib, whole (ribs 6-12), lean & fat, ¼" fat, roasted 3 oz	85	40.37	304.3	24.66	9.95	10.6	0.88	71.4	19.13	0	0	9.35

NDB#	Phosphorus	Iron	Sodium	Potassium	Magnesium	Zinc	Copper	Vitamin A	Thiamin	Riboflavin	Niacin	Vitamin B6	Folate	Vitamin B12	Vitamin C
	mg	mg	mg	mg	mg	mg	mg	IU	mg	mg	mg	mg	mcg	mcg	mg
11945	2.1	0.13	121.65	3.75	0.75	0.02	0.01	23.25	0	0	0.03	0	0.15	0	0.15
11943	2.04	0.2	1.68	18.96	0.72	0.02	0.01	318.6	0	0.01	0.07	0.03	0.72	0	10.19
02033	23.76	0.26	0.59	19.59	9.28	0.29	0.05	0	0.02	0	0.03	0.01	1.62	0	0.08
02034	2.57	0.53	0.41	10.26	3.36	0.05	0.01	39.48	0	0	0.04	0.01	2.07	0	0.18
02035	2.01	0.34	0.88	11.27	2.31	0.04	0.01	4.44	0	0	0.04	0.01	0.87	0	0.4
02036	0.84	0.35	0.59	11.46	2.64	0.04	0.01	37.54	0.01	0	0.01	0	0	0	0.73
02063	0.46	0.05	0.18	4.68	0.64	0.01	0	20.47	0	0	0.01	0	0.76	0	0.15
02037	1.76	0.08	1.04	12.07	1.85	0.01	0	3.71	0	0	0.01	0.01	0.65	0	0.57
02038	0.64	0.2	0.08	7.49	3	0.03	0.01	41.3	0.01	0	0.04	0.01	1.92	0	0.23
02047	0	0.06	6976.44	1.44	0.18	0.02	0.01	0	0	0	0	0	0	0	0
02039	1.96	0.53	0.34	14.71	5.27	0.06	0.01	71.82	0.01	0	0.06	0	0	0	0.7
02066	1.38	0.44	1.72	9.62	3.01	0.01	0.01	52.9	0	0.01	0.03	0.01	2.65	0	0
02041	5.01	0.52	1	48.31	5.55	0.06	0.01	67.2	0	0.02	0.14	0.02	4.38	0	0.8
02049	0.85	0.14	0.07	4.87	1.28	0.01	0	38.02	0	0	0.01	0	0.36	0	1.28
02042	2.81	1.73	0.77	11.4	3.09	0.09	0.01	53.2	0.01	0.01	0.07	0.02	3.84	0	0.7
02043	5.89	0.91	0.83	55.55	4.25	0.1	0.01	0	0	0.01	0.11	0.04	0.86	0	0.57
02050	0.78	0.02	1.17	19.24	1.56	0.01	0.01	0	0	0.01	0.06	0	0	0	0
02048	1.35	0.09	0.15	15	3.3	0	0.01	0	0	0	0	0	0	0	0

Meat

NDB#	Phosphorus	Iron	Sodium	Potassium	Magnesium	Zinc	Copper	Vitamin A	Thiamin	Riboflavin	Niacin	Vitamin B6	Folate	Vitamin B12	Vitamin C
13369	210.8	2.34	52.7	245.65	20.4	5.19	0.1	0	0.06	0.18	3.18	0.26	6.8	2.19	0
13034	187	2.64	51	209.1	16.15	5.81	0.11	0	0.06	0.2	2.7	0.24	7.65	2.51	0
13073	148.75	1.99	53.55	255.85	17	4.55	0.07	0	0.06	0.14	2.9	0.2	5.95	2.16	0

NDB#	Description & Serving	Grams	Water	Calories	Fat	Fat: Saturated	Fat: Monounsaturated	Fat: Polyunsaturated	Cholesterol	Protein	Carbohydrates	Fiber	Calcium
			g	kcal	g	g	g	g	mg	g	g	g	mg
13148	Shortribs, lean & fat, choice, braised 3 oz	85	30.36	400.35	35.68	15.13	16.05	1.3	79.9	18.33	0	0	10.2
13160	Bttm round, lean & fat, ¼" fat, all grds, braised 3 oz	85	44.32	233.75	14.37	5.41	6.25	0.54	81.6	24.36	0	0	5.1
13176	Eye of round, lean & fat, ¼" fat, roasted 3 oz	85	50.52	194.65	10.84	4.23	4.66	0.39	61.2	22.77	0	0	5.1
13184	Eye of round, lean, ¼" fat, roasted 3 oz	85	55.25	142.8	4.17	1.51	1.77	0.14	58.65	24.64	0	0	4.25
13238	Tenderloin, lean & fat, ¼" fat, broiled 3 oz	85	45.08	247.35	17.22	6.76	7.06	0.65	73.1	21.47	0	0	6.8
13298	Ground, extra lean, broiled, med 3 oz	85	48.67	217.6	13.88	5.46	6.08	0.52	71.4	21.59	0	0	5.95
13305	Ground, lean, broiled, med 3 oz	85	47.38	231.2	15.69	6.16	6.87	0.59	73.95	21.01	0	0	9.35
13312	Ground, reg, broiled, med 3 oz	85	55.25	142.8	17.59	6.91	7.7	0.65	76.5	24.64	0	0	4.25
13322	Heart, simmered 3 oz	85	54.47	148.75	4.78	1.43	1.06	1.16	164.05	24.47	0.36	0	5.1
13324	Kidneys, simmered 3 oz	85	58.51	122.4	2.92	0.93	0.63	0.63	328.95	21.66	0.82	0	14.45
13327	Liver, pan-fried 3 oz	85	47.33	184.45	6.8	2.27	1.38	1.45	409.7	22.71	6.67	0	9.35
13340	Tongue, simmered 3 oz	85	47.64	240.55	17.63	7.59	8.05	0.66	90.95	18.79	0.28	0	5.95
13347	Corned bf, brisket 3 oz	85	50.82	213.35	16.13	5.39	7.84	0.57	83.3	15.44	0.4	0	6.8
Lamb													
17014	Dom, leg, whole (shk & sirl), lean, ¼" fat, choice, roasted 3 oz	85	54.31	162.35	6.58	2.35	2.88	0.43	75.65	24.06	0	0	6.8
17025	Dom, loin, lean & fat, ¼" fat, choice, roasted 3 oz	85	44.63	262.65	20.05	8.7	8.23	1.59	80.75	19.17	0	0	15.3
17060	Dom, cubed for stew (leg & shoulder), lean, ¼" fat, braised 3 oz	85	47.8	189.55	7.48	2.68	3.01	0.69	91.8	28.64	0	0	12.75
17073	NZ, imp, frz, leg, whole (shk & sirl), lean & fat, roasted 3 oz	85	49.19	209.1	13.23	6.47	5.11	0.64	85.85	21.09	0	0	8.5
17075	NZ, imp, frz, leg, whole (shk & sirl), lean, roasted 3 oz	85	54.33	153.85	5.96	2.59	2.34	0.35	85	23.53	0	0	5.95
Veal													
17103	Leg, lean, roasted 3 oz	85	56.96	127.5	2.88	1.04	1.01	0.25	87.55	23.86	0	0	5.1
17109	Loin, lean, roasted 3 oz	85	54.9	148.75	5.9	2.19	2.12	0.48	90.1	22.37	0	0	17.85
17115	Rib, lean, roasted 3 oz	85	54.94	150.45	6.32	1.77	2.26	0.57	97.75	21.9	0	0	10.2
17143	Ground, broiled 3 oz	85	56.75	146.2	6.43	2.58	2.41	0.47	87.55	20.72	0	0	14.45

NDB#	Phosphorus	Iron	Sodium	Potassium	Magnesium	Zinc	Copper	Vitamin A	Thiamin	Riboflavin	Niacin	Vitamin B6	Folate	Vitamin B12	Vitamin C
	mg	mg	mg	mg	mg	mg	mg	IU	mg	mg	mg	mg	mcg	mcg	mg
13148	137.7	1.96	42.5	190.4	12.75	4.15	0.08	0	0.04	0.13	2.08	0.19	4.25	2.23	0
13160	208.25	2.65	42.5	239.7	18.7	4.17	0.1	0	0.06	0.2	3.17	0.28	8.5	2	0
13176	176.8	1.56	50.15	307.7	20.4	3.69	0.08	0	0.07	0.14	2.97	0.3	5.95	1.79	0
13184	192.1	1.66	52.7	335.75	22.95	4.03	0.09	0	0.08	0.14	3.19	0.32	5.95	1.84	0
13238	178.5	2.68	50.15	312.8	22.1	4.15	0.13	0	0.09	0.22	2.99	0.33	5.1	2.05	0
13298	136.85	2	59.5	266.05	17.85	4.63	0.06	0	0.05	0.23	4.22	0.23	7.65	1.84	0
13305	134.3	1.79	65.45	255.85	17.85	4.56	0.06	0	0.04	0.18	4.39	0.22	7.65	2	0
13312	192.1	1.66	52.7	335.75	22.95	4.4	0.07	0	0.03	0.16	4.9	0.23	7.65	2.49	0
13322	212.5	6.38	53.55	198.05	21.25	2.66	0.63	0	0.12	1.31	3.46	0.18	1.7	12.16	1.28
13324	260.1	6.21	113.9	152.15	15.3	3.59	0.58	1054.85	0.16	3.45	5.12	0.44	83.3	43.61	0.68
13327	391.85	5.34	90.1	309.4	19.55	4.63	3.8	30689.25	0.18	3.52	12.27	1.22	187	95.03	19.55
13340	120.7	2.88	51	153	14.45	4.08	0.19	0	0.03	0.3	1.83	0.14	4.25	5.02	0.43
13347	106.25	1.58	963.9	123.25	10.2	3.89	0.13	0	0.02	0.14	2.58	0.2	5.1	1.39	0
17014	175.1	1.8	57.8	287.3	22.1	4.2	0.1	0	0.09	0.25	5.39	0.14	19.55	2.24	0
17025	153	1.8	54.4	209.1	19.55	2.9	0.1	0	0.09	0.2	6.04	0.09	16.15	1.88	0
17060	174.25	2.38	59.5	221	23.8	5.59	0.12	0	0.06	0.2	5.06	0.1	17.85	2.32	0
7073	185.3	1.79	36.55	141.95	17	3.04	0.09	0	0.1	0.38	6.45	0.11	0.85	2.21	
17075	198.9	1.9	38.25	155.55	17.85	3.43	0.09	0	0.1	0.43	6.38	0.12	0	2.24	0
17103	200.6	0.77	57.8	334.05	23.8	2.62	0.11	0	0.05	0.28	8.57	0.26	13.6	1	0
17109	188.7	0.72	81.6	289	22.1	2.75	0.1	0	0.05	0.26	8.04	0.31	13.6	1.11	0
17115	175.95	0.82	82.45	264.35	20.4	3.82	0.09	0	0.05	0.25	6.38	0.23	11.9	1.34	0
17143	184.45	0.84	70.55	286.45	20.4	3.29	0.09	0	0.06	0.23	6.83	0.33	9.35	1.08	0

NDB#	Description & Serving	Grams	Water	Calories	Fat	Fat: Saturated	Fat: Monounsaturated	Fat: Polyunsaturated	Cholesterol	Protein	Carbohydrates	Fiber	Calcium
		g	kcal	g	g	g	g	mg	g	g	g	mg	

Pork

NDB#	Description & Serving	Grams	Water	Calories	Fat	Fat: Saturated	Fat: Monounsaturated	Fat: Polyunsaturated	Cholesterol	Protein	Carbohydrates	Fiber	Calcium
10011	Frsh, (ham), whole, lean, roasted 3 oz	85	51.56	179.35	8.02	2.81	3.78	0.72	79.9	25	0	0	5.95
10019	Frsh, (ham), shank half, lean, roasted 3 oz	85	51.37	182.75	8.93	3.09	4.27	0.77	78.2	23.98	0	0	5.95
10027	Frsh, loin, whole, lean, roasted 3 oz	85	51.87	177.65	8.19	2.98	3.67	0.65	68.85	24.33	0	0	15.3
10042	Frsh, center loin (chops), bone-in, lean, broiled 3 oz	85	51.98	171.7	6.86	2.51	3.09	0.49	69.7	25.66	0	0	26.35
10050	Frsh, center rib (chops), bone-in, lean, broiled 3 oz	85	48.41	186.15	8.28	2.94	3.78	0.53	68.85	26.15	0	0	26.35
10059	Frsh, sirloin (roasts), bone-in, lean, roasted 3 oz	85	51.46	183.6	8.75	3.08	3.84	0.74	73.1	24.49	0	0	17
10079	Frsh, shoulder, arm picnic, lean, roasted 3 oz	85	51.23	193.8	10.73	3.66	5.08	1.02	80.75	22.68	0	0	7.65
10089	Frsh, spareribs, lean & fat, braised 3 oz	85	34.36	337.45	25.76	9.45	11.46	2.32	102.85	24.7	0	0	39.95
10124	Cured, bacon, broiled, pan-fried or roasted 3 medium slices packed 20/lb raw, after cooking	19	2.46	109.44	9.36	3.31	4.5	1.1	16.15	5.79	0.11	0	2.28
10131	Cured, Canadian-style bacon, grilled 2 slices (6 per 6-oz pkg.)	46.5	28.69	86.03	3.92	1.32	1.88	0.38	26.97	11.27	0.63	0	4.65
10132	Cured, feet, pickled 1 lb	453.6	311.26	920.81	73.21	25.27	34.34	7.94	417.31	61.33	0.09	0	145.15
10134	Cured, ham, bnless, extra lean (approx 5% fat), roasted 3 oz	85	57.52	123.25	4.7	1.54	2.23	0.46	45.05	17.79	1.28	0	6.8
10136	Cured, ham, bnless, reg (approx 11% fat), roasted 3 oz	85	54.86	151.3	7.67	2.65	3.77	1.2	50.15	19.23	0	0	6.8
10153	Cured, ham, whole, lean, roasted 3 oz	85	55.91	133.45	4.68	1.56	2.15	0.54	46.75	21.29	0	0	5.95
10169	Cured, shoulder, arm picnic, lean, roasted 3 oz	85	54.28	144.5	5.98	2.01	2.75	0.69	40.8	21.2	0	0	9.35

Poultry: Chicken (broilers or fryers)

NDB#	Description & Serving	Grams	Water	Calories	Fat	Fat: Saturated	Fat: Monounsaturated	Fat: Polyunsaturated	Cholesterol	Protein	Carbohydrates	Fiber	Calcium
05030	Light meat, meat & skin, fried, batter ½ chicken, bone removed	188	94.43	520.76	29.03	7.75	11.98	6.77	157.92	44.27	17.86	0	37.6
05031	Light meat, meat & skin, fried, flour ½ chicken, bone removed	130	71.06	319.8	15.72	4.32	6.24	3.5	113.1	39.59	2.37	0.13	20.8
05032	Light meat, meat & skin, roasted ½ chicken, bone removed	132	79.87	293.04	14.32	4.03	5.62	3.05	110.88	38.31	0	0	19.8
05033	Light meat, meat & skin, stewed ½ chicken, bone removed	150	97.7	301.5	14.96	4.2	5.88	3.18	111	39.21	0	0	19.5
05035	Dark meat, meat & skin, fried, batter ½ chicken, bone bone removed	278	135.72	828.44	51.82	13.76	21.07	12.32	247.42	60.74	26.08	0	58.38

NDB#	Phosphorus	Iron	Sodium	Potassium	Magnesium	Zinc	Copper	Vitamin A	Thiamin	Riboflavin	Niacin	Vitamin B6	Folate	Vitamin B12	Vitamin C
	mg	mg	mg	mg	mg	mg	mg	IU	mg	mg	mg	mg	mcg	mcg	mg
10011	238.85	0.95	54.4	317.05	21.25	2.77	0.09	7.65	0.59	0.3	4.19	0.38	10.2	0.61	0.34
10019	236.3	0.94	54.4	306	21.25	2.93	0.09	6.8	0.54	0.29	4.15	0.39	5.1	0.6	0.34
10027	211.65	0.93	49.3	361.25	23.8	2.15	0.05	6.8	0.86	0.28	5.01	0.47	5.95	0.62	0.51
10042	204.85	0.72	51	318.75	22.95	2.02	0.04	6.8	0.98	0.26	4.71	0.4	5.1	0.63	0.34
10050	208.25	0.7	55.25	357	23.8	2.02	0.06	5.1	0.95	0.28	5.24	0.4	2.55	0.65	0.26
10059	193.8	0.95	53.55	311.1	21.25	2.18	0.07	5.95	0.68	0.28	4.72	0.36	5.1	0.66	0.26
10079	209.95	1.21	68	298.35	17	3.46	0.11	5.95	0.49	0.3	3.67	0.35	4.25	0.66	0.26
10089	221.85	1.57	79.05	272	20.4	3.91	0.12	8.5	0.35	0.32	4.65	0.3	3.4	0.92	0
10124	63.84	0.31	303.24	92.34	4.56	0.62	0.03	0	0.13	0.05	1.39	0.05	0.95	0.33	0
10131	137.64	0.38	718.89	181.35	9.77	0.79	0.03	0	0.38	0.09	3.22	0.21	1.86	0.36	0
10132	154.22	2.81	4186.73	1065.96	18.14	5.62	0.23	0	0.03	0.19	1.66	1.72	18.14	2.81	0
10134	166.6	1.26	1022.55	243.95	11.9	2.45	0.07	0	0.64	0.17	3.42	0.34	2.55	0.55	0
10136	238.85	1.14	1275	347.65	18.7	2.1	0.12	0	0.62	0.28	5.23	0.26	2.55	0.6	0
10153	192.95	0.8	1127.95	268.6	18.7	2.18	0.07	0	0.58	0.22	4.27	0.4	3.4	0.6	0
10169	206.55	0.92	1046.35	248.2	13.6	2.5	0.11	0	0.62	0.19	4.08	0.31	3.4	0.94	0
05030	315.84	2.37	539.56	347.8	41.36	1.99	0.11	148.52	0.21	0.28	17.21	0.73	11.28	0.53	0
05031	276.9	1.57	100.1	310.7	35.1	1.64	0.08	88.4	0.1	0.17	15.65	0.7	5.2	0.43	0
05032	264	1.5	99	299.64	33	1.62	0.07	145.2	0.08	0.16	14.7	0.69	3.96	0.42	0
05033	219	1.47	94.5	250.5	30	1.71	0.07	144	0.06	0.17	10.4	0.41	4.5	0.3	0
05035	403.1	4	820.1	514.3	55.6	5.78	0.22	286.34	0.33	0.61	15.59	0.7	25.02	0.75	0

NDB#	Description & Serving	Grams	Water	Calories	Fat	Fat: Saturated	Fat: Monounsaturated	Fat: Polyunsaturated	Cholesterol	Protein	Carbohydrates	Fiber	Calcium
		g	kcal	g	g	g	g	mg	g	g	g	mg	
05037	Dark meat, meat & skin, roasted ½ chicken, bone removed	167	97.91	422.51	26.35	7.3	10.34	5.83	151.97	43.37	0	0	25.05
05038	Dark meat, meat & skin, stewed ½ chicken, bone removed	184	115.9	428.72	26.97	7.47	10.58	5.96	150.88	43.24	0	0	25.76
05040	Light meat, meat only, fried 1 cup	140	84.2	268.8	7.76	2.13	2.76	1.76	126	45.95	0.59	0	22.4
05041	Light meat, meat only, roasted 1 cup, chopped or diced	140	90.66	242.2	6.31	1.78	2.16	1.37	119	43.27	0	0	21
05042	Light meat, meat only, stewed 1 cup, chopped or diced	140	95.23	222.6	5.59	1.57	1.89	1.22	107.8	40.43	0	0	18.2
05044	Dark meat, meat only, fried 1 cup	140	77.98	334.6	16.27	4.37	6.05	3.88	134.4	40.59	3.63	0	25.2
05045	Dark meat, meat only, roasted 1 cup, chopped or diced	140	88.28	287	13.62	3.72	4.98	3.16	130.2	38.32	0	0	21
05046	Dark meat, meat only, stewed 1 cup, chopped or diced	140	92.16	268.8	12.57	3.43	4.56	2.93	123.2	36.36	0	0	19.6
05028	Chicken, liver, all classes, simmered 1 cup, chopped or diced	140	95.63	219.8	7.63	2.58	1.88	1.26	883.4	34.1	1.23	0	19.6
05310	Cornish game hens, meat only, roasted ½ bird	110	79.09	147.4	4.26	1.09	1.36	1.03	116.6	25.63	0	0	14.3
Poultry: Duck													
05140	Duck, domesticated, meat & skin, roasted 1 cup, chopped or diced	140	72.58	471.8	39.69	13.54	18.06	5.11	117.6	26.59	0	0	15.4
05142	Duck, domesticated, meat only, roasted 1 cup, chopped or diced	140	89.91	281.4	15.68	5.84	5.18	2	124.6	32.87	0	0	16.8
Poultry: Goose													
05147	Goose, domesticated, meat & skin, roasted 1 cup, chopped or diced	140	72.73	427	30.69	9.62	14.35	3.53	127.4	35.22	0	0	18.2
05149	Goose, domesticated, meat only, roasted ½ goose	591	338.23	1406.58	74.88	26.95	25.65	9.1	567.36	171.21	0	0	82.74
Poultry: Turkey													
05192	Turkey, breast, meat & skin, roasted ½ breast, bone removed	864	546.22	1632.96	64.02	18.14	21.17	15.55	639.36	248.05	0	0	181.44
05194	Turkey, leg, meat & skin, roasted 1 leg, bone removed	546	334.1	1135.68	53.62	16.71	15.67	14.85	464.1	152.17	0	0	174.72
Luncheon meat													
07007	Bologna, beef 1 slice (4" dia × ⅛" thick)	23	12.72	71.76	6.56	2.78	3.17	0.25	13.34	2.81	0.18	0	2.76
07011	Bologna, turkey 2 slices	56.7	36.9	112.83	8.62	2.87	2.72	2.43	56.13	7.78	0.55	0	47.63
07017	Chicken roll, light meat 2 slices	56.7	38.9	90.15	4.18	1.15	1.68	0.91	28.35	11.07	1.39	0	24.38

NDB#	Phosphorus	Iron	Sodium	Potassium	Magnesium	Zinc	Copper	Vitamin A	Thiamin	Riboflavin	Niacin	Vitamin B6	Folate	Vitamin B12	Vitamin C
	mg	mg	mg	mg	mg	mg	mg	IU	mg	mg	mg	mg	mcg	mcg	mg
05037															
	280.56	2.27	145.29	367.4	36.74	4.16	0.13	335.67	0.11	0.35	10.62	0.52	11.69	0.48	0
05038															
	244.72	2.41	128.8	305.44	33.12	4.16	0.13	342.24	0.09	0.33	8.3	0.31	11.04	0.37	0
05040															
	323.4	1.6	113.4	368.2	40.6	1.78	0.08	42	0.1	0.18	18.71	0.88	5.6	0.5	0
05041															
	302.4	1.48	107.8	345.8	37.8	1.72	0.07	40.6	0.09	0.16	17.39	0.84	5.6	0.48	0
05042															
	222.6	1.3	91	252	30.8	1.67	0.06	37.8	0.06	0.16	10.91	0.46	4.2	0.32	0
05044															
	261.8	2.09	135.8	354.2	35	4.07	0.12	110.6	0.13	0.35	9.9	0.52	12.6	0.46	0
05045															
	250.6	1.86	130.2	336	32.2	3.92	0.11	100.8	0.1	0.32	9.17	0.5	11.2	0.45	0
05046															
	200.2	1.9	103.6	253.4	28	3.72	0.11	96.6	0.08	0.28	6.63	0.29	9.8	0.31	0
05028															
	436.8	11.86	71.4	196	29.4	6.08	0.52	22925	0.21	2.45	6.23	0.81	1078	27.15	22.12
05310															
	163.9	0.85	69.3	275	20.9	1.68	0.06	71.5	0.08	0.25	6.9	0.39	2.2	0.33	0.66
05140															
	218.4	3.78	82.6	285.6	22.4	2.6	0.32	294	0.24	0.38	6.76	0.25	8.4	0.42	0
05142															
	284.2	3.78	91	352.8	28	3.64	0.32	107.8	0.36	0.66	7.14	0.35	14	0.56	0
05147															
	378	3.96	98	460.6	30.8	3.67	0.37	98	0.11	0.45	5.84	0.52	2.8	0.57	0
05149															
	1826.19	16.96	449.16	2293.08	147.75	18.73	1.63	236.4	0.54	2.3	24.12	2.78	70.92	2.9	0
05192															
	1814.4	12.1	544.32	2488.32	233.28	17.54	0.41	0	0.49	1.13	54.99	4.15	51.84	3.11	0
05194															
	1086.54	12.56	420.42	1528.8	125.58	23.31	0.84	0	0.33	1.32	19.44	1.8	49.14	1.97	0
07007															
	20.24	0.38	225.63	36.11	2.76	0.5	0.01	0	0.01	0.03	0.55	0.03	1.15	0.33	0
07011															
	74.28	0.87	497.83	112.83	7.94	0.99	0.02	0	0.03	0.09	2	0.12	3.97	0.15	0
07017															
	89.02	0.55	331.13	129.28	10.77	0.41	0.02	46.49	0.04	0.07	3	0.12	1.13	0.09	0

NDB#	Description & Serving	Grams	Water	Calories	Fat	Fat, Saturated	Fat, Monounsaturated	Fat, Polyunsaturated	Cholesterol	Protein	Carbohydrates	Fiber	Calcium
		g	kcal	g	g	g	g	mg	g	g	g	mg	
07022	**Frankfurter, beef** 1 frankfurter (5 in long × ¾ in dia, 10 per pound) 45		24.62	141.75	12.83	5.42	6.13	0.62	27.45	5.4	0.81	0	9
07024	**Frankfurter, chicken** 1 frankfurter 45		25.89	115.65	8.77	2.49	3.82	1.82	45.45	5.82	3.06	0	42.75
07025	**Frankfurter, turkey** 1 frankfurter 45		28.35	101.7	7.97	2.65	2.51	2.25	48.15	6.43	0.67	0	47.7
07028	**Ham, sliced, extra lean (approx 5% fat)** 1 slice (6¼" × 4" × 1⁄16") 28.35		19.99	37.14	1.41	0.46	0.67	0.14	13.32	5.49	0.27	0	1.98
07029	**Ham, sliced, reg (approx 11% fat)** 1 slice (6¼" × 4" × 1⁄16") 28.35		18.33	51.6	3	0.96	1.4	0.34	16.16	4.98	0.88	0	1.98
07069	**Salami, bf & pork** 1 slice (4" dia × 1⁄8" thick) (10 per 8 oz package) 23		13.89	57.5	4.63	1.86	2.11	0.46	14.95	3.2	0.52	0	2.99
07070	**Salami, cooked, turkey** 2 slices 56.7		37.34	111.13	7.82	2.28	2.58	2	46.49	9.28	0.31	0	11.34
07071	**Salami, dry or hard, pork** 1 slice (3⅛" dia × 1⁄16" thick) 10		3.62	40.7	3.37	1.19	1.6	0.37	7.9	2.26	0.16	0	1.3
07079	**Turkey breast meat** 1 slice (3½" square; 8 per 6 oz package) 21		15.09	23.1	0.33	0.1	0.09	0.06	8.61	4.73	0	0	1.47
07081	**Turkey roll, light meat** 2 slices 56.7		40.57	83.35	4.09	1.15	1.42	0.99	24.38	10.6	0.3	0	22.68
07082	**Turkey roll, light & dark meat** 2 slices 56.7		39.78	84.48	3.96	1.16	1.3	1.01	31.19	10.29	1.21	0	18.14
	Nuts, seeds, and related products												
12061	**Almonds, dried, unblanched** 1 cup, sliced, unblanched 95		4.2	559.55	49.6	4.7	32.21	10.41	0	18.95	19.38	10.36	252.7
12063	**Almonds, dry roasted, unblanched, wo/salt** 1 cup whole kernels 138		4.14	810.06	71.21	6.75	46.24	14.94	0	22.54	33.35	18.91	389.16
12065	**Almonds, oil roasted, unblanched, wo/salt** 1 cup whole kernels 157		4.84	970.26	90.54	8.58	58.79	19	0	32.01	24.93	17.58	367.38
12071	**Almond paste** 1 oz 28.35		4	129.84	7.85	0.74	5.1	1.65	0	2.55	13.55	1.36	48.76
12078	**Brazil nuts, dried, unblanched** 1 cup, shelled (32 kernels) 140		4.68	918.4	92.71	22.62	32.22	33.78	0	20.08	17.92	7.56	246.4
12085	**Cashew nuts, dry roasted, wo/salt** 1 cup, halves and whole 137		2.33	786.38	63.5	12.55	37.42	10.74	0	20.97	44.79	4.11	61.65
12086	**Cashew nuts, oil roasted, wo/salt** 1 cup, halves and whole 130		5.08	748.8	21	62.67	12.38	36.94	10.6	0	37.08	4.94	53.3
12095	**Chestnuts, Chinese, roasted** 1 oz 28.35		11.4	67.76	0.22	0.03	0.11	0.06	0	1.27	14.84	0	5.39
12104	**Coconut meat, raw** 1 cup, shredded 80		37.59	283.2	26.79	23.76	1.14	0.29	0	2.66	12.18	7.2	11.2
12108	**Coconut meat, dried (desiccated), not swtnd** 1 oz 28.35		0.85	187.11	18.29	16.22	0.78	0.2	0	1.95	6.92	4.62	7.37

NDB#	Phosphorus	Iron	Sodium	Potassium	Magnesium	Zinc	Copper	Vitamin A	Thiamin	Riboflavin	Niacin	Vitamin B6	Folate	Vitamin B12	Vitamin C
	mg	mg	mg	mg	mg	mg	mg	IU	mg	mg	mg	mg	mcg	mcg	mg
07022	39.15	0.64	461.7	74.7	1.35	0.98	0.03	0	0.02	0.05	1.09	0.05	1.8	0.69	0
07024	48.15	0.9	616.5	37.8	4.5	0.47	0.02	58.5	0.03	0.05	1.39	0.14	1.8	0.11	0
07025	60.3	0.83	641.7	80.55	6.3	1.4	0.05	0	0.02	0.08	1.86	0.1	3.6	0.13	0
07028	61.8	0.22	405.12	99.23	4.82	0.55	0.02	0	0.26	0.06	1.37	0.13	1.13	0.21	0
07029	70.02	0.28	373.37	94.12	5.39	0.61	0.03	0	0.24	0.07	1.49	0.1	0.85	0.24	0
07069	26.45	0.61	244.95	45.54	3.45	0.49	0.05	0	0.05	0.09	0.82	0.05	0.46	0.84	0
07070	60.1	0.91	569.27	138.35	8.51	1.03	0.03	0	0.04	0.1	2	0.14	2.27	0.12	0
07071	22.9	0.13	226	37.8	2.2	0.42	0.02	0	0.09	0.03	0.56	0.06	0.2	0.28	0
07079	48.09	0.08	300.51	58.38	4.2	0.24	0.01	0	0.01	0.02	1.75	0.08	0.84	0.42	0
07081	103.76	0.73	277.26	142.32	9.07	0.88	0.02	0	0.05	0.13	3.97	0.18	2.27	0.14	0
07082	95.26	0.77	332.26	153.09	10.21	1.13	0.04	0	0.05	0.16	2.72	0.15	2.84	0.13	0
Nuts, seeds, and related products															
12061	494	3.48	10.45	695.4	281.2	2.77	0.89	0	0.2	0.74	3.19	0.11	55.77	0	0.57
12063	756.24	5.24	15.18	1062.6	419.52	6.76	1.69	0	0.18	0.83	3.89	0.1	88.04	0	0.97
12065	858.79	6.01	15.7	1072.31	477.28	7.69	1.92	0	0.2	1.55	5.5	0.13	100.17	0	1.1
12071	73.14	0.45	2.55	89.02	36.86	0.42	0.13	0	0.02	0.12	0.4	0.01	20.7	0	0.14
12078	840	4.76	2.8	840	315	6.43	2.48	0	1.4	0.17	2.27	0.35	5.6	0	0.98
12085	671.3	8.22	21.92	774.05	356.2	7.67	3.04	0	0.27	0.27	1.92	0.35	94.8	0	0
12086	553.8	5.33	22.1	689	331.5	6.18	2.82	0	0.55	0.23	2.34	0.33	88.01	0	0
12095	28.92	0.43	1.13	135.23	25.52	0.17	0.07	39.12	0.03	0.03	0.16	0.08	13.15	0	7
12104	90.4	1.94	16	284.8	25.6	0.88	0.35	0	0.05	0.02	0.43	0.04	21.12	0	2.64
12108	58.4	0.94	10.49	153.94	25.52	0.57	0.23	0	0.02	0.03	0.17	0.09	2.55	0	0.43

NDB#	Description & Serving	Grams	Water	Calories	Fat	Fat: Saturated	Fat: Monounsaturated	Fat: Polyunsaturated	Cholesterol	Protein	Carbohydrates	Fiber	Calcium
		g	kcal	g	g	g	g	mg	g	g	g	mg	
12115	Coconut cream, raw (liquid expressed from grated meat) 1 tablespoon	15	8.09	49.5	5.2	4.61	0.22	0.06	0	0.54	1	0.33	1.65
12121	Filberts or hazelnuts, dried, blanched 1 oz	28.35	0.54	190.51	19.08	1.4	14.95	1.83	0	3.61	4.53	1.81	55.28
12122	Filberts or hazelnuts, dry roasted, unblanched, wo/salt 1 oz	28.35	0.54	187.68	18.8	1.38	14.73	1.8	0	2.84	5.07	2.04	55.28
12123	Filberts or hazelnuts, oil roasted, unblanched, wo/salt 1 oz	28.35	0.34	187.11	18.03	1.33	14.13	1.73	0	4.04	5.43	1.81	55.57
12131	Macadamia nuts, dried 1 oz (11 whole kernels)	28.35	0.82	199.02	20.9	3.13	16.49	0.36	0	2.35	3.89	2.64	19.85
12133	Macadamia nuts, oil roasted, wo/salt 1 cup, whole or halves	134	2.24	962.12	102.54	15.35	80.91	1.77	0	9.73	17.29	12.46	60.3
12143	Pecans, dry roasted, wo/salt 1 oz	28.35	0.31	186.83	18.31	1.47	11.42	4.53	0	2.26	6.33	2.64	9.92
12144	Pecans, oil roasted, wo/salt 1 oz (15 halves)	28.35	1.19	194.2	20.19	1.62	12.58	5	0	1.97	4.55	1.9	9.64
12152	Pistachio nuts, dry roasted, wo/salt 1 cup	128	2.68	775.68	67.61	8.56	45.64	10.22	0	19.11	35.24	13.82	89.6
12166	Sesame butter, tahini, from roasted & toasted kernels (most common type) 1 tablespoon	15	0.46	89.25	8.06	1.13	3.05	3.53	0	2.55	3.18	1.4	63.9
12537	Sunflower seed kernels, dry roasted, w/salt 1 cup	128	1.54	744.96	63.74	6.68	12.17	42.09	0	24.74	30.81	11.52	89.6
12023	Sesame seeds, whole, dried 1 tablespoon	9	0.42	51.57	4.47	0.63	1.69	1.96	0	1.6	2.11	1.06	87.75
12036	Sunflower seed kernels, dried 1 cup, with hulls, edible yield	46	2.47	262.2	22.8	2.39	4.35	15.06	0	10.48	8.63	4.83	53.36
12154	Walnuts, black, dried 1 cup, chopped	125	5.45	758.75	70.73	4.54	15.91	46.87	0	30.44	15.13	6.25	72.5

Seafood

Fish

NDB#	Description & Serving	Grams	Water	Calories	Fat	Fat: Saturated	Fat: Monounsaturated	Fat: Polyunsaturated	Cholesterol	Protein	Carbohydrates	Fiber	Calcium
15187	Bass, freshwater, mxd sp, cooked, dry heat 3 oz	85	58.47	124.1	4.02	0.85	1.56	1.16	73.95	20.55	0	0	87.55
15188	Bass, striped, cooked, dry heat 3 oz	85	62.36	105.4	2.54	0.55	0.72	0.85	87.55	19.32	0	0	16.15
15189	Bluefish, cooked, dry heat 3 oz	85	53.24	135.15	4.62	1	1.95	1.15	64.6	21.84	0	0	7.65
15009	Carp, cooked, dry heat 3 oz	85	59.19	137.7	6.09	1.18	2.54	1.56	71.4	19.43	0	0	44.2
15235	Catfish, channel, farmed, cooked, dry heat 3 oz	85	60.84	129.2	6.82	1.52	3.53	1.18	54.4	15.91	0	0	7.65
15012	Caviar, black & red, granular 1 tablespoon	16	7.6	40.32	2.86	0.65	0.74	1.18	94.08	3.94	0.64	0	44
15016	Cod, Atlantic, cooked, dry heat 3 oz	85	64.53	89.25	0.73	0.14	0.11	0.25	46.75	19.41	0	0	11.9

NDB#	Phosphorus	Iron	Sodium	Potassium	Magnesium	Zinc	Copper	Vitamin A	Thiamin	Riboflavin	Niacin	Vitamin B6	Folate	Vitamin B12	Vitamin C
	mg	mg	mg	mg	mg	mg	mg	IU	mg	mg	mg	mg	mcg	mcg	mg
12115	18.3	0.34	0.6	48.75	4.2	0.14	0.06	0	0	0	0.13	0.01	3.45	0	0.42
12121	91.57	0.96	0.85	130.98	83.92	0.71	0.44	19.56	0.15	0.03	0.33	0.18	21.12	0	0.28
12122	91.57	0.96	0.85	130.98	83.92	0.71	0.44	19.56	0.06	0.06	0.79	0.18	21.12	0	0.28
12123	92.42	0.97	0.85	131.83	84.48	0.71	0.45	19.85	0.06	0.06	0.79	0.18	21.29	0	0.28
12131	38.56	0.68	1.42	104.33	32.89	0.48	0.08	0	0.1	0.03	0.61	0.06	4.45	0	0
12133	268	2.41	9.38	440.86	156.78	1.47	0.4	12.06	0.29	0.15	2.71	0.27	21.31	0	0
12143	86.18	0.62	0.28	104.9	37.71	1.61	0.35	37.71	0.09	0.03	0.26	0.06	11.54	0	0.57
12144	83.35	0.6	0.28	101.78	36.57	1.56	0.34	36.57	0.09	0.03	0.25	0.05	11.17	0	0.57
12152	609.28	4.06	7.68	1241.6	166.4	1.74	1.55	304.64	0.54	0.31	1.8	0.33	75.65	0	9.34
12166	109.8	1.34	17.25	62.1	14.25	0.69	0.24	10.05	0.18	0.07	0.82	0.02	14.66	0	0
12537	1478.4	4.86	998.4	1088	165.12	6.77	2.34	0	0.14	0.31	9.01	1.03	303.87	0	1.79
12023	56.61	1.31	0.99	42.12	31.59	0.7	0.37	0.81	0.07	0.02	0.41	0.07	8.7	0	0
12036	324.3	3.11	1.38	316.94	162.84	2.33	0.81	23	1.05	0.12	2.07	0.35	104.6	0	0.64
12154	580	3.84	1.25	655	252.5	4.28	1.28	370	0.27	0.14	0.86	0.69	81.88	0	4

Seafood

NDB#	Phosphorus	Iron	Sodium	Potassium	Magnesium	Zinc	Copper	Vitamin A	Thiamin	Riboflavin	Niacin	Vitamin B6	Folate	Vitamin B12	Vitamin C
15187	217.6	1.62	76.5	387.6	32.3	0.71	0.1	97.75	0.07	0.08	1.29	0.12	14.45	1.96	1.79
15188	215.9	0.92	74.8	278.8	43.35	0.43	0.03	88.4	0.1	0.03	2.17	0.29	8.5	3.75	0
15189	247.35	0.53	65.45	405.45	35.7	0.88	0.06	390.15	0.06	0.08	6.16	0.39	1.7	5.29	0
15009	451.35	1.35	53.55	362.95	32.3	1.62	0.06	27.2	0.12	0.06	1.79	0.19	14.71	1.25	1.36
15235	208.25	0.7	68	272.85	22.1	0.89	0.1	42.5	0.36	0.06	2.14	0.14	5.95	2.38	0.68
15012	56.96	1.9	240	28.96	48	0.15	0.02	298.88	0.03	0.1	0.02	0.05	8	3.2	0
15016	117.3	0.42	66.3	207.4	35.7	0.49	0.03	39.1	0.07	0.07	2.14	0.24	6.89	0.89	0.85

NDB#	Description & Serving	Grams	Water	Calories	Fat	Fat: Saturated	Fat: Monounsaturated	Fat: Polyunsaturated	Cholesterol	Protein	Carbohydrates	Fiber	Calcium
		g	kcal	g	g	g	g	mg	g	g	g	mg	
15192	Cod, Pacific, cooked, dry heat 3 oz	85	64.6	89.25	0.69	0.09	0.09	0.27	39.95	19.51	0	0	7.65
15229	Cuttlefish, mxd sp, cooked, moist heat 3 oz	85	51.95	134.3	1.19	0.2	0.14	0.23	190.4	27.61	1.39	0	153
15194	Dolphinfish, cooked, dry heat 3 oz	85	60.54	92.65	0.77	0.2	0.13	0.18	79.9	20.16	0	0	16.15
15195	Drum, freshwater, cooked, dry heat 3 oz	85	60.3	130.05	5.37	1.22	2.39	1.26	69.7	19.12	0	0	65.45
15026	Eel, mxd sp, cooked, dry heat 1 oz, boneless	28.35	16.81	66.91	4.24	0.86	2.61	0.34	45.64	6.7	0	0	7.37
15029	Flatfish (flounder & sole sp), cooked, dry heat 3 oz	85	62.19	99.45	1.3	0.31	0.2	0.55	57.8	20.54	0	0	15.3
15032	Grouper, mxd sp, cooked, dry heat 3 oz	85	62.36	100.3	1.11	0.25	0.23	0.34	39.95	21.11	0	0	17.85
15034	Haddock, cooked, dry heat 3 oz	85	63.11	95.2	0.79	0.14	0.13	0.26	62.9	20.6			35.7
15035	Haddock, smoked 1 oz, boneless	28.35	20.26	32.89	0.27	0.05	0.04	0.09	21.83	7.15	0	0	13.89
15037	Halibut, Atlantic & Pacific, cooked, dry heat 3 oz	85	60.94	119	2.5	0.35	0.82	0.8	34.85	22.69	0	0	51
15041	Herring, Atlantic, pickled 1 oz, boneless	28.35	15.65	74.28	5.1	0.68	3.39	0.48	3.69	4.02	2.73	0	21.83
15042	Herring, Atlantic, kippered 1 oz, boneless	28.35	16.92	61.52	3.51	0.79	1.45	0.83	23.25	6.97	0	0	23.81
15047	Mackerel, Atlantic, cooked, dry heat 3 oz	85	45.28	222.7	15.14	3.55	5.96	3.66	63.75	20.27	0	0	12.75
15201	Mackerel, Pacific & jack, mxd sp, cooked, dry heat 1 oz, boneless	28.35	17.5	56.98	2.87	0.82	0.96	0.71	17.01	7.29	0	0	8.22
15203	Monkfish, cooked, dry heat 3 oz	85	66.73	82.45	1.66	0	0	0	27.2	15.78	0	0	8.5
15056	Mullet, striped, cooked, dry heat 3 oz	85	59.94	127.5	4.13	1.22	1.17	0.78	53.55	21.09	0	0	26.35
15061	Perch, mxd sp, cooked, dry heat 3 oz	85	62.26	99.45	1	0.2	0.17	0.4	97.75	21.13	0	0	86.7
15063	Pike, northern, cooked, dry heat 3 oz	85	62.02	96.05	0.75	0.13	0.17	0.22	42.5	20.99	0	0	62.05
15204	Pike, walleye, cooked, dry heat 3 oz	85	62.45	101.15	1.33	0.27	0.32	0.49	93.5	20.86	0	0	119.85
15205	Pollock, Atlantic, cooked, dry heat 3 oz	85	61.23	100.3	1.07	0.14	0.12	0.53	77.35	21.18	0	0	65.45
15067	Pollock, walleye, cooked, dry heat 3 oz	85	62.95	96.05	0.95	0.2	0.15	0.45	81.6	19.98	0	0	5.1
15069	Pompano, Florida, cooked, dry heat 3 oz	85	53.52	179.35	10.32	3.82	2.82	1.24	54.4	20.14	0	0	36.55

NDB#	Phosphorus	Iron	Sodium	Potassium	Magnesium	Zinc	Copper	Vitamin A	Thiamin	Riboflavin	Niacin	Vitamin B6	Folate	Vitamin B12	Vitamin C
	mg	mg	mg	mg	mg	mg	mg	IU	mg	mg	mg	mg	mcg	mcg	mg
15192	189.55	0.28	77.35	439.45	26.35	0.43	0.03	27.2	0.02	0.04	2.11	0.39	6.8	0.88	2.55
15229	493	9.21	632.4	541.45	51	2.94	0.85	573.75	0.01	1.47	1.86	0.23	20.4	4.59	7.23
15194	155.55	1.23	96.05	453.05	32.3	0.5	0.05	176.8	0.02	0.07	6.31	0.39	5.1	0.59	0
15195	196.35	0.98	81.6	300.05	32.3	0.72	0.25	166.6	0.07	0.18	2.43	0.29	14.45	1.96	0.85
15026	78.53	0.18	18.43	98.94	7.37	0.59	0.01	1073.61	0.05	0.01	1.27	0.02	4.9	0.82	0.51
15029	245.65	0.29	89.25	292.4	49.3	0.54	0.02	32.3	0.07	0.1	1.85	0.2	7.82	2.13	0
15032	121.55	0.97	45.05	403.75	31.45	0.43	0.04	140.25	0.07	0.01	0.32	0.3	8.67	0.59	0
15034	204.85	1.15	73.95	339.15	42.5	0.41	0.03	53.55	0.03	0.04	3.94	0.29	11.31	1.18	0
15035	71.16	0.4	216.31	117.65	15.31	0.14	0.01	20.7	0.01	0.01	1.44	0.11	4.34	0.45	0
15037	242.25	0.91	58.65	489.6	90.95	0.45	0.03	152.15	0.06	0.08	6.05	0.34	11.73	1.16	0
15041	25.23	0.35	246.65	19.56	2.27	0.15	0.03	244.09	0.01	0.04	0.94	0.05	0.68	1.21	0
15042	92.14	0.43	260.25	126.72	13.04	0.39	0.04	36.29	0.04	0.09	1.25	0.12	3.88	5.3	0.28
15047	236.3	1.33	70.55	340.85	82.45	0.8	0.08	153	0.14	0.35	5.82	0.39	1.28	16.15	0.34
15201	45.36	0.42	31.19	147.7	10.21	0.24	0.03	13.32	0.04	0.15	3.02	0.11	0.57	1.2	0.6
15203	217.6	0.35	19.55	436.05	22.95	0.45	0.03	39.1	0.02	0.06	2.17	0.24	6.8	0.88	0.85
15056	207.4	1.2	60.35	389.3	28.05	0.75	0.12	119.85	0.09	0.09	5.36	0.42	8.33	0.21	1.02
15061	218.45	0.99	67.15	292.4	32.3	1.22	0.16	27.2	0.07	0.1	1.62	0.12	4.93	1.87	1.45
15063	239.7	0.6	41.65	281.35	34	0.73	0.06	68.85	0.06	0.07	2.38	0.11	14.71	1.96	3.23
15204	228.65	1.42	55.25	424.15	32.3	0.67	0.19	68.85	0.27	0.17	2.38	0.12	14.45	1.96	0
15205	240.55	0.5	93.5	387.6	73.1	0.51	0.05	34	0.05	0.19	3.39	0.28	2.55	3.13	0
15067	409.7	0.24	98.6	328.95	62.05	0.51	0.05	64.6	0.06	0.06	1.4	0.06	3.06	3.57	0
15069	289.85	0.57	64.6	540.6	26.35	0.59	0.07	102	0.58	0.13	3.23	0.2	14.71	1.02	0

NDB#	Description & Serving	Grams	Water	Calories	Fat	Fat. Saturated	Fat Monounsaturated	Fat Polyunsaturated	Cholesterol	Protein	Carbohydrates	Fiber	Calcium
		g	kcal	g	g	g	g	mg	g	g	g	mg	
15207	Roe, mxd sp, cooked, dry heat 1 oz	28.35	16.62	57.83	2.33	0.53	0.6	0.97	135.8	8.11	0.54	0	7.94
15232	Roughy, orange, cooked, dry heat 3 oz	85	58.74	75.65	0.77	0.02	0.52	0.01	22.1	16.02	0	0	32.3
15075	Sablefish, smoked 3 oz	85	51.12	218.45	17.12	3.58	9.01	2.28	54.4	15	0	0	42.5
15179	Salmon, chinook, smoked (lox), reg 3 oz	85	61.2	99.45	3.67	0.79	1.72	0.85	19.55	15.54	0	0	9.35
15209	Salmon, Atlantic, wild, cooked, dry heat 3 oz	85	50.68	154.7	6.91	1.07	2.29	2.77	60.35	21.62	0	0	12.75
15210	Salmon, chinook, cooked, dry heat 3 oz	85	55.76	196.35	11.37	2.73	4.88	2.26	72.25	21.86	0	0	23.87
15211	Salmon, chum, cooked, dry heat 3 oz	85	58.17	130.9	4.11	0.92	1.68	0.98	80.75	21.95	0	0	11.9
15212	Salmon, pink, cooked, dry heat 3 oz	85	59.23	126.65	3.76	0.61	1.02	1.47	56.95	21.73	0	0	14.45
15086	Salmon, sockeye, cooked, dry heat 3 oz	85	52.56	183.6	9.32	1.63	4.5	2.05	73.95	23.21	0	0	5.95
15088	Sardine, Atlantic, canned in oil, drained sol w/bone 1 oz	28.35	16.9	58.97	3.25	0.43	1.1	1.46	40.26	6.98	0	0	108.3
15092	Sea bass, mxd sp, cooked, dry heat 3 oz	85	61.32	105.4	2.18	0.56	0.46	0.81	45.05	20.09	0	0	11.05
15215	Shad, American, cooked, dry heat 3 oz	85	50.34	214.2	15	0	0	0	81.6	18.45	0	0	51
15100	Smelt, rainbow, cooked, dry heat 3 oz	85	61.87	105.4	2.64	0.49	0.7	0.96	76.5	19.21	0	0	65.45
15102	Snapper, mxd sp, cooked, dry heat 3 oz	85	59.8	108.8	1.46	0.31	0.27	0.5	39.95	22.36	0	0	34
15106	Sturgeon, mxd sp, smoked 3 oz	85	53.13	147.05	3.74	0.88	2	0.37	68	26.52	0	0	14.45
15109	Surimi 3 oz	85	64.89	84.15	0.77	0.15	0.12	0.39	25.5	12.9	5.82	0	7.65
15111	Swordfish, cooked, dry heat 3 oz	85	58.44	131.75	4.37	1.2	1.68	1	42.5	21.58	0	0	5.1
15116	Trout, rainbow, wild, cooked, dry heat 3 oz	85	59.93	127.5	4.95	1.38	1.48	1.56	58.65	19.48	0	0	73.1
15118	Tuna, fresh, bluefin, cooked, dry heat 3 oz	85	50.23	156.4	5.34	1.37	1.75	1.57	41.65	25.42	0	0	8.5
15221	Tuna, yellowfin, fresh, cooked, dry heat 3 oz	85	53.39	118.15	1.04	0.26	0.17	0.31	49.3	25.47	0	0	17.85
15222	Turbot, European, cooked, dry heat 3 oz	85	59.88	103.7	3.21	0	0	0	52.7	17.49	0	0	19.55
15131	Whitefish, mxd sp, smoked 1 oz, boneless	28.35	20.08	30.62	0.26	0.06	0.08	0.08	9.36	6.63	0	0	5.1

NDB#	Phosphorus	Iron	Sodium	Potassium	Magnesium	Zinc	Copper	Vitamin A	Thiamin	Riboflavin	Niacin	Vitamin B6	Folate	Vitamin B12	Vitamin C
	mg	mg	mg	mg	mg	mg	mg	IU	mg	mg	mg	mg	mcg	mcg	mg
15207	146	0.22	33.17	80.23	7.37	0.36	0.04	85.9	0.08	0.27	0.62	0.05	26.08	3.27	4.65
15232	217.6	0.2	68.85	327.25	32.3	0.82	0.15	68.85	0.1	0.16	3.11	0.29	6.8	1.96	0
15075	188.7	1.44	626.45	400.35	62.9	0.37	0.03	346.8	0.11	0.1	4.51	0.33	16.75	1.7	0
15179	139.4	0.72	1700	148.75	15.3	0.26	0.2	74.8	0.02	0.09	4.01	0.24	1.62	2.77	0
15209	217.6	0.88	47.6	533.8	31.45	0.7	0.27	37.4	0.23	0.41	8.57	0.8	24.65	2.59	0
15210	315.35	0.77	51	429.25	103.	0.48	0.05	421.6	0.04	0.13	8.54	0.39	29.75	2.44	3.49
15211	308.55	0.6	54.4	467.5	23.8	0.51	0.06	96.9	0.08	0.19	7.25	0.39	4.25	2.94	0
15212	250.75	0.84	73.1	351.9	28.05	0.6	0.08	115.6	0.17	0.06	7.25	0.2	4.25	2.94	0
15086	234.6	0.47	56.1	318.75	26.35	0.43	0.06	177.65	0.18	0.15	5.67	0.19	4.25	4.93	0
15088	138.92	0.83	143.17	112.55	11.06	0.37	0.05	63.5	0.02	0.06	1.49	0.05	3.35	2.53	0
15092	210.8	0.31	73.95	278.8	45.05	0.44	0.02	181.05	0.11	0.13	1.62	0.39	4.93	0.26	0
15215	296.65	1.05	55.25	418.2	32.3	0.4	0.07	102	0.16	0.26	9.15	0.39	14.45	0.12	0
15100	250.75	0.98	65.45	316.2	32.3	1.8	0.15	49.3	0.01	0.12	1.5	0.14	3.91	3.37	0
15102	170.85	0.2	48.45	443.7	31.45	0.37	0.04	97.75	0.05	0	0.29	0.39	4.93	2.98	1.36
15106	238.85	0.79	628.15	322.15	39.95	0.48	0.04	793.05	0.08	0.08	9.44	0.23	17	2.47	0
15109	239.7	0.22	121.55	95.2	36.55	0.28	0.03	56.1	0.02	0.02	0.19	0.03	1.36	1.36	0
15111	286.45	0.88	97.75	313.65	28.9	1.25	0.14	116.45	0.04	0.1	10.02	0.32	1.96	1.72	0.94
15116	228.65	0.32	47.6	380.8	26.35	0.43	0.05	42.5	0.13	0.08	4.9	0.29	16.15	5.36	1.7
15118	277.1	1.11	42.5	274.55	54.4	0.65	0.09	2142	0.24	0.26	8.96	0.45	1.87	9.25	0
15221	208.25	0.8	39.95	483.65	54.4	0.57	0.07	57.8	0.43	0.05	10.15	0.88	1.7	0.51	0.85
15222	140.25	0.39	163.2	259.25	55.25	0.24	0.04	34	0.06	0.08	2.28	0.21	7.65	2.16	1.45
15131	37.42	0.14	288.89	119.92	6.52	0.14	0.09	53.87	0.01	0.03	0.68	0.11	2.07	0.92	0

NDB#	Description & Serving	Grams	Water	Calories	Fat	Fat: Saturated	Fat: Monounsaturated	Fat: Polyunsaturated	Cholesterol	Protein	Carbohydrates	Fiber	Calcium
		g	kcal	g	g	g	g	mg	g	g	g	mg	

Shellfish

NDB#	Description & Serving	Grams	Water	Calories	Fat	Fat: Saturated	Fat: Monounsaturated	Fat: Polyunsaturated	Cholesterol	Protein	Carbohydrates	Fiber	Calcium
15156	Abalone, mxd sp, cooked, fried 3 oz — 85		51.09	160.65	5.76	1.4	2.33	1.42	79.9	16.69	9.39	0	31.45
15159	Clam, mxd sp, cooked, moist heat 20 small clams — 190		120.92	281.2	3.71	0.36	0.33	1.05	127.3	48.55	9.75	0	174.8
15137	Crab, Alaska king, cooked, moist heat 1 leg — 134		103.92	129.98	2.06	0.18	0.25	0.72	71.02	25.93	0	0	79.06
15140	Crab, blue, cooked, moist heat 1 cup (not packed) — 135		104.53	137.7	2.39	0.31	0.38	0.92	135	27.27	0	0	140.4
15226	Crab, dungeness, cooked, moist heat 1 crab — 127		93.1	139.7	1.57	0.21	0.27	0.52	96.52	28.35	1.21	0	74.93
15227	Crab, queen, cooked, moist heat 3 oz — 85		63.84	97.75	1.28	0.16	0.28	0.46	60.35	20.16	0	0	28.05
15243	Crayfish, mxd sp, farmed, cooked, moist heat 3 oz — 85		68.68	73.95	1.11	0.18	0.21	0.35	116.45	14.89	0	0	43.35
15148	Lobster, northern, cooked, moist heat 3 oz — 85		64.63	83.3	0.5	0.09	0.14	0.08	61.2	17.43	1.09	0	51.85
15165	Mussel, blue, cooked, moist heat 3 oz — 85		51.98	146.2	3.81	0.72	0.86	1.03	47.6	20.23	6.28	0	28.05
15167	Oyster, eastern, wild, raw 6 medium — 84		71.53	57.12	2.07	0.65	0.26	0.81	44.52	5.92	3.28	0	37.8
15169	Oyster, eastern, wild, cooked, moist heat 6 medium — 42		29.53	57.54	2.06	0.65	0.26	0.81	44.1	5.92	3.28	0	37.8
15244	Oyster, eastern, wild, cooked, dry heat 6 medium — 59		49.15	42.48	1.12	0.32	0.14	0.48	28.91	4.87	2.83	0	26.55
15171	Oyster, Pacific, raw 3 oz — 85		69.75	68.85	1.96	0.43	0.3	0.76	42.5	8.03	4.21	0	6.8
15231	Oyster, Pacific, cooked, moist heat 3 oz — 85		54.5	138.55	3.91	0.87	0.61	1.52	85	16.07	8.42	0	13.6
15173	Scallop, mxd sp, cooked, breaded & fried 2 large scallops — 31		18.12	66.65	3.39	0.83	1.39	0.89	18.91	5.6	3.14	0	13.02
15151	Shrimp, mxd sp, cooked, moist heat 4 large — 22		17	21.78	0.24	0.06	0.04	0.1	42.9	4.6	0	0	8.58
15176	Squid, mxd sp, cooked, fried 3 oz — 85		54.86	148.75	6.36	1.6	2.34	1.82	221	15.25	6.62	0	33.15

Vegetables and vegetable juices

NDB#	Description & Serving	Grams	Water	Calories	Fat	Fat: Saturated	Fat: Monounsaturated	Fat: Polyunsaturated	Cholesterol	Protein	Carbohydrates	Fiber	Calcium
11008	Artichokes (globe or French), cooked, boiled, drained, wo/salt 1 medium artichoke — 120		100.76	60	0.19	0.04	0.01	0.08	0	4.18	13.42	6.48	54
11011	Asparagus, raw 1 small spear (5" long or less) — 12		11.09	2.76	0.02	0.01	0	0.01	0	0.27	0.54	0.25	2.52

NDB#	Phosphorus	Iron	Sodium	Potassium	Magnesium	Zinc	Copper	Vitamin A	Thiamin	Riboflavin	Niacin	Vitamin B6	Folate	Vitamin B12	Vitamin C
	mg	mg	mg	mg	mg	mg	mg	IU	mg	mg	mg	mg	mcg	mcg	mg
15156	184.45	3.23	502.35	241.4	47.6	0.81	0.19	4.25	0.19	0.11	1.62	0.13	4.59	0.59	1.53
15159	642.2	53.12	212.8	1193.2	34.2	5.19	1.31	1083	0.29	0.81	6.37	0.21	54.72	187.89	41.99
15137	375.2	1.02	1436.48	351.08	84.42	10.21	1.58	38.86	0.07	0.07	1.8	0.24	68.34	15.41	10.18
15140	278.1	1.23	376.65	437.4	44.55	5.7	0.87	8.1	0.14	0.07	4.46	0.24	68.58	9.86	4.46
15226	222.25	0.55	480.06	518.16	73.66	6.95	0.93	132.08	0.07	0.26	4.6	0.22	53.34	13.18	4.57
15227	108.8	2.45	587.35	170	53.55	3.05	0.53	147.05	0.08	0.21	2.45	0.15	35.7	8.82	6.12
15243	204.85	0.94	82.45	202.3	28.05	1.26	0.49	42.5	0.04	0.07	1.42	0.11	9.35	2.64	0.43
15148	157.25	0.33	323	299.2	29.75	2.48	1.65	73.95	0.01	0.06	0.91	0.07	9.44	2.64	0
15165	242.25	5.71	313.65	227.8	31.45	2.27	0.13	258.4	0.26	0.36	2.55	0.09	64.26	20.4	11.56
15167	113.4	5.59	177.24	131.04	39.48	76.28	3.74	84	0.08	0.08	1.16	0.05	8.4	16.35	3.11
15169	85.26	5.04	177.24	118.02	39.9	76.28	3.18	75.6	0.08	0.08	1.04	0.05	5.88	14.71	2.52
15244	80.24	2.55	143.96	99.12	27.14	43.42	2.04	0	0.05	0.05	0.99	0.06	10.62	16.4	2.42
15171	137.7	4.34	90.1	142.8	18.7	14.13	1.34	229.5	0.06	0.2	1.71	0.04	8.5	13.6	6.8
15231	206.55	7.82	180.2	256.7	37.4	28.25	2.28	413.1	0.11	0.38	3.08	0.08	12.75	24.48	10.88
15173	73.16	0.25	143.84	103.23	18.29	0.33	0.02	23.25	0.01	0.03	0.47	0.04	5.64	0.41	0.71
15151	30.14	0.68	49.28	40.04	7.48	0.34	0.04	48.18	0.01	0.01	0.57	0.03	0.77	0.33	0.48
15176	213.35	0.86	260.1	237.15	32.3	1.48	1.8	29.75	0.05	0.39	2.21	0.05	4.51	1.04	3.57
Vegetables and vegetable juices															
11008	103.2	1.55	114	424.8	72	0.59	0.28	212.4	0.08	0.08	1.2	0.13	61.2	0	12
11011	6.72	0.1	0.24	32.76	2.16	0.06	0.02	69.96	0.02	0.02	0.14	0.02	15.36	0	1.58

NDB#	Description & Serving	Grams	Water	Calories	Fat	Fat: Saturated	Fat: Monounsaturated	Fat: Polyunsaturated	Cholesterol	Protein	Carbohydrates	Fiber	Calcium
		g		kcal	g	g	g	g	mg	g	g	g	mg
11027	Bamboo shoots, cooked, boiled, drained, wo/salt 1 cup (½" slices)	120	115.1	14.4	0.26	0.06	0.01	0.12	0	1.84	2.3	1.2	14.4
11053	Beans, snap, green, cooked, boiled, drained, wo/salt 1 cup	125	111.53	43.75	0.35	0.08	0.01	0.18	0	2.36	9.86	4	57.5
11081	Beets, cooked, boiled, drained ½ cup slices	85	74	37.4	0.15	0.02	0.03	0.05	0	1.43	8.47	1.7	13.6
11090	Broccoli, raw 1 cup, flowerets	71	64.39	19.88	0.25	0.04	0.02	0.12	0	2.12	3.72	2.13	34.08
11099	Brussels sprouts, cooked, boiled, drained, wo/salt ½ cup	78	68.11	30.42	0.4	0.08	0.03	0.2	0	1.99	6.76	2.03	28.08
11109	Cabbage, raw 1 cup, shredded	70	64.51	17.5	0.19	0.02	0.01	0.09	0	1.01	3.8	1.61	32.9
11110	Cabbage, cooked, boiled, drained, wo/salt ½ cup shredded	75	70.2	16.5	0.32	0.04	0.02	0.15	0	0.77	3.35	1.73	23.25
11112	Cabbage, red, raw 1 cup, shredded	70	64.09	18.9	0.18	0.02	0.01	0.09	0	0.97	4.28	1.4	35.7
11113	Cabbage, red, cooked, boiled, drained, wo/salt ½ cup shredded	75	70.2	15.75	0.15	0.02	0.01	0.07	0	0.79	3.48	1.5	27.75
11115	Cabbage, savoy, cooked, boiled, drained, wo/salt 1 cup, shredded	145	133.4	34.8	0.13	0.02	0.01	0.06	0	2.61	7.84	4.06	43.5
11117	Cabbage, Chinese (pak-choi), cooked, boiled, drained, wo/salt 1 cup, shredded	170	162.44	20.4	0.27	0.04	0.02	0.13	0	2.65	3.03	2.72	158.1
11124	Carrots, raw 1 cup, grated	110	96.57	47.3	0.21	0.03	0.01	0.08	0	1.13	11.15	3.3	29.7
11960	Carrots, baby, raw 1 medium	10	8.98	3.8	0.05	0.01	0	0.03	0	0.08	0.82	0.18	2.3
11125	Carrots, cooked, boiled, drained, wo/salt ½ cup slices	78	68.16	35.1	0.14	0.03	0.01	0.07	0	0.85	8.17	2.57	24.18
11135	Cauliflower, raw 1 cup	100	91.91	25	0.21	0.03	0.01	0.1	0	1.98	5.2	2.5	22
11136	Cauliflower, cooked, boiled, drained, wo/salt ½ cup (1" pieces)	62	57.66	14.26	0.28	0.04	0.02	0.13	0	1.14	2.55	1.67	9.92
11965	Cauliflower, green, raw 1 cup	64	57.47	19.84	0.19	0.03	0.02	0.09	0	1.89	3.9	2.05	21.12
11967	Cauliflower, green, cooked, no salt ⅕ head	90	80.52	28.8	0.28	0.04	0.03	0.12	0	2.74	5.65	2.97	28.8
11143	Celery, raw 1 cup, diced	120	113.57	19.2	0.17	0.04	0.03	0.08	0	0.9	4.38	2.04	48
11148	Chard, Swiss, cooked, boiled, drained, wo/salt 1 cup, chopped	175	162.14	35	0.14	0.02	0.03	0.05	0	3.29	7.25	3.68	101.5
11151	Chicory, witloof, raw ½ cup	45	42.53	7.65	0.05	0.01	0	0.02	0	0.41	1.8	1.4	8.55
11162	Collards, cooked, boiled, drained, wo/salt 1 cup, chopped	190	174.53	51.3	0.36	0.05	0.03	0.17	0	2.57	11.65	5.32	43.7
11168	Corn, swt, yellow, cooked, boiled, drained, wo/salt 1 baby ear	8	5.57	8.64	0.1	0.02	0.03	0.05	0	0.27	2.01	0.22	0.16

NDB#	Phosphorus	Iron	Sodium	Potassium	Magnesium	Zinc	Copper	Vitamin A	Thiamin	Riboflavin	Niacin	Vitamin B6	Folate	Vitamin B12	Vitamin C
	mg	mg	mg	mg	mg	mg	mg	IU	mg	mg	mg	mg	mcg	mcg	mg
11027	24	0.29	4.8	639.6	3.6	0.56	0.1	0	0.02	0.06	0.36	0.12	2.76	0	0
11053	48.75	1.6	3.75	373.75	31.25	0.45	0.13	832.5	0.09	0.12	0.77	0.07	41.63	0	12.13
11081	32.3	0.67	65.45	259.25	19.55	0.3	0.06	29.75	0.02	0.03	0.28	0.06	68	0	3.06
11090	46.86	0.62	19.17	230.75	17.75	0.28	0.03	1094.82	0.05	0.08	0.45	0.11	50.41	0	66.17
11099	43.68	0.94	16.38	247.26	15.6	0.26	0.06	560.82	0.08	0.06	0.47	0.14	46.8	0	48.36
11109	16.1	0.41	12.6	172.2	10.5	0.13	0.02	93.1	0.04	0.03	0.21	0.07	30.1	0	22.54
11110	11.25	0.13	6	72.75	6	0.07	0.01	99	0.04	0.04	0.21	0.08	15	0	15.08
11112	29.4	0.34	7.7	144.2	10.5	0.15	0.07	28	0.04	0.02	0.21	0.15	14.49	0	39.9
11113	21.75	0.26	6	105	8.25	0.11	0.05	20.25	0.03	0.02	0.15	0.11	9.45	0	25.8
11115	47.85	0.55	34.8	266.8	34.8	0.33	0.08	1289.05	0.07	0.03	0.03	0.22	67.14	0	24.65
11117	49.3	1.77	57.8	630.7	18.7	0.29	0.03	4365.6	0.05	0.11	0.73	0.28	69.02	0	44.2
11124	48.4	0.55	38.5	355.3	16.5	0.22	0.05	30941.9	0.11	0.06	1.02	0.16	15.4	0	10.23
11960	3.8	0.08	3.5	27.9	1.2	0.02	0	197.2	0	0.01	0.09	0.01	3.3	0	0.84
11125	23.4	0.48	51.48	177.06	10.14	0.23	0.1	19152.12	0.03	0.04	0.39	0.19	10.84	0	1.79
11135	44	0.44	30	303	15	0.28	0.04	19	0.06	0.06	0.53	0.22	57	0	46.4
11136	19.84	0.2	9.3	88.04	5.58	0.11	0.02	10.54	0.03	0.03	0.25	0.11	27.28	0	27.47
11965	39.68	0.47	14.72	192	12.8	0.41	0.03	97.28	0.05	0.07	0.47	0.14	36.48	0	56.38
11967	51.3	0.65	20.7	250.2	17.1	0.57	0.04	126.9	0.06	0.09	0.61	0.19	36.9	0	65.34
11143	30	0.48	104.4	344.4	13.2	0.16	0.04	160.8	0.06	0.05	0.39	0.1	33.6	0	8.4
11148	57.75	3.96	313.25	960.75	150.5	0.58	0.29	5493.25	0.06	0.15	0.63	0.15	15.05	0	31.5
11151	11.7	0.11	0.9	94.95	4.5	0.07	0.02	13.05	0.03	0.01	0.07	0.02	16.65	0	1.26
11162	15.2	0.3	30.4	248.9	13.3	0.21	0.06	5181.3	0.04	0.1	0.55	0.1	11.4	0	22.99
11168	8.24	0.05	1.36	19.92	2.56	0.04	0	17.36	0.02	0.01	0.13	0	3.71	0	0.5

NDB#	Description & Serving	Grams	Water	Calories	Fat	Fat, Saturated	Fat, Monounsaturated	Fat, Polyunsaturated	Cholesterol	Protein	Carbohydrates	Fiber	Calcium
		g		kcal	g	g	g	g	mg	g	g	g	mg
11203	Cress, garden, raw 1 cup	50	44.7	16	0.35	0.01	0.12	0.11	0	1.3	2.75	0.55	40.5
11205	Cucumber, with peel, raw ½ cup slices	52	49.93	6.76	0.07	0.02	0	0.03	0	0.36	1.44	0.42	7.28
11210	Eggplant, cooked, boiled, drained, wo/salt 1 cup (1" cubes)	99	90.85	27.72	0.23	0.04	0.02	0.09	0	0.82	6.57	2.48	5.94
11213	Endive, raw ½ cup, chopped	25	23.45	4.25	0.05	0.01	0	0.02	0	0.31	0.84	0.78	13
11234	Kale, cooked, boiled, drained, wo/salt 1 cup, chopped	130	118.56	41.6	0.52	0.07	0.04	0.25	0	2.47	7.32	2.6	93.6
11242	Kohlrabi, cooked, boiled, drained, wo/salt 1 cup, sliced	165	149	47.85	0.18	0.02	0.01	0.09	0	2.97	11.04	1.82	41.25
11247	Leeks (bulb & lower leaf-portion), cooked, boiled, drained, wo/salt ¼ cup chopped or diced	26	23.61	8.06	0.05	0.01	0	0.03	0	0.21	1.98	0.26	7.8
11250	Lettuce, butterhead (incl Boston & bibb types), raw 1 cup, shredded or chopped	55	52.57	7.15	0.12	0.02	0	0.06	0	0.71	1.28	0.55	17.6
11251	Lettuce, cos or romaine, raw ½ cup shredded	28	26.57	4.48	0.06	0.01	0	0.03	0	0.45	0.66	0.48	10.08
11252	Lettuce, iceberg (incl crisphead types), raw 1 cup, shredded or chopped	55	52.74	6.6	0.1	0.01	0	0.06	0	0.56	1.15	0.77	10.45
11253	Lettuce, looseleaf, raw ½ cup shredded	28	26.32	5.04	0.08	0.01	0	0.04	0	0.36	0.98	0.53	19.04
11260	Mushrooms, raw 1 cup, whole	96	88.14	24	0.4	0.05	0.01	0.16	0	2.01	4.46	1.15	4.8
11950	Mushrooms, enoki, raw 1 large	5	4.47	1.7	0.02	0	0	0.01	0	0.12	0.35	0.13	0.05
11268	Mushrooms, shiitake, dried 1 mushroom	3.6	0.34	10.66	0.04	0.01	0.01	0.01	0	0.34	2.71	0.41	0.4
11269	Mushrooms, shiitake, cooked, wo/salt 1 cup (pieces)	145	121.05	79.75	0.32	0.08	0.1	0.04	0	2.26	20.71	3.05	4.35
11279	Okra, cooked, boiled, drained, wo/salt 8 pods (3" long)	85	76.42	27.2	0.14	0.04	0.02	0.04	0	1.59	6.13	2.13	53.55
11282	Onions, raw 1 cup, chopped	160	143.49	60.8	0.26	0.04	0.04	0.1	0	1.86	13.81	2.88	32
11283	Onions, cooked, boiled, drained, wo/salt 1 cup	210	184.51	92.4	0.4	0.07	0.06	0.15	0	2.86	21.32	2.94	46.2
11291	Onions, spring (incl tops & bulb), raw 1 tablespoon, chopped	6	5.39	1.92	0.01	0	0	0	0	0.11	0.44	0.16	4.32
11297	Parsley, raw 1 cup	60	52.63	21.6	0.47	0.08	0.18	0.07	0	1.78	3.8	1.98	82.8
11299	Parsnips, cooked, boiled, drained, wo/salt ½ cup slices	78	60.62	63.18	0.23	0.04	0.09	0.04	0	1.03	15.23	3.12	28.86
11305	Peas, green, cooked, boiled, drained, wo/salt 1 cup	160	124.59	134.4	0.35	0.06	0.03	0.16	0	8.58	25.02	8.8	43.2

NDB#	Phosphorus	Iron	Sodium	Potassium	Magnesium	Zinc	Copper	Vitamin A	Thiamin	Riboflavin	Niacin	Vitamin B6	Folate	Vitamin B12	Vitamin C
	mg	mg	mg	mg	mg	mg	mg	IU	mg	mg	mg	mg	mcg	mcg	mg
11203	38	0.65	7	303	19	0.12	0.09	4650	0.04	0.13	0.5	0.12	40.2	0	34.5
11205	10.4	0.14	1.04	74.88	5.72	0.1	0.02	111.8	0.01	0.01	0.11	0.02	6.76	0	2.76
11210	21.78	0.35	2.97	245.52	12.87	0.15	0.11	63.36	0.08	0.02	0.59	0.09	14.26	0	1.29
11213	7	0.21	5.5	78.5	3.75	0.2	0.02	512.5	0.02	0.02	0.1	0.01	35.5	0	1.63
11234	36.4	1.17	29.9	296.4	23.4	0.31	0.2	9620	0.07	0.09	0.65	0.18	17.29	0	53.3
11242	74.25	0.66	34.65	561	31.35	0.51	0.22	57.75	0.07	0.03	0.64	0.25	19.97	0	89.1
11247	4.42	0.29	2.6	22.62	3.64	0.02	0.02	11.96	0.01	0.01	0.05	0.03	6.32	0	1.09
11250	12.65	0.17	2.75	141.35	7.15	0.09	0.01	533.5	0.03	0.03	0.17	0.03	40.32	0	4.4
11251	12.6	0.31	2.24	81.2	1.68	0.07	0.01	728	0.03	0.03	0.14	0.01	38	0	6.72
11252	11	0.28	4.95	86.9	4.95	0.12	0.02	181.5	0.03	0.02	0.1	0.02	30.8	0	2.15
11253	7	0.39	2.52	73.92	3.08	0.08	0.01	532	0.01	0.02	0.11	0.02	13.94	0	5.04
11260	99.84	1.19	3.84	355.2	9.6	0.7	0.47	0	0.1	0.43	3.95	0.09	20.26	0	3.36
11950	5.65	0.04	0.15	19.05	0.8	0.03	0	0.35	0	0.01	0.18	0	1.5	0	0.60
11268	10.58	0.06	0.47	55.22	4.75	0.28	0.19	0	0.01	0.05	0.51	0.03	5.88	0	0.13
11269	42.05	0.64	5.8	169.65	20.3	1.93	1.3	0	0.05	0.25	2.18	0.23	30.31	0	0.44
11279	47.6	0.38	4.25	273.7	48.45	0.47	0.07	488.75	0.11	0.05	0.74	0.16	38.85	0	13.86
11282	52.8	0.35	4.8	251.2	16	0.3	0.1	0	0.07	0.03	0.24	0.19	30.4	0	10.24
11283	73.5	0.5	6.3	348.6	23.1	0.44	0.14	0	0.09	0.05	0.35	0.27	31.5	0	10.92
11291	2.22	0.09	0.96	16.56	1.2	0.02	0	23.1	0	0	0.03	0	3.84	0	1.13
11297	34.8	3.72	33.6	332.4	30	0.64	0.09	3120	0.05	0.06	0.79	0.05	91.2	0	79.8
11299	53.82	0.45	7.8	286.26	22.62	0.2	0.11	0	0.06	0.04	0.56	0.07	45.4	0	10.14
11305	187.2	2.46	4.8	433.6	62.4	1.9	0.28	955.2	0.41	0.24	3.23	0.35	101.28	0	22.72

NDB#	Description & Serving	Grams	Water	Calories	Fat	Fat: Saturated	Fat Monounsaturated	Fat Polyunsaturated	Cholesterol	Protein	Carbohydrates	Fiber	Calcium
		g	kcal	g	g	g	g	mg	g	g	g	mg	
11333	Peppers, sweet, green, raw 1 cup, chopped	149	137.36	40.23	0.28	0.04	0.02	0.15	0	1.33	9.58	2.68	13.41
11951	Peppers, sweet, yellow, raw 10 strips	52	47.85	14.04	0.11	0	0	0	0	0.52	3.29	0.47	5.72
11363	Potatoes, baked, flesh, wo/salt 1 potato (2⅓" × 4¾")	156	117.66	145.08	0.16	0.04	0	0.07	0	3.06	33.63	2.34	7.8
11364	Potatoes, baked, skin, wo/salt 1 potato skin	58	27.44	114.84	0.06	0.02	0	0.02	0	2.49	26.72	4.58	19.72
11365	Potatoes, boiled, cooked in skin, flesh, wo/salt 1 potato (2½" dia, sphere)	136	104.69	118.32	0.14	0.04	0	0.06	0	2.54	27.38	2.45	6.8
11423	Pumpkin, cooked, boiled, drained, wo/salt 1 cup, mashed	245	229.54	49	0.17	0.09	0.02	0.01	0	1.76	11.98	2.7	36.75
11952	Radicchio, raw 1 cup, shredded	40	37.26	9.2	0.1	0.02	0	0.04	0	0.57	1.79	0.36	7.6
11429	Radishes, raw 1 cup, slices	116	110.01	19.72	0.63	0.03	0.02	0.05	0	0.7	4.16	1.86	24.36
11436	Rutabagas, cooked, boiled, drained, wo/salt 1 cup, mashed	240	213.31	93.6	0.53	0.07	0.06	0.23	0	3.1	20.98	4.32	115.2
11458	Spinach, cooked, boiled, drained, wo/salt 1 cup	180	164.18	41.4	0.47	0.08	0.01	0.19	0	5.35	6.75	4.32	244.8
11477	Squash, summer, zucchini, incl skin, raw 1 cup, sliced	113	107.67	15.82	0.16	0.03	0.01	0.07	0	1.31	3.28	1.36	16.95
11480	Squash, summer, zucchini, incl skin, frz, cooked, boiled, drained, wo/salt 1 cup	223	211.27	37.91	0.29	0.06	0.02	0.12	0	2.56	7.94	2.9	37.91
11483	Squash, winter, acorn, cooked, baked, wo/salt 1 cup, cubes	205	169.95	114.8	0.29	0.06	0.02	0.12	0	2.3	29.89	9.02	90.2
11486	Squash, winter, butternut, cooked, baked, wo/salt 1 cup, cubes	205	179.99	82	0.18	0.04	0.01	0.08	0	1.85	21.5	0	84.05
11490	Squash, winter, hubbard, cooked, baked, wo/salt 1 cup, cubes	205	174.46	102.5	1.27	0.26	0.09	0.53	0	5.08	22.16	0	34.85
11493	Squash, winter, spaghetti, cooked, boiled, drained, or baked, wo/salt 1 cup	155	143.07	44.95	0.4	0.1	0.03	0.2	0	1.02	10.01	2.17	32.55
11496	Succotash (corn & limas), cooked, boiled, drained, wo/salt 1 cup	192	131.27	220.8	1.54	0.28	0.3	0.73	0	9.73	46.81	8.64	32.64
11508	Sweet potato, cooked, baked in skin, wo/salt 1 large	180	131.13	185.4	0.2	0.04	0.01	0.09	0	3.1	43.69	5.4	50.4
11510	Sweet potato, cooked, boiled, wo/skin, wo/salt 1 medium	151	109.99	158.55	0.45	0.1	0.02	0.2	0	2.49	36.66	2.72	31.71
11529	Tomatoes, red, ripe, raw, year round average 1 cup, chopped or sliced	180	168.77	37.8	0.59	0.08	0.09	0.24	0	1.53	8.35	1.98	9
11530	Tomatoes, red, ripe, cooked, boiled, wo/salt 2 medium	246	226.71	66.42	1.01	0.14	0.15	0.42	0	2.63	14.34	2.46	14.76
11565	Turnips, cooked, boiled, drained, wo/salt 1 cup, mashed	230	215.28	41.4	0.18	0.02	0.01	0.1	0	1.63	11.27	4.6	50.6
11591	Watercress, raw 1 cup, chopped	34	32.34	3.74	0.03	0.01	0	0.01	0	0.78	0.44	0.51	40.8

NDB#	Phosphorus	Iron	Sodium	Potassium	Magnesium	Zinc	Copper	Vitamin A	Thiamin	Riboflavin	Niacin	Vitamin B6	Folate	Vitamin B12	Vitamin C
	mg	mg	mg	mg	mg	mg	mg	IU	mg	mg	mg	mg	mcg	mcg	mg
11333	28.31	0.69	2.98	263.73	14.9	0.18	0.1	941.68	0.1	0.04	0.76	0.37	32.78	0	133.06
11951	12.48	0.24	1.04	110.24	6.24	0.09	0.06	123.76	0.01	0.01	0.46	0.09	13.52	0	95.42
11363	78	0.55	7.8	609.96	39	0.45	0.34	0	0.16	0.03	2.18	0.47	14.2	0	19.97
11364	58.58	4.08	12.18	332.34	24.94	0.28	0.47	0	0.07	0.06	1.78	0.36	12.53	0	7.83
11365	59.84	0.42	5.44	515.44	29.92	0.41	0.26	0	0.14	0.03	1.96	0.41	13.6	0	17.68
11423	0.56	0.22	2650.9	73.5	1.4	2.45	563.5	22.05	0.08	0.19	1.01	0.11	20.83	0	11.52
11952	16	0.23	8.8	120.8	5.2	0.25	0.14	10.8	0.01	0.01	0.1	0.02	24	0	3.2
11429	20.88	0.34	27.84	269.12	10.44	0.35	0.05	9.28	0.01	0.05	0.35	0.08	31.32	0	26.45
11436	134.4	1.27	48	782.4	55.2	0.84	0.1	1346.4	0.2	0.1	1.72	0.24	36	0	45.12
11458	100.8	6.43	126	838.8	156.6	1.37	0.31	14742	0.17	0.42	0.88	0.44	262.44	0	17.64
11477	36.16	0.47	3.39	280.24	24.86	0.23	0.06	384.2	0.08	0.03	0.45	0.1	24.97	0	10.17
11480	55.75	1.07	4.46	432.62	28.99	0.45	0.1	963.36	0.09	0.09	0.86	0.1	17.39	0	8.25
11483	92.25	1.91	8.2	895.85	88.15	0.35	0.18	877.4	0.34	0.03	1.81	0.4	38.34	0	22.14
11486	55.35	1.23	8.2	582.2	59.45	0.27	0.13	14352.05	0.15	0.03	1.99	0.25	39.36	0	30.96
11490	47.15	0.96	16.4	733.9	45.1	0.31	0.09	12371.75	0.15	0.1	1.14	0.35	33.21	0	19.48
11493	21.7	0.53	27.9	181.35	17.05	0.31	0.05	170.5	0.06	0.03	1.26	0.15	12.4	0	5.43
11496	224.64	2.92	32.64	787.2	101.76	1.21	0.34	564.48	0.32	0.18	2.55	0.22	62.98	0	15.74
11508	99	0.81	18	626.4	36	0.52	0.37	39279.6	0.13	0.23	1.09	0.43	40.68	0	44.28
11510	40.77	0.85	19.63	277.84	15.1	0.41	0.24	25751.54	0.08	0.21	0.97	0.37	16.76	0	25.82
11529	43.2	0.81	16.2	399.6	19.8	0.16	0.13	1121.4	0.11	0.09	1.13	0.14	27	0	34.38
11530	76.26	1.38	27.06	686.34	34.44	0.27	0.23	1827.78	0.17	0.14	1.84	0.23	31.98	0	56.09
11565	43.7	0.51	115	310.5	18.4	0.46	0.15	0	0.06	0.05	0.69	0.15	21.16	0	26.68
11591	20.4	0.07	13.94	112.2	7.14	0.04	0.03	1598	0.03	0.04	0.07	0.04	3.13	0	14.62

Index

BUSINESS, CAREERS & PERSONAL FINANCE

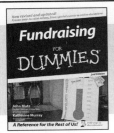

0-7645-9847-3

0-7645-2431-3

Also available:
- Business Plans Kit For Dummies
0-7645-9794-9
- Economics For Dummies
0-7645-5726-2
- Grant Writing For Dummies
0-7645-8416-2
- Home Buying For Dummies
0-7645-5331-3
- Managing For Dummies
0-7645-1771-6
- Marketing For Dummies
0-7645-5600-2

- Personal Finance For Dummies
0-7645-2590-5*
- Resumes For Dummies
0-7645-5471-9
- Selling For Dummies
0-7645-5363-1
- Six Sigma For Dummies
0-7645-6798-5
- Small Business Kit For Dummies
0-7645-5984-2
- Starting an eBay Business For Dummies
0-7645-6924-4
- Your Dream Career For Dummies
0-7645-9795-7

HOME & BUSINESS COMPUTER BASICS

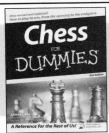

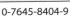

0-470-05432-8

0-471-75421-8

Also available:
- Cleaning Windows Vista For Dummies
0-471-78293-9
- Excel 2007 For Dummies
0-470-03737-7
- Mac OS X Tiger For Dummies
0-7645-7675-5
- MacBook For Dummies
0-470-04859-X
- Macs For Dummies
0-470-04849-2
- Office 2007 For Dummies
0-470-00923-3

- Outlook 2007 For Dummies
0-470-03830-6
- PCs For Dummies
0-7645-8958-X
- Salesforce.com For Dummies
0-470-04893-X
- Upgrading & Fixing Laptops For Dummies
0-7645-8959-8
- Word 2007 For Dummies
0-470-03658-3
- Quicken 2007 For Dummies
0-470-04600-7

FOOD, HOME, GARDEN, HOBBIES, MUSIC & PETS

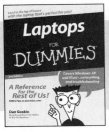

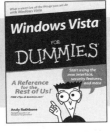

0-7645-8404-9

0-7645-9904-6

Also available:
- Candy Making For Dummies
0-7645-9734-5
- Card Games For Dummies
0-7645-9910-0
- Crocheting For Dummies
0-7645-4151-X
- Dog Training For Dummies
0-7645-8418-9
- Healthy Carb Cookbook For Dummies
0-7645-8476-6
- Home Maintenance For Dummies
0-7645-5215-5

- Horses For Dummies
0-7645-9797-3
- Jewelry Making & Beading For Dummies
0-7645-2571-9
- Orchids For Dummies
0-7645-6759-4
- Puppies For Dummies
0-7645-5255-4
- Rock Guitar For Dummies
0-7645-5356-9
- Sewing For Dummies
0-7645-6847-7
- Singing For Dummies
0-7645-2475-5

INTERNET & DIGITAL MEDIA

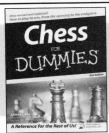

0-470-04529-9

0-470-04894-8

Also available:
- Blogging For Dummies
0-471-77084-1
- Digital Photography For Dummies
0-7645-9802-3
- Digital Photography All-in-One Desk Reference For Dummies
0-470-03743-1
- Digital SLR Cameras and Photography For Dummies
0-7645-9803-1
- eBay Business All-in-One Desk Reference For Dummies
0-7645-8438-3
- HDTV For Dummies
0-470-09673-X

- Home Entertainment PCs For Dummies
0-470-05523-5
- MySpace For Dummies
0-470-09529-6
- Search Engine Optimization For Dummies
0-471-97998-8
- Skype For Dummies
0-470-04891-3
- The Internet For Dummies
0-7645-8996-2
- Wiring Your Digital Home For Dummies
0-471-91830-X

Available wherever books are sold. For more information or to order direct: U.S. customers visit www.dummies.com or call 1-877-762-2974.
U.K. customers visit www.wileyeurope.com or call 0800 243407. Canadian customers visit www.wiley.ca or call 1-800-567-4797.

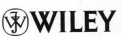

SPORTS, FITNESS, PARENTING, RELIGION & SPIRITUALITY

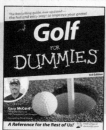

0-471-76871-5

0-7645-7841-3

Also available:
- Catholicism For Dummies
  0-7645-5391-7
- Exercise Balls For Dummies
  0-7645-5623-1
- Fitness For Dummies
  0-7645-7851-0
- Football For Dummies
  0-7645-3936-1
- Judaism For Dummies
  0-7645-5299-6
- Potty Training For Dummies
  0-7645-5417-4
- Buddhism For Dummies
  0-7645-5359-3

- Pregnancy For Dummies
  0-7645-4483-7 †
- Ten Minute Tone-Ups For Dummies
  0-7645-7207-5
- NASCAR For Dummies
  0-7645-7681-X
- Religion For Dummies
  0-7645-5264-3
- Soccer For Dummies
  0-7645-5229-5
- Women in the Bible For Dummies
  0-7645-8475-8

TRAVEL

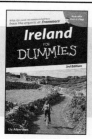

0-7645-7749-2

0-7645-6945-7

Also available:
- Alaska For Dummies
  0-7645-7746-8
- Cruise Vacations For Dummies
  0-7645-6941-4
- England For Dummies
  0-7645-4276-1
- Europe For Dummies
  0-7645-7529-5
- Germany For Dummies
  0-7645-7823-5
- Hawaii For Dummies
  0-7645-7402-7

- Italy For Dummies
  0-7645-7386-1
- Las Vegas For Dummies
  0-7645-7382-9
- London For Dummies
  0-7645-4277-X
- Paris For Dummies
  0-7645-7630-5
- RV Vacations For Dummies
  0-7645-4442-X
- Walt Disney World & Orlando
  For Dummies
  0-7645-9660-8

GRAPHICS, DESIGN & WEB DEVELOPMENT

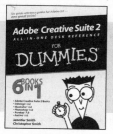

0-7645-8815-X

0-7645-9571-7

Also available:
- 3D Game Animation For Dummies
  0-7645-8789-7
- AutoCAD 2006 For Dummies
  0-7645-8925-3
- Building a Web Site For Dummies
  0-7645-7144-3
- Creating Web Pages For Dummies
  0-470-08030-2
- Creating Web Pages All-in-One Desk
  Reference For Dummies
  0-7645-4345-8
- Dreamweaver 8 For Dummies
  0-7645-9649-7

- InDesign CS2 For Dummies
  0-7645-9572-5
- Macromedia Flash 8 For Dummies
  0-7645-9691-8
- Photoshop CS2 and Digital
  Photography For Dummies
  0-7645-9580-6
- Photoshop Elements 4 For Dummies
  0-471-77483-9
- Syndicating Web Sites with RSS Feeds
  For Dummies
  0-7645-8848-6
- Yahoo! SiteBuilder For Dummies
  0-7645-9800-7

NETWORKING, SECURITY, PROGRAMMING & DATABASES

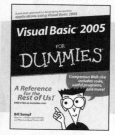

0-7645-7728-X

0-471-74940-0

Also available:
- Access 2007 For Dummies
  0-470-04612-0
- ASP.NET 2 For Dummies
  0-7645-7907-X
- C# 2005 For Dummies
  0-7645-9704-3
- Hacking For Dummies
  0-470-05235-X
- Hacking Wireless Networks
  For Dummies
  0-7645-9730-2
- Java For Dummies
  0-470-08716-1

- Microsoft SQL Server 2005 For Dummies
  0-7645-7755-7
- Networking All-in-One Desk Reference
  For Dummies
  0-7645-9939-9
- Preventing Identity Theft For Dummies
  0-7645-7336-5
- Telecom For Dummies
  0-471-77085-X
- Visual Studio 2005 All-in-One Desk
  Reference For Dummies
  0-7645-9775-2
- XML For Dummies
  0-7645-8845-1

HEALTH & SELF-HELP

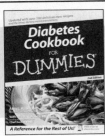

0-7645-8450-2

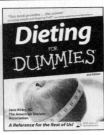

0-7645-4149-8

Also available:

- Bipolar Disorder For Dummies
  0-7645-8451-0
- Chemotherapy and Radiation
  For Dummies
  0-7645-7832-4
- Controlling Cholesterol For Dummies
  0-7645-5440-9
- Diabetes For Dummies
  0-7645-6820-5* †
- Divorce For Dummies
  0-7645-8417-0 †

- Fibromyalgia For Dummies
  0-7645-5441-7
- Low-Calorie Dieting For Dummies
  0-7645-9905-4
- Meditation For Dummies
  0-471-77774-9
- Osteoporosis For Dummies
  0-7645-7621-6
- Overcoming Anxiety For Dummies
  0-7645-5447-6
- Reiki For Dummies
  0-7645-9907-0
- Stress Management For Dummies
  0-7645-5144-2

EDUCATION, HISTORY, REFERENCE & TEST PREPARATION

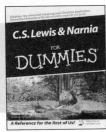

0-7645-8381-6

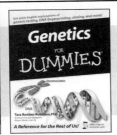

0-7645-9554-7

Also available:

- The ACT For Dummies
  0-7645-9652-7
- Algebra For Dummies
  0-7645-5325-9
- Algebra Workbook For Dummies
  0-7645-8467-7
- Astronomy For Dummies
  0-7645-8465-0
- Calculus For Dummies
  0-7645-2498-4
- Chemistry For Dummies
  0-7645-5430-1
- Forensics For Dummies
  0-7645-5580-4

- Freemasons For Dummies
  0-7645-9796-5
- French For Dummies
  0-7645-5193-0
- Geometry For Dummies
  0-7645-5324-0
- Organic Chemistry I For Dummies
  0-7645-6902-3
- The SAT I For Dummies
  0-7645-7193-1
- Spanish For Dummies
  0-7645-5194-9
- Statistics For Dummies
  0-7645-5423-9

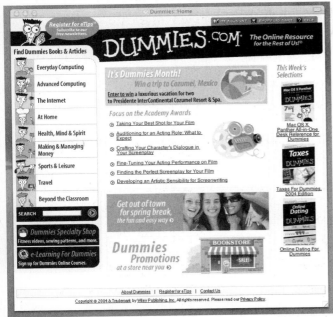

Get smart @ dummies.com®

- **Find a full list of Dummies titles**
- **Look into loads of FREE on-site articles**
- **Sign up for FREE eTips e-mailed to you weekly**
- **See what other products carry the Dummies name**
- **Shop directly from the Dummies bookstore**
- **Enter to win new prizes every month!**

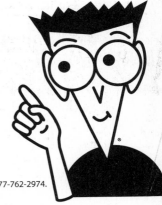

* Separate Canadian edition also available
† Separate U.K. edition also available

Available wherever books are sold. For more information or to order direct: U.S. customers visit www.dummies.com or call 1-877-762-2974.
U.K. customers visit www.wileyeurope.com or call 0800 243407. Canadian customers visit www.wiley.ca or call 1-800-567-4797.

Do More with Dummies

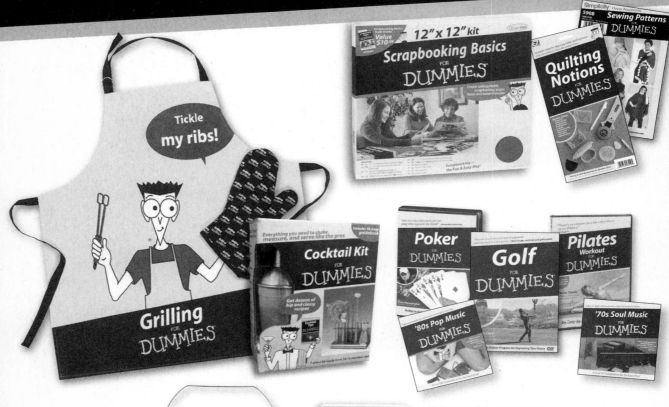

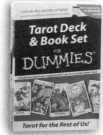

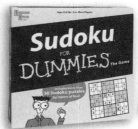

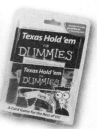

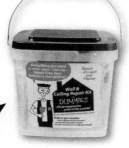

Instructional DVDs • Music Compilations
Games & Novelties • Culinary Kits
Crafts & Sewing Patterns
Home Improvement/DIY Kits • and more!

Check out the Dummies Specialty Shop at www.dummies.com for more information!

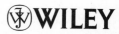